A VIDEO ATLAS OF
NEUROMUSCULAR DISORDERS

A VIDEO ATLAS OF NEUROMUSCULAR DISORDERS

Second Edition

Aziz Shaibani, MD, FACP, FAAN, FANA

DIRECTOR, NERVE AND MUSCLE CENTER OF TEXAS, HOUSTON, TEXAS
CLINICAL PROFESSOR OF MEDICINE, BAYLOR COLLEGE OF MEDICINE
ADJUNCT PROFESSOR OF NEUROLOGY,
KANSAS UNIVERSITY MEDICAL CENTER

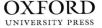

OXFORD
UNIVERSITY PRESS

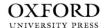

Oxford University Press is a department of the University of Oxford. It furthers the University's objective of excellence in research, scholarship, and education by publishing worldwide. Oxford is a registered trade mark of Oxford University Press in the UK and certain other countries.

Published in the United States of America by Oxford University Press
198 Madison Avenue, New York, NY 10016, United States of America.

Library of Congress Cataloging-in-Publication Data
Names: Shaibani, Aziz, author.
Title: A video atlas of neuromuscular disorders / Aziz Shaibani.
Description: Second edition. | Oxford ; New York : Oxford University Press, [2018] |
Includes bibliographical references and index.
Identifiers: LCCN 2017038929 (print) | LCCN 2017039984 (ebook) |
ISBN 9780190661311 (updf) | ISBN 9780190661328 (epub) | ISBN 9780190661304 (alk. paper)
Subjects: | MESH: Neuromuscular Diseases—physiopathology |
Neurologic Manifestations | Atlases | Case Reports
Classification: LCC RC925.5 (ebook) |
LCC RC925.5 (print) | NLM WE 17 | DDC 616.7/44—dc23
LC record available at https://lccn.loc.gov/2017038929

9 8 7 6 5 4 3 2 1
Printed by Sheridan Books, Inc., United States of America

CONTENTS

FOREWORD TO THE FIRST EDITION

I t is a pleasure to write a foreword for Dr. Aziz Shaibani's *Video Atlas of Neuromuscular Disorders*. Why do we need another book on neuromuscular disease? We currently have several successful textbooks in the market that cover muscle and nerve disorders. The answer is that Dr. Shaibani has put together a truly unique volume that fills a niche not currently covered. His book provides a large number of outstanding videos of patients who exhibit signs of neuromuscular problems that we all encounter in our clinics.

Dr. Shaibani is uniquely qualified to author such a scholarly contribution. Dr. Shaibani completed his neurology residency and neuromuscular fellowship at the Baylor School of Medicine. He immediately established a premier neuromuscular practice in the center of the largest medical center in the world, Texas Medical Center. Despite the fact that there were neuromuscular programs at several universities in Houston, Dr. Shaibani's practice has thrived and continues to expand. This, of course, is because Dr. Shaibani is a master clinician in the field of neuromuscular disease, and patients come to him from throughout the United States as well as internationally for his expert opinion and care. He continues to be closely affiliated with the academic neurology and internal medicine programs in the University of Texas and Baylor College of Medicine.

In addition, we have developed extremely close ties with Dr. Shaibani at our own University of Kansas Medical Center, where he holds a position of adjunct professor of neurology, because of our many collaborative academic and research projects. Dr. Shaibani is an active member of important national neuromuscular organizations such as the Muscle Study Group and the Western ALS Study Group. He has been an investigator in dozens of important neuromuscular research clinical trials.

But back to this video atlas. Clearly Professor Shaibani has accomplished what many of us have hoped we would do in our busy neuromuscular practices. He has taken the time and effort to meticulously video record the patients he sees in his practice if they exhibit any typical or even atypical neurology signs as a manifestation of their disorder. It is clear watching these videos that they are done in real time, in the office, and without sophisticated equipment. In this way, he has managed to give us multiple examples of a disease manifestation such as myotonia, its variants, or facioscapulohumeral muscular dystrophy, in its various forms, as some of the many, many examples. It should be noted that all patients have given written permission for Dr. Shaibani to use these videos for publication.

I've also realized there is some degree of variability as well as some degree of consistency in the manifestations of neuromuscular disease that we observe in patients. What Professor Shaibani has done is amazing in that he has recorded multiple presentations of these neurologic signs for us to compare and examine. The video atlas is organized in chapters of the various neuromuscular disorders. Each series of videos has an accompanying brief, well-written summary of the disease and the various signs that will be demonstrated on the videos. Accurate and usable references are supplied.

This video atlas, I am sure, will become popular with a wide range of learners. Of course, neurology residents and neuromuscular fellows, clinical neurophysiology fellows, and junior faculty and practitioners of neuromuscular medicine will clearly benefit by seeing multiple examples of neuromuscular clinical signs. I believe that early learners, such as undergraduates, medical students, and perhaps research PhDs will benefit by being able to see these examples for perhaps the first and only time in their careers. Finally, I do believe that experienced neuromuscular practitioners, such as myself and my many colleagues, will find great value in having these videos as a resource for teaching various learners. I think we will all be a bit envious that we did not take the time and effort to collect videos so extensively in this fashion.

So, I would like to give a huge "congratulations" to Dr. Aziz Shaibani for his remarkable efforts in putting together this *Video Atlas of Neuromuscular Disorders*. I know from many conversations with Aziz that this was a true labor of love that took him many years to create. We in the neuromuscular community are most appreciative of Dr. Shaibani for having provided us with this unique academic contribution to our field. I hope Aziz keeps recording videos in his practice and that future editions will be forthcoming with time. I know this atlas will be a great success.

Richard J. Barohn, MD
Gertrude and Dewey Ziegler Professor and Chair, Department of Neurology
University Distinguished Professor
University of Kansas Medical Center
Kansas City, Kansas

FOREWORD TO THE FIRST EDITION

I t is truly an honor for me to write the foreword for this neuromuscular video atlas edited by Dr. Aziz Shaibani. Dr. Shaibani is the Director of the Nerve and Muscle Center of Texas and a Clinical Professor of Medicine at Baylor College of Medicine and Adjunct Professor of Neurology at the University of Kansas. I've known Dr. Shaibani for two decades, since I too was in Texas. He has an extensive experience evaluating and treating patients with neuromuscular diseases and in training medical students, residents, and fellows. Over the years, he has videotaped patient examinations and has created a catalog of rare and common neurological signs in patients with a wide range of neuromuscular disorders.

In this atlas, Dr. Shaibani presents 280 of these video cases. The videos include patients describing their symptoms and pertinent neuromuscular examination. Each video is accompanied by a clinical synopsis of the case, and in some cases EMG videos and figures of biopsies. Each case is followed by a question and answer section for the viewers (e.g., guess the next test, correct diagnosis, or treatment), a discussion, and references. As is apparent in this video atlas, Dr. Shaibani is an astute clinician and an excellent teacher. It is one thing to read about various neuromuscular signs and disorders in textbooks, but another to actually see them. Thus, I enthusiastically recommend this video atlas for neurologists and physiatrists who evaluate patients with neuromuscular conditions. I congratulate Dr. Shaibani for his valuable contribution to the field.

Anthony Amato, MD
Vice Chairman
Department of Neurology
Chief, Neuromuscular Division
Brigham and Women's Hospital
Professor of Neurology
Harvard Medical School
Boston, Massachusetts

PREFACE TO THE SECOND EDITION

The first edition of *Video Atlas of Neuromuscular Disorders* achieved a high level of interest among neuromuscular experts and trainees alike and won two prestigious awards: The first prize of the British Medical Association award in the category of Neurobiology, and the 2015 Prose Award in clinical practice of medicine. This confirmed the main claim of the atlas—namely, that the descriptive era in neuromuscular diseases has been replaced by visual illustrations, mostly in the form of videos. Oxford University Press contacted me less than two years after the publication of the first edition to inquire about creating a second edition.

In this edition, the text has been updated to reflect new advances in the diagnosis (especially in the field of genetics) and treatment (at least three neuromuscular drugs were approved by the U.S. Food and Drug Administration since the first edition) and 50 new video cases have been added, with better-quality recording and biopsy images.

The aim of the book remains unchanged: to provide teaching videos that display different manifestations of neuromuscular diseases.

Aziz Shaibani, MD
Houston, 2018

PREFACE TO THE FIRST EDITION

The idea for this atlas is derived from an appreciation for the need of a new method of learning in the age of electronic communications and reduced attention span. Instead of spending time to reconstruct mental images of complicated neuromuscular cases from a lengthy and often dry text, this video atlas will allow viewers to spend that time to figure out the diagnostic and therapeutic challenges of these cases—an intellectual process that is intended to enforce clinical skills, which are invaluable for the profession of medicine.

Two hundred sixty-four video cases are artistically produced to express the manifestations of different neuromuscular diseases. Each case is described and is followed by one or more multiple-choice questions (MCQs). One page is dedicated to highlight salient points about the topic and to provide an update for the experts.

The book is divided into 28 chapters, each containing several cases. The chapters are not related to each other, and they can be read separately according to the interest of the reader. Each case is separately "clickable" from the index of cases at the beginning of each chapter. The material reflects information about common and rare neuromuscular disorders such as myasthenia gravis, amyotrophic lateral sclerosis (ALS), muscular dystrophy, chronic inflammatory demyelinating polyneuropathy (CIDP), stiff person syndrome (SPS), myopathies, and neuropathies.

The descriptions and MCQs make the book ideal for medical students, neurology residents, and subspecialty fellows who are preparing for their board examinations, while the updates are more suited to address issues at the level of neuromuscular specialists and practicing neurologists.

This book is by no means a textbook in neuromuscular disorders, but rather a "sharpener" of neuromuscular skills and decision-making for those who already have acquired the basic necessary medical knowledge.

A book is, after all, a personal experience. The text material of this book reflects our experience and knowledge in neuromuscular medicine. I have chosen to emphasize certain aspects of neuromuscular medicine and ignore others, depending on my appreciation of their significance. Whenever references are used, they have been cited after each case. I also relied on two major resources: *Neuromuscular Disorders* by Anthony Amato and James Russell, and the website of the neuromuscular disease center at Washington University (http://neuromuscular.wustl.edu/).

Aziz Shaibani, MD

ACKNOWLEDGMENTS

I would like to profusely thank the following colleagues for their critical review of cases from the atlas: Sendra Ajroud-Driss, MD, Brent Beson, MD, David Gehret, MD, Melanie Doerflinger Glenn, MD, James Howard, MD, Viktoriya Irodenko, MD, Liberty Jenkin, MD, Vikas Kumar, MD, Todd Levine, MD, Teerin Liewluck, MD, Jau-Shin Lou, MD, Blanca Marky, MD, Matt Mayer, MD, Tahseen Mozaffar, MD, Sabrina Paganoni, MD, Michael Pulley, MD, Devon Rubin, MD, David Saperstein, MD, Sona Shah, MD, Maryam Tahmasbi Sohi, MD, Rabie Tawil, MD, Steven Vernino, MD, and the rest of Rick's real neuromuscular friends (www.rrnmf.com).

Special thanks go to Duaa Jabari, MD, Nawar Hussin, MD, and Hayan Ibraheem, MD for their technical support, and to Randolph Evans, MD, for encouragement and review.

I would like to thank the referring physicians for their confidence in our center, and I thank the patients, the primary source of information, for allowing us to publish their videos for educational purposes.

Finally, the time to prepare this work was taken away from family time, and I would like to thank my wife Arwa and our children, Ahmad, Senan, and Rami, for allowing me to do so.

Aziz Shaibani, MD

GAIT DISORDERS

CASE 1.1: BILATERAL FOOT DROP

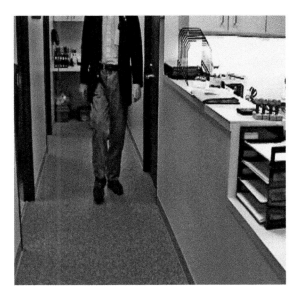

VIDEO 1.1

A 67-year-old man presented with a 3-year history of gradually worsening gait imbalance, feet numbness, and hand grip weakness. Gait is shown in Video 1.1. Examination also showed moderate impairment of sensation to vibration and proprioception in the feet and diffuse areflexia. Proximal strength was normal. Nerve conduction studies (NCSs) revealed that distal motor latencies of the bilateral peroneal and tibial nerves were 9–11 milliseconds with mild asymmetry. Their median and ulnar counterparts were 6–7 milliseconds. Compound muscle action potential (CMAP) amplitudes were preserved, and the sural responses were absent. F waves were mildly prolonged. Cerebrospinal fluid (CSF) protein was 110 mg/dl. The immunoglobin G (IgG) synthesis rate was increased. Immunofixation protein electrophoresis (IFPE) revealed immunoglobin M (IgM) lambda spikes.

The diagnosis would be supported by abnormal:

1. Myelin-associated glycoprotein (MAG) antibody titer
2. Sulfatide antibody titer
3. Charcot-Marie-Tooth (CMT) mutation analysis
4. Blood lead level
5. Porphyrins in the urine

DIAGNOSIS

- Video gait analysis: Weak ankle dorsiflexion results in decreased toe clearance and foot "slap" during heel strike. Compensation often occurs through excessive hip flexion during the swing phase, referred to as a *steppage gait pattern.*
- Foot drop may result from any insult at the level of the deep peroneal nerve, common peroneal nerve, sciatic nerve, lumbosacral (LS) plexus, nerve roots, motor neurons, neuromuscular junction (NMJ), muscles, spinal cord, and brain.
- Preservation of the ankle invertors is against L5 radiculopathy and in favor of peroneal neuropathy since ankle invertors are tibially innervated.
- Painful asymmetrical foot drop is typically seen in vasculitis.
- Painless asymmetrical foot drop with preserved ankle reflexes is typically seen in amyotrophic lateral sclerosis (ALS), myasthenia gravis (MG), and distal myopathies. Foot drop may be the first presenting feature of ALS.
- Chronic inflammatory demyelinating polyneuropathy (CIDP) patients may present with foot drop, especially distal acquired demyelinating sensorimotor neuropathy (DADSAM), which is associated with MAG antibodies and is refractory to treatment.
- Facioscapulohumeral muscular dystrophy (FSHD) may present with foot drop. Preservation or hypertrophy of the extensor digitorum brevis (EDB) muscle distinguishes myopathic from neurogenic foot drop.
- The presence of wrist drop with foot drop should suggest MG or lead poisoning.
- The most common presentation of CMT 1A is tripping and falls due to poor clearance of toes, secondary to foot drop with minimal sensory symptoms.
- Foot drop should not be confused with dystonic and spastic ankle flexion, such as in hereditary spastic paraplegia (HSP) and focal ankle dystonia. In these cases, a careful examination fails to reveal weakness of the ankle extensors, ankle reflexes are brisk, and the tone is increased in the plantar flexors.
- Copper deficiency may present with an ALS-like picture (progressive atrophy and fasciculations), plus distal sensory impairment and leucopenia. A remote gastrectomy and the usage of zinc-rich denture fixative (e.g., Fixodent) are strong risk factors.
- In this case, the progressive distal asymmetrical demyelinating features with high CSF proteins and monoclonal gammopathy strongly raised the possibility of DADSAM.

CASE 1.2: GAIT IMBALANCE AND APRAXIA OF EYELID OPENING

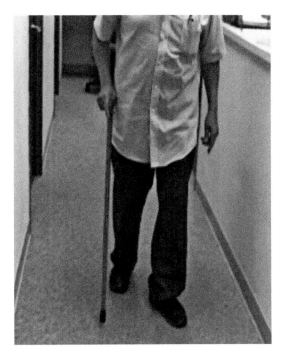

VIDEO 1.2

A 75-year-old man presented with a 4-year history of falls, which prompted his referral for neuromuscular evaluation. The symptoms were much more pronounced on the right side. Gradually, he became aphasic. He had no urinary incontinence. Cognition was difficult to evaluate due to aphasia. Brain magnetic resonance imaging (MRI) revealed mild asymmetrical cortical atrophy.

This picture is typically seen in:

1. Polyneuropathy
2. Parkinson disease
3. Normal pressure hydrocephalus (NPH)
4. Corticobasal degeneration
5. Progressive supranuclear palsy (PSP)

DIAGNOSIS

- Video gait analysis: Shuffling gait is characterized by markedly decreased stride length and a flat foot sliding forward during initial contact. This patient's gait also demonstrates increased lateral trunk sway and decreased reciprocal arm swing. Notice how many steps it takes to change direction 180 degrees.
- There are several areas of overlap between movement disorders and neuromuscular disorders, resulting in consultation of a neuromuscular specialist on patients with movement disorder. Examples of such an overlap:
  - Some movement disorders are associated with neuromuscular disorders such as restless leg syndrome with neuropathy.
  - Both disorders may coexist in patients only by coincidence; many of these diseases are especially common in the elderly, such as neuropathy and Parkinson disease.
  - Deceptive presentations, such as dropped head syndrome, which may be confused with camptocormia or Parkinsonian posture. Sensory ataxia may be confused with the gait apraxia of NPH or shuffling gait of Parkinson disease.
- Neuromuscular specialists should be aware of different manifestations and associations of movement disorders in order to detect them when referred to a neuromuscular clinic.
- Gait imbalance is a common cause of a referral to a neuromuscular clinic:
  - Gait is a complicated process that requires the integrity of many central and peripheral mechanisms for its maintenance, such as nerves, muscles, corticospinal tracts, cerebellum, basal ganglion, and cerebral cortex.
  - Normal gait also requires nonneurological elements such as skeleton, vision, and vestibular apparatus.
  - Gait examination is an integral part of the examination of the nervous system; without it, the examination is never complete.
- Corticobasal degeneration in this case is suggested by the clinical and radiological asymmetry, aphasia, gait apraxia, dementia, and apraxia of the eyelid opening.
- PSP is another tautopathy that is commonly confused with this Parkinson-plus syndrome, and both can cause disorder of extraocular movements (EOMs) and gait. However, in PSP, there is predominant loss of downward gaze, midbrain atrophy, and little if any asymmetry.

CASE 1.3: SENSORY ATAXIA

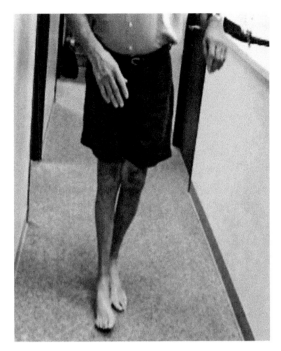

VIDEO 1.3

A 62-year-old man presented with a 1-year history of loss of balance and difficulty rising out of a deep chair. Examination is shown in the video. In addition, he had proximal arm and leg weakness, diffuse areflexia, and no family history of significance. NCS: motor nerve conduction velocity (NCV): 30 milliseconds. F-latencies: 70s. Distal motor latencies (DMLs): 8 milliseconds. CSF protein was 150 mg/dl with increased IgG index.

Although findings of high foot arches, hammertoes, and thin legs suggested CMT, the rest of the picture is consistent with:

1. Vasculitic neuropathy (NP)
2. CIDP
3. Diabetic polyneuropathy (DPN)
4. Amyloid neuropathy
5. Alcohol-related neuropathy

DIAGNOSIS

- Painless, progressive sensory ataxia with ankle dorsiflexor weakness and areflexia is very suggestive of CIDP.
- Increased IgG index in the CSF signifies increased intrathecal IgG synthesis, which in turn supports a primary inflammatory process in the peripheral or central nervous system.
- High foot arches can be congenital, and in that case, they may be a marker of a congenital or hereditary neuromuscular disorder such as congenital myopathy, muscular dystrophy, and CMT, or acquired due to chronic weakness of the ankle extensors, leading to unopposed action of the ankle plantar flexors. In that case, they are markers for chronic neuropathies such as CIDP. Hammertoes strongly support the former.
- CIDP may present with predominantly sensory findings such as sensory ataxia.
- CIDP is probably more common in CMT patients, and there is a suggestion that CMT may alter the antigenicity of the myelin. A similar argument is made for the inflammatory component of Duchenne muscular dystrophy (DMD) and hence a justification for steroid therapy.
- Gait disorder, autoimmunity, late-onset polyneuropathy (GALOP) is a variant of CIDP that is associated with IgM antibodies, mostly against sulfatide moiety (in 80% of cases), and it is usually refractory, but may respond to cyclophosphamide, plasmapheresis, or both.
- Sensory ataxia with preserved or brisk knee reflexes strongly argues against CIDP and suggests axonal neuropathy like vasculitis or dorsal myelopathy, such as that due to multiple sclerosis (MS), copper deficiency, or B_{12} deficiency.
- Ataxia is the last and least responsive of CIDP symptoms to therapy, and patients' expectations are to be lowered from the start.
- Ataxic, predominantly sensory neuropathy is typically seen in Sjogren syndrome and paraneoplastic syndromes.

CASE 1.4: SPASTIC GAIT

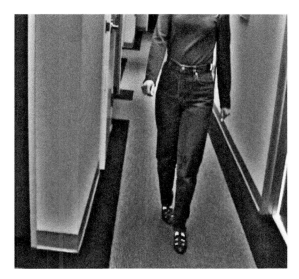

VIDEO 1.4

A 32-year-old woman presented with stiff legs, which she developed at the age of 15. She had no family history of significance or sensory symptoms. Gradually, she developed the gait shown in Video 1.4. Her deep tendon reflexes (DTRs) were 3/4. MRIs of the brain and spinal cord were normal. CSF examination was normal. Spasticity improved with institution of intrathecal Baclofen pump.

These findings are consistent with:

1. HSP
2. Cerebral palsy
3. MS
4. CMT disease
5. Multisystem atrophy

DIAGNOSIS

- Video gait analysis: The patient's spastic gait pattern is apparent from increased adductor tone, resulting in scissoring or crossing of the legs, as well as increased plantar flexor tone, resulting in toe walking and excessive inversion at the ankle.
- HSP is a hereditary disorder in which multiple identified genetic mutations (at least 30) correlate with a fairly homogeneous phenotypic syndrome characterized by spastic paraparesis.
- Patients with HSP are referred to neuromuscular clinics due to:
  - Suspicion of progressive lateral sclerosis, a variant of ALS characterized by progressive upper motor neuron (UMN) signs such as spasticity and hyperreflexia.
  - Suspicion of polyneuropathy due to gait imbalance and mild impairment of vibratory sensation in the feet.
- As in most hereditary neuromuscular disorders, the absence of a positive family history does not exclude the disorder.
- Some HSP variants, such as those caused by mutations of spastic paraplegia genes (SPGs) 9, 10, 14, 15, 20, 22, 26, and 30, may display lower motor neuron (LMN) signs, further complicating differentiation from ALS.
- Slow progression, high foot arches, and mild sensory impairment in the feet due to dorsal column dysfunction favor HSP, while involvement of the arms and bulbar muscles favor primary lateral sclerosis (PLS).
- Mutation analysis can detect 60% of the autosomal-dominant (AD) cases, but there is a high false negative rate. A total of 10% of sporadically affected individuals turn out to have diagnostic dominant mutations. Whole exome sequencing will hopefully increase diagnostic yield.

CASE 1.5: PAINFUL LEG SPASMS

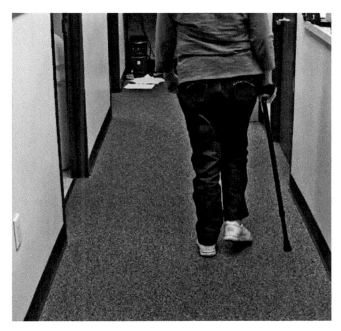

VIDEO 1.5

A 59-year-old woman presented with a 5-year history of progressive leg stiffness, painful spasms, and loss of balance. She had progressive visual failure and hearing impairment as well. Eye examination revealed mild optic atrophy, and mild sensory impairment in the feet was also detected. She has one healthy child and several healthy sisters. No gait abnormality is reported in the parents. MRI of the brain and spinal cord, CSF examination, and electromyography (EMG) were normal. B_{12} level and copper level were normal. Very long chain fatty acid levels were normal.

The most appropriate test at this point is mutation analysis for:

1. Autosomal-recessive (AR) HSP
2. AD HSP
3. ABCD gene mutations
4. Proteolipid protein gene mutations
5. SOD gene mutations

DIAGNOSIS

- The lack of affected children or siblings suggests an AR disease.
- The optic atrophy and hearing loss suggest mitochondrial dysfunction.
- SPG 7 (paraplegin) mutations account for 4% of paraplegin mutations.
- SPG encodes a mitochondrial protein, and therefore the manifestations are protean, including optic atrophy and hearing loss.
- HSP differential diagnosis:
  - Adrenomyeloneuropathy
  - Spinocerebellar ataxia (SCA)
  - Cerebral palsy
  - PLS
  - Tropical spastic paraplegia
  - Compressive myelopathies: meningioma
- HSP is generally classified as pure or complicated.
  - In pure HSP, symptoms are generally limited to gradual weakening of the legs and impaired sensation in the feet.
  - In complicated HSP, a rare disorder, additional symptoms may include the following:
    - Peripheral neuropathy
    - Epilepsy
    - Ataxia
    - Optic neuropathy
    - Retinopathy
    - Dementia
    - Ichthyosis
    - Mental retardation
    - Deafness
    - Problems with speech, swallowing, or breathing
  - Some of these additional symptoms may be related to a separate disorder, such as diabetic neuropathy or epilepsy, rather than being directly caused by HSP.

CASE 1.6: LATERAL PELVIC TILTING

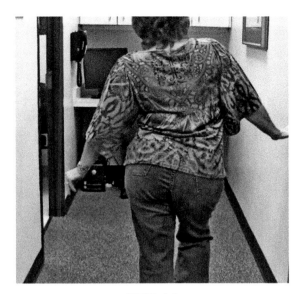

VIDEO 1.6

A 44-year-old woman presented with difficulty arising out of a chair, noticed 10 years earlier, which had gradually gotten worse. She had no sensory symptoms. A maternal cousin had a similar gait difficulty. She had no dysphagia or skin rash but had proximal weakness in the arms and legs with loss of reflexes. The creatine kinase (CK) level was 430 IU/L, and EMG revealed high-amplitude, long-duration units with a firing frequency of 25 Hz in the proximal and distal muscles of the legs and arms.

This gait abnormality can be seen in:

1. Myopathies
2. Spinal muscular atrophy (SMA)
3. Congenial MG
4. Stiff person syndrome
5. Myelopathies

DIAGNOSIS

- Video gait analysis: Pelvic drop is a sign of proximal muscle weakness in the gluteus medius, which typically activates in the standing leg to hold the pelvis neutral. Exaggerated lumbar lordosis is also noted. In more advanced disease, Trendelenburg or lateral trunk movement is used to compensate for the underlying weakness.
- Lateral pelvic tilting is a postural strategy to save energy and is a feature of chronic proximal weakness, especially when it starts at an early age.
- Although traditionally, it is reported as classical for muscular dystrophies, particularly DMD, it may be produced by chronic neurogenic proximal weakness, such as in SMA types 3 and 4 and in congenital MG.
- It has been observed that in cases of SMA, the initial postural adjustment involves pelvic rotation, while in DMD, it involves knee flexion. However, in the later stages of the disease, it may be difficult to distinguish them clinically. Even the Gowers' maneuver may be produced by SMA.
- SMA is a group of disorders characterized by chronic and inherited degeneration of motor neurons. Unlike hereditary ALS, there are no UMN signs. Progressive muscular atrophy is a variant of ALS. It is more progressive than most SMAs, and it is rarely hereditary.
- Most SMA cases are caused by mutation of the survival motor neuron (SMN) gene on chromosome 5q13.2. The SMN protein inhibits the apoptosis of motor neurons. These mutations are AR. Non-5q SMA is a large group of disorders and can be AD or AR.
- Non-5q SMAs are classified by age of onset and distribution of weakness; soon, classification according to molecular genetics will prevail.
  - Adult-onset SMAs are:
    - Proximal SMA: 30% AD, normal life expectancy, may have tongue fasciculations and tremors.
    - Distal SMA.
  - Kennedy disease: bulbar and proximal weakness, with sensory symptoms and elevated CK due to severe muscle cramps.
  - Scapuloperoneal SMA: asymmetric weakness of shoulder girdle and peroneal muscles leading to scapular winging and bilateral foot drop. It may be confused with FSHD.
- Nusinersen was approved by the U.S. Food and Drug Administration (FDA) in December 2016 to treat SMA caused by SMN gene mutations. It is administered intrathecally. It is an antisense oligonucleotide that increases the production of full-length SMN proteins by binding to a specific sequence in the intron downsream of exon 7 of the SMN2 messenger RNA (mRNA) script.

SUGGESTED READINGS

Armanda S, Mercier M, Watelain E, et al. A comparison of gait in spinal muscular atrophy, type II, and Duchenne muscular dystrophy. *Gait Post.* 2005;21:369–378.

U.S. Food and Drug Administration (FDA). FDA approves first drug for spinal muscular atrophy. www.fda.gov/newsevents/newsroom/pressannouncements/ucm534611.htm

CASE 1.7: BIZARRE GAIT

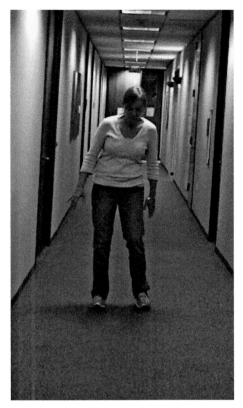

VIDEO 1.7

A 46-year-old woman presented with acute left arm and leg weakness, which she noticed one morning right after she woke up. Urgent brain MRI was negative. Intravenous (IV) solumedrol reversed it. A few days later, she could not lift her legs; however, her examination revealed normal strength. She had a normal CK level and EMG. She had no sensory or reflex changes. Her gait was demonstrated.

This gait abnormality is most likely due to:

1. Functional gait disorder (FGD)
2. Sensory ataxia
3. Cerebellar ataxia
4. Myelopathy
5. Stroke

DIAGNOSIS

- FGD is common and affects mostly females.
- Gait patterns are variable and may change from one pattern to another.
- The most important clue is that the gait disorder does not conform to the description of a recognizable organic pattern and biomechanical methods of compensation.
- Falls are rare, and good strength is often demonstrated.
- Provoking factors such as stress are commonly missed, and most patients are surprised when they are told of the possible role of stress.
- Common pattern of FGDs:
  - Hemiparesis: leg dragging
  - Paraparesis: dragging of both feet
  - Ataxia
  - Dystonia
  - Myoclonus
  - Slapping
  - Robotic
  - Hesitant
  - Sudden buckling without falls
  - Waddling
  - Shaking

CASE 1.8: PROXIMAL AND DISTAL WEAKNESS

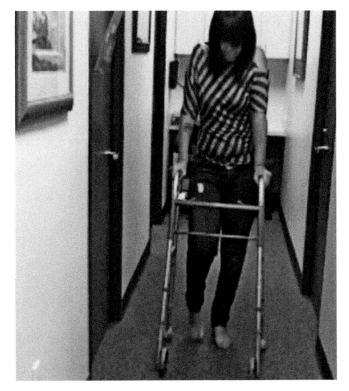

VIDEO 1.8

A 36-year-old woman presented with a 14-year history of difficulty arising out of a chair. She then had gait difficulty (as shown in Video 1.8), and she progressed to a walker within 5 years. The CK level was 6,300 IU/L, and EMG revealed evidence of irritative chronic myopathy. There was no relevant family history. The muscle biopsy, shown in Figure 1.8.1, also showed variation of fiber size (20–120 μ), fiber necrosis, split fibers, and increased internal nuclei. She did not respond to steroids, intravenous immunoglobulin (IVIG), or methotrexate.

Which of the following is (are) consistent with dysferlinopathy:

1. Proximal and distal weakness
2. Chronic course
3. Very high CK level
4. Mild endomysial inflammation
5. No response to anti-inflammatory agents

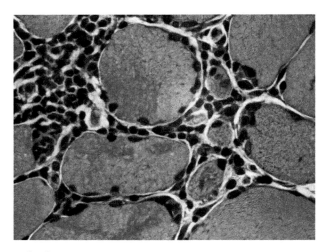

FIGURE 1.8.1 Endomysial inflammation.

DIAGNOSIS

- Waddling is a feature of chronic myopathies, more so for dystrophic types. It is associated with the exaggeration of lumbar lordosis.
- Slapping due to bilateral foot drop and poor knee extension further complicates this gait.
- The chronicity and age of onset suggest a dystrophic process. More than 20 times the normal CK level and dystrophic biopsy support this notion.
- Proximal and distal weakness with inflammatory and dystrophic myopathic changes is typically seen in dysferlinopathy.
- The other dystrophic myopathies that are associated with inflammatory pathology are DMD and FSHD.
- Dysferlin is an integral protein of the muscle membrane and is a target of at least 450 mutations, leading to different phenotypes. It is an AR disease.
- A total of 6.5% of unclassified myopathies in muscle biopsies showed dysferlinopathy.
- Posterior leg muscles are affected early, leading to difficulty walking on the toes. In the Miyoshi variant (allelic to LGMD 2B), distal leg muscles are the main target of pathology, resulting in atrophy in the calves. No cardiac involvement is reported. Calf atrophy is typically seen, but hypertrophy is also reported.
- Sometimes (6% of cases), asymptomatic hyper-CKemia is the only finding.
- Western blot (WB) analysis reveals that dysferlin is reduced to 0%–20% in LGMD 2B and to 0 in Miyoshi myopathy.
- The disease is slowly progressive.
- Dysferlin is present in the white blood cells (WBCs) and WB analysis on (WBC) is as sensitive as muscle biopsy.

CASE 1.9: LURCHING WITHOUT FALLS

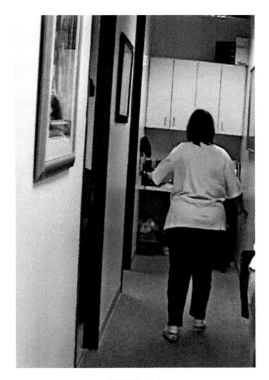

VIDEO 1.9

A 25-year-old woman who was recently divorced and had lost her job presented with the gait abnormality demonstrated in Video 1.9. She felt mild pressure, like headache and chest tightness. DTRs were brisk, but she had no weakness or sensory symptoms. At times, she felt like a lump in her throat was interfering with her swallowing.

This gait is likely due to:

1. Myelopathy
2. Cerebellar disorder
3. Neuropathy
4. Functional disorder
5. Trauma to the head

DIAGNOSIS

- A hysterical gait may present with monoplegia, monoparesis, hemiparesis, paraplegia, or paraparesis.
- With hysterical gait, there tends to be no leg circumduction, hyperreflexia, or Babinski sign.
- Characteristic features of a patient with hysterical gait include sudden buckling of the knees (usually without falls), swaying with the eyes closed, with a buildup of sway amplitude and improvement with distraction.
- Patients with a hysterical gait tend to drag the foot when walking rather than lift it.
- Hysterical gaits can be dramatic, with patients lurching wildly in all directions, thus demonstrating a remarkable ability to make rapid postural adjustments. In contrast, patients with true paraparesis or paraplegia tend to fall frequently.
- An unusual and illusive presentation of hysterical gait is known as *astasia-abasia*. In this condition, the patient is unable to turn or walk but retains normal use of the legs while lying in bed. However, atrophy of the vermis and frontal gait disorders (gait apraxia) can have similar presentation.

SUGGESTED READING

Shaibani A, Shabbagh MN. Pseudoneurologic syndromes: recognition and diagnosis. *Am Fam Phys*. 1998 May 15;57(10):2485–2494.

CASE 1.10: ATAXIA AND DYSDIADOCHOKINESIA

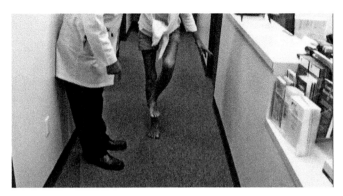

VIDEO 1.10

A 45-year-old woman presented with progressive gait imbalance for 18 months. She had also lost 30 pounds. She had no sensory, visual, or bulbar symptoms. She heavily drank alcohol 2 years earlier. She had partial pancreatectomy 3 years earlier. Examination is shown in the video. She had normal strength, DTRs, feet sensation, and strength. MRI of the brain showed mild vermal atrophy. CSF examination was negative for oligoclonal bands (OCBs). Abdominal ultrasound (US) showed a right ovarian mass.

Which of the following antibodies is likely to be elevated?

1. Anti-Yo (anti-Purkinje cell antibodies)
2. Anti-Hu
3. Anti-Ma2
4. Anti–glutamate acid decarboxylase (GAD)
5. Antigliadin

DIAGNOSIS

- Patients with ataxia may be referred for neuromuscular evaluation.
- Cerebellar ataxia is less sensitive to loss of visual cues than sensory ataxia; therefore, the Romberg sign is typically negative.
- The steps are uncoordinated and overshoot rather than hesitant and trying to find the ground.
- Other cerebellar dysfunction features are common, like nystagmus, dysmetria, dysdiadochokinesia, dysarthria, diplopia, and hyporeflexia.
- Progressive cerebellar ataxia has many causes:
  - Progressive MS: Demyelinating enhancing plaques are seen in the MRI of the brain, particularity the cerebellum. CSF examination shows OCBs in 80% of cases.
  - Paraneoplastic cerebellar degeneration (PCD): This is usually subacute and is associated with weight loss and other paraneoplastic syndromes such as sensory neuropathy.
  - Hereditary SCA may exacerbate spontaneously or by stress or medications, simulating a progressive picture.
  - Space-occupying lesions are to be ruled out by appropriate imaging.
  - Toxic factors such as medications and ethanol intoxication.
- PCD:
  - Cerebellar dysfunction occurs due to remote effects of cancer. Molecular mimicry is the presumed mechanism.
  - PCD may precede the diagnosis of cancer by 2–5 years.
  - Ovary, uterus, breast, and lungs are the main sources. Chest X-ray and abdominal US are the most important tests in a patient with progressive cerebellar features.
  - Anti-Hu antibodies react with all neurons, but anti-Yo antibodies react only with Purkinje cells in the cerebellum.
  - Patients with anti-Yo antibodies have ovarian or breast cancer 90% of times.
  - Anti-Ri antibodies are reported in paraneoplastic encephalitis and opsoclonus in association with breast cancer and lung cancer.

CASE 1.11: GAIT DIFFICULTY WITH NORMAL EMG

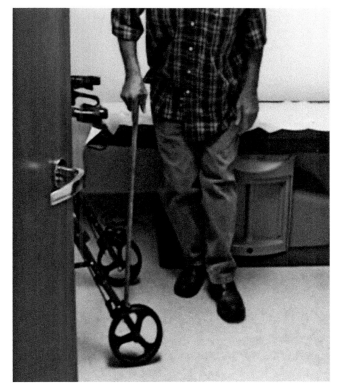

VIDEO 1.11

A 64-year-old diabetic man presented with a 2-year history of gait difficulty. He had chronic foot numbness and polyarthralgia. EMG of the proximal leg muscles and CK were both normal.

Which of the following tests is the most appropriate test?

1. Imaging of the hips/ortho consult
2. Muscle biopsy
3. Brain MRI
4. EMG of the arms
5. Aspiration of the hip joint

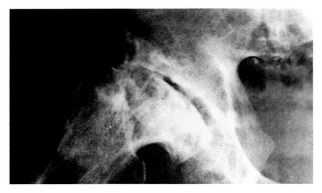

FIGURE 1.11.1 X-ray of the right hip joint revealed severe arthritis.

DIAGNOSIS

- Nonneurological disorders may be referred to neuromuscular clinics because they mimic neuromuscular (NM) disorders. Gait imbalance is the most common source of such referrals.
- This patient had a history of chronic arthritis and gradually developed restriction of hip range of motion (ROM). His examination demonstrated severe limitation of passive range of motion for hip flexion and abduction. The lack of pain (silent arthritis) was likely due to diabetic neuropathy. He also had bilateral knee arthritis, which explains his knee bending during attempted walking.
- While he had foot numbness and absent ankle reflexes suggestive of diabetic neuropathy, this gait was not neuropathic.
- His referring physician suspected myopathy. Normal CK occurs in 30% of myopathies, but a normal needle examination of weak muscles strongly argues against myopathic or neurogenic weakness.
- Detailed and careful needle exploration of several weak muscles is necessary. Normal duration, amplitude, number of phases, and recruitment pattern of motor units in multiple-tested tracks and muscles should argue against a neuromuscular etiology. In these cases, central or nonneurological causes should be entertained.
- In chronic myopathies, motor unit estimation may be needed because compensation may lead to an apparently normal EMG picture.
- The hip X-ray/MRI of this patient (see Figure 1.11.1) showed severe arthritis. Bilateral total hip replacement (THR) reversed his gait, but maximum improvement took a year.

CASE 1.12: WIDE-BASED GAIT

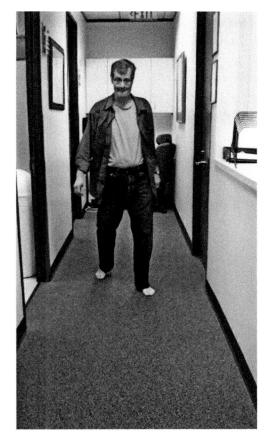

VIDEO 1.12

A 61-year-old man presented with a 10-year history of gait instability and mild foot numbness. He was a reformed alcohol drinker. In addition to what is shown in Video 1.12, examination revealed mild sensory impairment in the feet and absent ankle reflexes. There was no muscle weakness. He had a distant cousin who was wheelchair-bound due to gait imbalance. Nerve conduction study was normal.

The most likely diagnosis is:

1. Hereditary cerebellar ataxia
2. Sensorimotor neuropathy
3. HSP
4. PCD
5. Alcohol-related cerebellar atrophy

DIAGNOSIS

- Wide-based gait is a feature of vermal dysfunction, while the Romberg sign signifies sensory ataxia. Therefore, this patient displays evidence of both cerebellar and sensory ataxias.
- The chronicity of the symptoms argues against paraneoplastic syndrome and suggests either alcohol-related cerebellar degeneration or hereditary cerebellar degeneration (HCD). Positive family history argues for the latter.
- Normal NCS suggests that the sensory ataxia is due to a preganglionic lesion, which is common in HCD.
- It is imperative to examine ataxic patients for other cerebellar findings, such as nystagmus, dysmetria, dysarthria, and dysdiadochokinesia, and to examine the dimensions of the cerebellum in the brain MRI.
- There are more than 40 types of HCD, the discussion of which is beyond the scope of this book.
- Generally, hereditary cerebellar ataxia (HCA) is classified into AD and AR. Friedreich's ataxia is the most common among the recessive ones.
- Sensory neuropathy is common in HCA types 1, 2, and 3 and in Friedreich ataxia.
- Fasciculations are characteristic of HCA type 3.
- It is important to determine the genetic type of ataxia to do proper genetic counseling.
- An estimated 50%–60% of the dominant hereditary ataxias can be identified with highly accurate and specific molecular genetic testing for *SCA1, SCA2, SCA3, SCA6, SCA7, SCA8, SCA10, SCA12, SCA17*, and *DRPLA*; all have trinucleotide repeat expansions in the pertinent genes.

SUGGESTED READING

Bird TD. Hereditary ataxia overview. *GeneRev*. February 27, 2014.

CASE 1.13: MAGNETIC GAIT

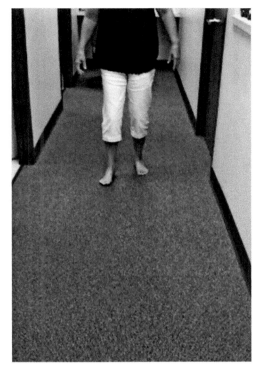

VIDEO 1.13

A 70-year-old woman presented with a 6-month history of falls and urinary incontinence. Her family noticed impaired recent memory. She had no sensory symptoms, and her examination revealed normal strength and coordination. Brain MRI revealed enlarged ventricles. CSF opening pressure was 100 mm/Hg. Removal of 30 ml of CSF improved gait for a few days.

The gait is characterized by:

1. Waddling
2. High steppage
3. Low steppage
4. Being apractic
5. Being ataxic

DIAGNOSIS

- Gait disorders in the elderly are frequent referrals to neuromuscular clinics. Peripheral neuropathy is common in this age group, and the finding of sensory impairment in the feet is the most common cause of referral as a possible cause of the gait abnormality.
- Many in the field believe that NPH is an underdiagnosed cause of treatable dementia and frequent falls in the elderly.
- The gait is characterized by difficulty making the first steps, as if the feet are glued to the ground (gait apraxia).
- There is no single reliable diagnostic test, and the same symptoms can be produced by ischemic brain disease.
- Improvement of gait and neuropsychological performance after a high-volume spinal tap is the most reliable indicator of the need for a ventriculoperitoneal shunt (VPS).
- Intrathecal injection of radionucleotide (cisternogram) to measure the appearance of the isotopes in the cerebral convexities 24–48 later has a controversial diagnostic value.

CASE 1.14: PROGRESSIVE ATAXIA

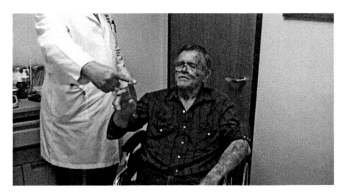

VIDEO 1.14

A 74-year-old man presented with a 6-month history of falls and slurring of speech. He had lost 15 pounds. He was a chronic smoker and had a history of diabetic neuropathy. MRI of the brain was normal. EMG revealed moderate axonal sensorimotor neuropathy. MRI of cervical spines revealed cervical cord compression by osteophytes with intramedullary signal abnormality. A chest X-ray showed a right pulmonary nodule.

The clinical picture is highly suggestive of:

1. Diabetic polyneuropathy
2. Cervical myelopathy
3. PCD
4. Paraneoplastic myopathy
5. Limbic encephalopathy

DIAGNOSIS

- Patients with cerebellar ataxia may be referred to neuromuscular clinics due to suspicion of ataxic neuropathy, particularly if they have a concomitant neuropathy, usually diabetic or alcohol-related.
- The Romberg sign greatly favors sensory ataxia, as opposed to cerebellar ataxia, because patients with proprioceptive loss rely on vision to compensate for loss of balance.
- Both cerebellar and sensory ataxias may occur simultaneously as a part of the same paraneo-plastic syndrome or due to unrelated causes.
- Weight loss and history of smoking are strong risk factors for PCD.
- Cancers commonly associated with PCD:
  - Small-cell lung cancer (SCLC)
  - Ovarian cancer
  - Breast cancer
  - Hodgkin lymphoma
- The main target of this autoimmune attack is the Purkinje cells in the cerebellum.
- Cerebellar ataxia may precede the other manifestations of cancer by up to 2 years.
- Paraneoplastic antibodies are more useful to reveal an association with malignancy than to define the exact type of the malignancy, as many of them can be present in several types of paraneoplastic syndromes.
- Hu antibodies are more commonly seen in paraneoplastic sensory neuronopathy, but they are also reported in PCD. Small-cell lung cancer is the main source.
- Reversible neuronal (Tr) antibodies are associated with lymphoma.
- Yo antibodies are associated with ovarian and breast cancer.
- The prognosis is guarded and largely depends on the underlying malignancy.

CASE 1.15: FREQUENT FALLS

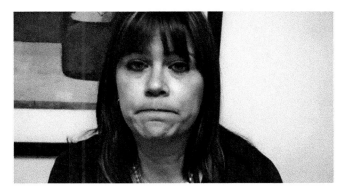

VIDEO 1.15

A lady presented with frequent falls.

These episodes are consistent with:

1. Syncope
2. Vestibular neuritis
3. Cardiac arrhythmia
4. Periodic paralysis
5. Psychogenic etiology

DIAGNOSIS

- Sudden and transient loss of muscle tone without alteration of consciousness or vertigo is called a *drop attack.*
- These patients are referred to neuromuscular clinics after negative investigations for central nervous system disorders such as:
  - Brain stem ischemic
  - Hydrocephalus
  - Colloid cyst of the third ventricle
  - Atonic seizures
- The closest neuromuscular disorder to these attacks is periodic paralysis, familial or nonfamilial, hypokalemic or hyperkalemic.
- However, periodic familial paralysis is not that brief, and it does not happen that often without trigger factors such as exercise or a high-carbohydrate diet.
- Cataplexy is usually associated with narcolepsy. Her multiple sleep latency tests were negative.
- Syncope is associated with altered consciousness.
- Dysautonomia was ruled out by a negative autonomic reflex test.
- Cardiac arrhythmias cause blurred consciousness. Her long-term holter was negative, even though she had several attacks during the recording.
- Brain stem ischemia was ruled out by brain MRI. She had no risk factors.
- Vestibular disorders were ruled out by electronystagmography (ENG) and vestibular evaluation.
- She had a history of severe anxiety attacks. Panic attacks were not likely since she denied a sense of apprehension or chest tightness or palpitation.
- The most common cause of drop attacks in the elderly is carotid sinus hypersensitivity.
- Psychogenic etiology is suspected. The problem was corrected after her anxiety was treated and the source of stress was eliminated.

CASE 1.16: CHRONIC PROGRESSIVE GAIT DISORDER WITH OPHTHALMOPLEGIA

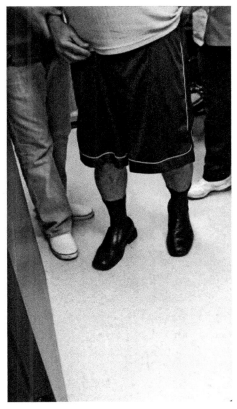

VIDEO 1.16

A 59-year-old man presented with a 3-year history of gait difficulty and frequent falls. His wife noticed clumsiness of the right arm, increased emotionality, and impairment of memory. He also developed slurring of speech. Brain MRI showed mild atrophy of the right frontoparietal lobes. Sensorimotor examination was limited by dementia and impersistence.

The most likely diagnosis is:

1. Parkinson disease
2. PSP
3. Corticobasal degeneration (CBD)
4. Multisystem atrophy (MSA)–P
5. MSA-C

DIAGNOSIS

- Patients with ophthalmoplegia and gait instability are referred to neuromuscular clinics for suspicion of mitochondrial syndromes.
- This patient had ophthalmoplegia, severe shuffling and hesitation of gait, rigidity, hyper-reflexia, hypomimia, and dysarthria.
- The first step in evaluating ophthalmoplegia is to determine if it is central or peripheral by performing the Doll's eye movement test. In this case, it was central.
- The first test in evaluating neuropathy is by examining foot sensation and ankle reflexes. In this case, the reflexes were brisk and the foot sensation was hard to evaluate.
- Supranuclear ophthalmoplegia is an important finding in many movement disorders. A certain degree of impairment is seen in most patients with neurodegenerative disorders with careful testing. However, it is grossly clinically detectable in only a few patients.
- PSP is notorious for causing falls due to impairment of the downward gaze. In this case, gaze is impaired in all directions.
- Clinical and radiological asymmetry, dementia, and apraxia are important features of CBD, which can also cause ophthalmoplegia and Parkinsonism.
- In this case, the abnormal gait and hypomimia suggested PD initially. However, the gait rhythm has a lower frequency than that of PD.
- Gait apraxia that is seen in NPH is a misnomer and should not be confused with leg apraxia of CBD, which is not as well studied as upper extremities apraxia. In this case, these is no leg apraxia, as the patient could not stride across a line drawn on the floor.
- Although CBD and PSP are pathologically distinct, it may be impossible to distinguish them clinically or radiologically.

SUGGESTED READING

Hashimoto AK, Hashimoto T, Tamaru F, Ueno E, Yanagisawa N. Analysis of gait disturbance in a patient with corticobasal degeneration (in Japanese). *Rinsho Shinkeigaku*. 1995 Feb;35(2):153–157.

CASE 1.17: SPASTIC GAIT

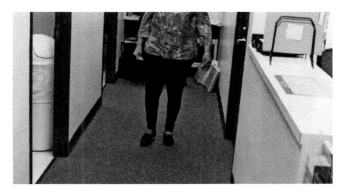

VIDEO 1.17

A 59-year-old woman presented with an 8-year history of loss of balance, falls, stiffness of the right leg, and foot numbness. She had no urinary symptoms. She had no past history of focal neurological deficit. Her symptoms progressed, and she started using a cane. In addition to what is demonstrated in Video 1.17, her examination showed impaired sensation to vibration and proprioception in the feet. Cervical MRI revealed no spinal cord compression. EMG/NCS was normal.

The most appropriate next diagnostic step in this case is:

1. Brain MRI and CSF examination
2. Epidermal nerve fiber density analysis
3. Nerve biopsy
4. Autonomic reflex testing
5. Therapeutic trial with steroids

DIAGNOSIS

- Patients with ataxia are referred for neuromuscular evaluation for neuropathy. Many of these patients turn out to have a nonneuromuscular syndrome, such as:
  - Sensory ataxia due to myelopathy such as B_{12} or copper deficiency or MS.
  - Cerebellar ataxia such as HCD, paraneoplastic cerebellar degeneration.
  - Gait apraxia such as normal-pressure hydrocephalus.
  - Spastic gait without sensory ataxia, such as HSP.
  - Movement disorders like Parkinson disease and Parkinson-plus syndrome.
- In a patient with sensory ataxia and decreased sensation in the feet, the following should direct the attention to the spinal cord:
  - More impairment of proprioception than vibration in the feet
  - Ankle hyperreflexia
  - Positive Babinski sign: it is a good habit to check plantar responses whenever foot numbness is associated with normal or brisk ankle reflexes
  - Increased muscle tone in the legs (spastic gait)
  - Urinary urgency (although this could be due to dysautonomia)
- A skin biopsy has no practical utility in these cases. The lack of pain and the predominance of vibratory loss argue against small fiber involvement.
- This patient had multiple 3–8-mm nonenhancing periventricular white matter lesions in the brain MRI and 4 OCBs in the CSF that did not exist in the serum.
- Progressive MS can be difficult to diagnose and, unfortunately, response to the currently available preventive therapies for relapsing-remitting multiple sclerosis (RRMS) is poor in chronic progressive MS.

CASE 1.18: SENSORY ATAXIA WITH BRISK ANKLE REFLEXES

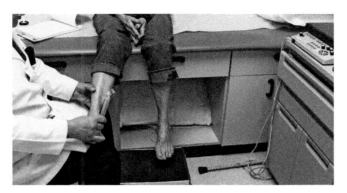

VIDEO 1.18

A 70-year-old woman presented with progressive gait instability. She had subtotal gastrectomy 10 years earlier. She used dentures. Cervical and thoracic MRIs were normal. NCS revealed mild axonal sensorimotor neuropathy. The serum B_{12} level was normal. Her peripheral WBC was 3.2 cells/mcL.

The most appropriate testing at this point is to check:

1. Copper level
2. Bone marrow aspiration
3. CSF protein
4. Selenium level
5. Zinc level

DIAGNOSIS

- Severe impairment of foot sensation to proprioception and vibration with brisk ankle and knee reflexes suggests dorsal myelopathy. Compressive causes of myelopathy were ruled out by MRIs of cervical and thoracic spines. Other causes of noncompressive dorsal myelopathies were ruled out, including B_{12} deficiency. NCS also showed axonal sensorimotor neuropathy. We are dealing with a case of myeloneuropathy.
- Small fiber neuropathy is usually associated with foot pain instead of sensory ataxia, normal reflexes, and normal NCS.
- There have been an increasing number of myeloneuropathy cases reported in association with copper deficiency.
- Risk factors:
  - Remote gastrectomy: Copper is absorbed in the stomach and proximal jejunum.
  - Usage of high zinc–content fixative for dentures. The high zinc content competes with copper and drives its level down.
  - Poor nutritional status.
- Leucopenia is common in copper deficiency, and it is an important diagnostic clue in neurological cases.
- Copper deficiency may also present with muscle atrophy and fasciculations similar to ALS.
- The myeloneuropathy may improve with oral or IV copper replacement, but residual deficit is common. Hematological abnormalities are more amenable to correction.
- The exact role of copper in neural growth and regeneration is not cleIt is important that copper and B_{12} levels are checked in all cases of noncompressive myelopathies.
- Studies have shown that the prevalence of micronutrient deficiency after bariatiric surgery continues to increase while monitoring of patients is decreasing (reference 1).
- All patients with gastrectomy and gastric bypass surgery should be supplemented with vitamins consistently starting right after surgery and be monitored for years.

SUGGESTED READING

Parrott J., Frank L, Rabena R, Craggs-Dino L, Isom KA, Greiman L, et al. American Society for Metabolic and Bariatric Surgery Integrated Health Nutritional Guidelines for the Surgical Weight Loss Patient 2016 update: micronutrients. *Surg Obes Relat Dis.* 2017 Jan 19.

CASE 1.19: FAMILIAL GAIT SPASTICITY

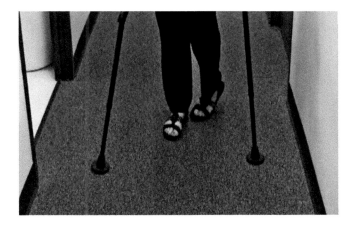

VIDEO 1.19

A 72-year-old woman presented with a 10-year history of slowly progressive gait imbalance. EMG revealed mild sensory neuropathy. She had two brothers with similar symptoms. B_{12} and copper levels were normal. Testing for HSP AD and AR mutations were negative. MRI of the cervical and spinal cord was normal.

The following tests are appropriate except:

1. Serum very-long-chain fatty acid (VLCFA) level
2. Examination of the affected brothers
3. ATP-binding cassette, subfamily D (ALD), member 1 (*ABCD1*) gene mutation
4. Serum fasting cortisol level
5. Serum zinc level

DIAGNOSIS

- Video 1.19 demonstrated and examination showed spastic gait, hyperreflexia, positive Babinski signs, and sensory ataxia.
- The VLCFA level was very high, and pathogenic *ABCD1* mutation was found.
- X-linked adrenomyeloneuropathy is an important but rare cause of chronic progressive myeloneuropathy in adults, and heterozygous cases that affect women are even rarer.
- It is caused by mutation of the *ABCD1* gene. It codes for the adrenoleukodystrophy protein, which is an important component of the peroxisomal membrane and allows the passage of VLCFA to the perioxisomes.
- More than 650 mutations are found in this gene.
- Symptoms start in the second to fourth decades, with spastic paraparesis and sensory ataxia and hyperreflexia. Associated axonal neuropathy and dysautonomia are common. Adrenal insufficiency occurs in 70% of cases, leading to skin pigmentation, hypotension, gastrointestinal (GI) upset, and generalized weakness. Cortisone level is low.
- The female carries display symptoms at age 20–55 years as late-onset myelopathy. Adrenal insufficiency is rare despite a low corticosteroid reserve.
- Steroid replacement is effective for adrenal insufficiency, but there is no cure for myelopathy.
- All noncompressive myelopathies should be tested for VLCFA level and if high, for *ABCD1* mutations, especially if there is a family history of affected males and features of adrenal insufficiency.
- Although it is an X-linked disease, women may be affected later in life and are usually misdiagnosed as MS or familial spastic paraparesis.
- This disease is allelic, with adrenal leukodystrophy that affects children.

CASE 1.20: ATAXIA AND NIGHT BLINDNESS

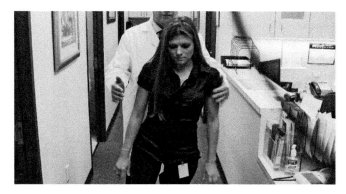

VIDEO 1.20

A 32-year-old woman presented with visual impairment since childhood; she was diagnosed with retinitis pigmentosa. A few years later, she developed loss of balance and foot numbness; she was diagnosed with neuropathy. She continued to get worse. MRIs of the brain and spinal cord were negative. She had a sister with similar symptoms and a brother who was diagnosed with CMT. The retinal exam is shown in Figure 1.20.1. EMG revealed mild sensory neuropathy.

Mutation of which of the following genes may explain this picture?

1. *MT-ATP6* gene
2. *FLVCR1* gene
3. *PHYH* gene
4. *TTPA* gene
5. *SCA-2* gene

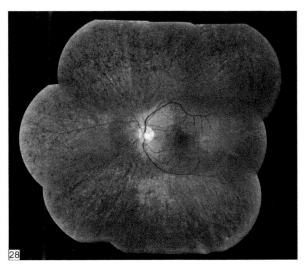

FIGURE 1.20.1 Fundoscopic examination.

TABLE 1.20.1 Genetic Conditions Associated with Ataxia, Neuropathy, and Retinitis Pigmentosa

Disease	Chromosome	Gene	Inheritance
• NARP	• mtDNA	• *MT-ATP6*	• Maternal
• Polyneuropathy, hearing loss, ataxia, retinitis pigmentosa, and cataract (PHARC)	• 20p11.21	• *ABHD12*	• AR
• Ataxia with isolated vitamin E deficiency	• 8q12.3	• *TTPA*	• AR
• Refsum disease	• 10p13	• *PHYH*	• AR
• Abetalipoproteinemia	• 4q23	• *MTP*	• AR
• Congenital disorder of glycosylation type IA (CDG1A)	• 16p13.2	• PMM2	• AR
• SCA-2	• 12q24.12	• SCA2	• AD
• PCARP	• 1q32.2	• FLVCR1	• AR

DIAGNOSIS

- Video 1.20 demonstrated and examination showed severe impairment of proprioception and vibration sensation in the feet and mild loss of pinprick (PP) sensation, absent ankle and knee jerks, and sensory ataxia. Fundoscopic examination revealed retinitis pigmentosa (Figure 1.20.1).
- These listed possibilities have to be considered in patients with ataxia, neuropathy, and retinitis pigmentosa (Table 1.20.1).
- Nerve conduction study revealed sensory neuropathy.
- In this case, most of the following possibilities were ruled out:
  - Genetic testing for neuropathy, ataxia, and retinitis pigmentosa (NARP) was negative.
  - Phytanic acid level was normal.
  - The patients did not have cerebellar ataxia or hearing loss.
  - The transferrin glycosylation pattern was normal.
  - Serum lactate and pyruvate levels were normal.
  - Mitochondrial genome was entirely normal.
  - Vitamin E and abetalipoprotin B levels were normal.
- Sequencing of feline leukemia virus subgroup C cellular receptor (FLVCR1) revealed two pathogenic mutations.
- Posterior column ataxia, with retinitis pigmentosa (PCARP) is an AR disorder characterized by ataxia, neuropathy, and retinitis pigmentosa. Mutation of the *FLVCR1* gene is reported at least in four families to cause this syndrome. The gene is mapped to 1q32.
- *FLVCR1* is a heme exporter. Its role in causing neurological damage is not clear.

SUGGESTED READINGS

Ishiura H, Fukuda Y, Mitsui J, et al. Posterior column ataxia with retinitis pigmentosa in a Japanese family with a novel mutation in FLVCR1. *Neurogenet.* 2011;12:117–121.

Shaibani A, Wong LJ, Wei Zhang V, Lewis RA, Shinawi M. Autosomal recessive posterior column ataxia with retinitis pigmentosa caused by novel mutations in the FLVCR1 gene. *Int J Neurosci.* 2015 Jan;125(1):43–49.

CASE 1.21: NEUROPATHY AND NYSTAGMUS

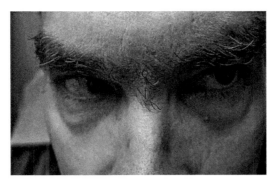

VIDEO 1.21

A 50-year-old man presented with gait imbalance since age 20. As he grew up, he had to turn his head to different directions to see, despite preservation of EOM. A neuroophthalmological consultation concluded that he had oculomotor apraxia (OMA). Progressively, he relied on a wheelchair for mobility. Brain MRI showed cerebellar atrophy. He also had numbness of the feet, and the NCS revealed axonal sensorimotor neuropathy. CK level was 780 IU/L, and alpha-fetoprotein was elevated in the blood.

These findings are typically seen in:

1. Friedreich's ataxia
2. Ataxia with OMA
3. SCA-1
4. Machado-Joseph disease (MCD)
5. SCA and sensory neuropathy

DIAGNOSIS

- This patient was referred for a neuromuscular consultation because of progressive ataxia and neuropathy. Sensory ataxia due to neuropathy often compounds cerebellar ataxia and increases the risk of falling and the need for assistance. The differential diagnosis of neuropathy and cerebellar ataxia includes:
  - SCAs:
    - AD
      - ▸ SCA1: Neuropathy occurs in 42% of cases. Risk of neuropathy increases with the CAG repeat number.
      - ▸ SCA2: Neuropathy occurs in 80% of cases.
      - ▸ SCA3: Neuropathy occurs in 54% of cases. The risk of neuropathy increases with a lower number of Cytosine Adenin Guanin (CAG) repeats.
    - AR
  - Toxin: alcohol, phenytoin
  - Mitochondrial syndromes: neuropathy, ataxia, retinitis pigmentosa (NARP), Dejerine–Sottas disease, and mitochondrial neurogastrointestinal encephalopathy (MNGIE)
  - CMT disease
  - Paraneoplastic syndromes
- Ataxia with OMA type 2:
  - AR ataxia.
  - 50% of patients have difficulty moving their eyes horizontally and moving them quickly, despite absence of defect of controlled, voluntary, and purposeful eye movement (OMA).
  - Usually, ataxia starts at age 15 and functional ambulation is lost 10 years later.
  - It is more common in French Canadians.
  - Neuropathy is usually severe and axonal.
  - Responsible mutation is in the *SETX* gene.
  - High CK and alpha fetoprotein levels are typical.

CASE 1.22: PROGRESSIVE BENDING

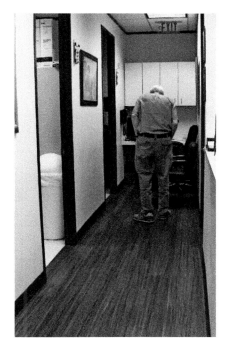

VIDEO 1.22

An 81-year-old man with severe disability resulting from the symptom shown in Video 1.22. He had normal DTRs and strength of the extremities. Symptoms did not fluctuate. There was no diplopia or ptosis. The EMG showed no proximal muscle abnormalities. There was scattered fibrillations limited to the thoracic paraspinal muscles. RST of the left spinal accessory nerve was negative. The CK level was 661 IU/L. The AChR antibody titre was normal. MRI of the thoracic spines is shown in Figure 1.22.1.

The thoracic flexion shown in the video is likely due to:

1. Kyphosis
2. Dystonia
3. Axial myopathy
4. MG
5. ALS

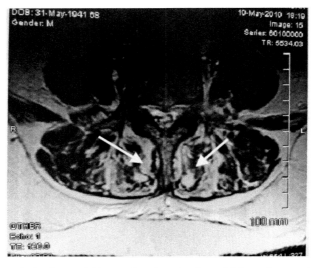

FIGURE 1.22.1 MRI cervical spines, axial image showing atrophy and fatty replacement of the paraspinal muscles.

DIAGNOSIS

- Progressive postural flexion of the thoracolumbar spine upon standing and walking and flattening upon lying down (camptocormia, bent spine syndrome) are consistent with axial muscular weakness rather than skeletal deformity, such as kyphosis, or movement disorders like dystonia, which do not correct with lying down.
- The patient also has mild incidental senile ptosis. The lack of fluctuation and ocular or bulbar symptoms argue against MG, and the restriction of denervation to the TPS muscles argues against ALS. Mild CK elevation is not specific.
- Spontaneous discharges (fibrillations and positive sharp waves) in the thoracic paraspinal muscles are nonspecific and can be seen in denervating conditions such as ALS and myopathic conditions such as axial myopathy, acid maltase deficiency, and inflammatory myopathy. Also, it can be secondary to the flexion deformity itself, causing accelerated degeneration of the thoracic paraspinal muscles with fatty replacement.
- MRI of the thoracic spines show severe atrophy and fatty replacement of the paraspinal muscles (Fig. 1.22.1).
- Axial muscle weakness (neuromuscular paraspinal disorder) can be mimicked by Parkinson disease, dystonia, and psychogenic causes. The first two diseases cause spinal flexion by rigidity of the abdominal muscles.
  - Axial muscle weakness can be associated with MG, ALS, and different myopathies. Most of the time, it remains restricted to the paraspinal muscles (axial myopathy).
    - The average age of onset is 65 years, and pain due to dysfunctional posturing is common.

- Unfortunately, most cases turn out to be due to senile paraspinal muscular degeneration and fatty replacement, for which no treatment is available.

SUGGESTED READING

Shinjo SK, Ramos Torres SC, Radu AS. Camptocormia: A rare axial myopathy disease. *Clinics*. 2008 Jun;63(3):416–417.

PTOSIS

CASE 2.1: CHRONIC FIXED PTOSIS

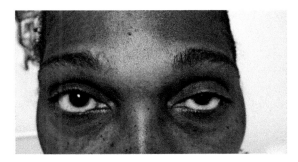

VIDEO 2.1

A 50-year-old African-American female presented with history of systemic lupus erythematosus (SLE) and a 20-year history of bilateral fixed ptosis with no diplopia or dysphagia. She had a sister with ptosis as well.

Chronic nonprogressive fixed ptosis is most likely due to:

1. Myasthenia gravis (MG)
2. Congenital ptosis
3. Oculopharyngeal muscular dystrophy (OPMD)
4. Congenital myasthenic syndrome (CMS)
5. Chronic progressive external ophthalmoplegia (CPEO)

DIAGNOSIS

- Drooping of upper eyelid (ptosis) is an important finding of many neuromuscular disorders.
- The upper eyelids are lifted by:
  - A skeletal muscle called levator palpebrae superioris (LPS) that is supplied by the oculomotor nerve.
  - A smooth muscle called Muller muscle that is supplied by sympathetic fibers originating from stellate ganglion.
    - Orbicularis oculi (OO) muscles are supplied by the facial nerves, and their function is to close the eyes. Weakness of OO does not lead to ptosis, but results in impaired closure of the eyelids.
- Ptosis may result from:
  - Congenital weakness of LPS
  - Disruption of sympathetic flow to the Muller muscle (Horner's syndrome)
  - Disruption of the oculomotor nerve (like diabetic third cranial nerve palsy)
  - Neuromuscular transmission disorders
  - Muscle diseases (OPMD, myotonic dystrophy, etc.)
- Congenital ptosis:
  - Is bilateral in 25% of cases, nonprogressive, and nonfluctuating. It can be asymmetrical.
  - Other family members may have mild and undetected ptosis.
  - Lid creases are absent or very high. (A lid crease originates from fusion of the LPS tendon with the pretarsal plate, and if LPS is congenitally absent, there will be no crease.)
  - Amblyopia and strabismus are common.
  - 5% of patients have weakness of superior rectus due to shared embryology with LPS.
- In evaluation of ptosis, it is often useful to examine an old photo (driver's license photo, for example). Patients may have had ptosis for a long time, which they considered normal. It is also beneficial to examine photos of family members to detect a familial pattern of ptosis.

CASE 2.2: OPHTHALMOPLEGIA AND PROXIMAL WEAKNESS

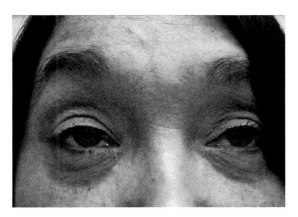

VIDEO 2.2

A 65-year-old woman presented with the demonstrated findings since childhood. Acetylcholine receptor (AChR) antibody titer was negative. There was a significant decremental response to 2 Hz repetitive facial nerve stimulation (RNS). Repetitive compound muscle action potentials (CMAPs) were noted during motor nerve conduction study. The patient responded to Fluoxetine 80 mg a day.

Which of the following CMSs applies to this case?

1. Slow channel syndrome
2. Dok-7 mutation
3. Acetylcholinesterase (AChE) deficiency
4. Choline acetyltransferase deficiency
5. Fast channel syndrome

DIAGNOSIS

- Video 2.2 demonstrated bilateral ptosis and severe fixed ophthalmoplegia and proximal weakness.
- CMSs are due to genetic mutations in genes that encode for proteins at the neuromuscular junction.
- They may be classified as presynaptic, synaptic, and postsynaptic.
- The most common CMSs include:
  - Presynaptic CMS: choline acetyltransferase deficiency. It often causes a severe phenotype, with episodes of apnea.
  - Synaptic CMS: AChE deficiency. It results in overactivation of the neuromuscular junctions, as well as autonomic ganglia. Thus, the pupils are often nonreactive in these patients. Electrodiagnostic testing may show a repetitive CMAP.
  - Postsynaptic CMS: AChR subunit mutations (including alpha, beta, delta, and epsilon), muscle-specific kinase (MuSK), rapsyn, and Dok-7. Mutation of AChR subunits may result in three different physiological effects:
    - AChR deficiency: fatal or severe
    - Early AChR closure (fast channel)
    - Prolonged AChR opening (slow channel)
- Epsilon mutation is not fatal because expression of the fetal gamma-AChR subunit will partially rescue the phenotype.
- Fast channel is a milder defect that would result in partially attenuated receptor response to acetylcholine (ACh). The phenotype may be improved with AChE inhibitors (e.g., pyridostigmine) and 3,4-diaminopyridine.
- Patients with slow channel syndrome demonstrate a repetitive CMAP on electrodiagnostic testing. Due to prolonged opening of these channels, agents that partially block the AChR, such as quinine, quinidine, or fluoxetine, often provide symptomatic improvement.
- Mutations in Dok-7 and rapsyn have been demonstrated to exhibit a later onset limb-girdle distribution weakness.

SUGGESTED READING

Engel AG, Shen XM, Selcen D, Sine SM. Congenital myasthenic syndromes: pathogenesis, diagnosis, and treatment. *Lancet Neurol.* 2015 May;14(5):461.

CASE 2.3: DELAYED EYE OPENING

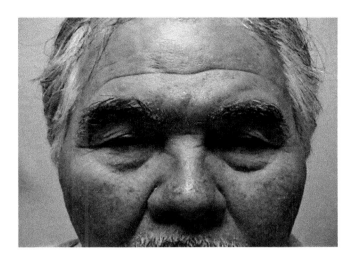

VIDEO 2.3

A 60-year-old man presented with a 4-year history of falls. In addition to what was shown in Video 2,3, he had a normal Doll's eye movement and cerebellar ataxia.

The most likely diagnosis is:

1. Parkinson disease
2. Multisystem atrophy-P
3. Progressive supranuclear palsy (PSP)
4. CPEO
5. Multisystem atrophy–C

DIAGNOSIS

- Examination revealed supranuclear ophthalmoplegia, eyelid apraxia, hypomimia, and mild cerebellar ataxia.
- Apraxia of lid opening (ALO) is a nonparalytic motor abnormality characterized by difficulty initiating the act of lid elevation after lid closure, despite preservation of muscle strength.
- These patients are referred to neuromuscular clinics because they are suspected of having ptosis and along with ophthalmoplegia, MG, and mitochondrial disease are suspected.
- Delayed eye opening after voluntary closure is not a feature of ptosis. Relief of apraxia by sensory cues such as touching the face is characteristic. This phenomenon of *geste antagoniste* might be useful in distinguishing ALO from myotonia of eyelids.
- The lack of forceful closure differentiates ALO from blepharospasm. However, 10% of blepharospasm patients may display features of ALO as well. This explains the lack of response to botulinum toxin (BT) in some cases of blepharospasm.
- ALO is a feature of many neurodegenerative disorders such as Parkinson disease, Huntington disease, corticobasal degeneration, and PSP.
- Doll's eye movement was preserved in this case, which is indicative of supranuclear nature.
- Axial rigidity and frequent falls are suggestive of PSP. Impairment of downward gaze may have been present early in the course and was replaced by a total ophthalmoplegia as the disease progressed.
- Like PSP, corticobasal degeneration is a tauopathy, but it is usually associated with features of cortical dysfunction such as aphasia, dementia, and alien hand syndrome.

CASE 2.4: PTOSIS IN THE ELDERLY

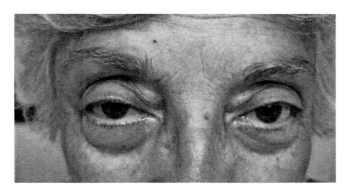

VIDEO 2.4

A 70-year-old woman presented with a long-standing, nonfluctuating bilateral ptosis without diplopia.

The most likely diagnosis is:

1. Hyperthyroidism
2. Ocular MG
3. Dermatochalasis
4. Oculopharyngeal muscular dystrophy
5. Levator dehiscence

DIAGNOSIS

- Elderly people with droopy eyelids are often referred to neuromuscular clinics, especially when their chronic ptosis starts impairing their vision. It is common that patients do not think much about chronic ptosis and consider it to be normal. The appearance of other age-related symptoms, such as declined vision, dryness of eyes, and decreased swallowing due to dryness, are prompting factors for evaluation.
- The most accurate measurement of ptosis is marginal reflex distance (MRD), which is the distance between the lower eyelid margin and the center of pupillary light reflex with the eye in the primary gaze. MRD of more than 2 mm or an asymmetry of more than 2 mm indicates ptosis.
- Ptosis is a common presentation to both emergency rooms and neurology clinics, and it has a wide variety of causes, ranging from serious ones like posterior communicating artery aneurysm to benign ones like dehiscence of the LPS.
- The upper eyelid normally covers 20% of the cornea. The position of the eyelid is affected by gaze (drooping slightly with lateral gaze, elevated with upward gaze, and drooping with downward gaze) and by the state of arousal (elevated with full arousal and drooping with drowsiness).
- Levator dehiscence is the most common cause of lowered eyelids and occurs mostly in the elderly.
  - The eye crease is created by insertion of the LPS to the pretarsal plate and is normally less than 5 mm.
  - When the LPS tendon is disinserted from the tarsal plate, the eyelid droops and becomes thin, but maintains a normal range of motion.
  - Such a disinsertion of the LPS may be caused by trauma to the eye such as eye surgery (cataract extraction) or nonsurgical trauma as simple as eye rubbing.
  - Hard contact lenses can also cause it. In these cases, the ptosis appears acutely, leading to an alarm in the family, but most of the time, a history of chronic drooping is present.
  - High skin crease (more than 7 mm) is a characteristic feature. Typically, the eyelid has a normal range of motion.
  - Failure to diagnose this condition may lead to unnecessary investigations. Correction is simple, by surgical shortening of the LPS or insertion of a tendon sling. Ptosis props are rarely useful.

CASE 2.5: UNIDIRECTIONAL DIPLOPIA

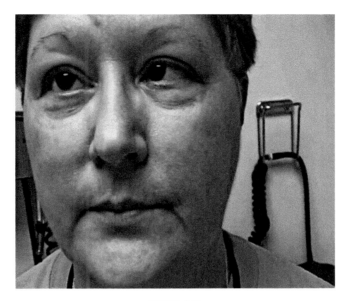

VIDEO 2.5

A 48-year-old woman presented with acute horizontal right gaze diplopia with no ptosis or diurnal variation.

Which muscle is weak, as detected by the demonstrated test?

1. Right medial rectus (MR)
2. Right lateral rectus (LR)
3. Left MR
4. Right LR
5. Right superior oblique (SO)

DIAGNOSIS

- The red lens diplopia test utilizes diplopia as a test of localization of the weak eye muscle. The test is most valuable in interpreting horizontal diplopia.
- The red lens over one eye enables the clinician to identify the eye to which the red image belongs. By convention, the red lens is placed in front of the right eye (red is right). Hence, the red image always belongs to the right eye.
- One can replace the red lens with eye closure (by asking the patient to close one eye to determine the source of double images).
- The most important principle of the test is that the outer image is always the false image.
- If a muscle of one eye is weak, that eye cannot keep up with the normal eye. The normal eye keeps the object focused on its fovea, and therefore in the center of its visual field. But the weak eye loses the foveal fixation, and the visual image of the object strikes the retina peripheral to the fovea. Therefore, the outer image is always the false image.
- The distance between these two images increases as the eyes move farther into the field of action of the weak muscle because the image in the normal eye continues to be focused on the fovea.
- The visual image in the weak eye moves farther from the fovea. The image that is displaced farthest in the direction of the gaze belongs to the eye with the paralyzed muscle.
- The test is done by holding a pin light 60–90 cm in front of the patient's eyes and asking the patient to fixate on the light; move the light into each of the six diagnostic positions of gaze. If the patient has diplopia, he or she will see two lights: one red and one white. This test can be interpreted as follows (with the red lens over the right eye):
  1. When the patient looks to the right and:
     a. Describes the red image to the right of the white image (the red image is the outer image), there is paralysis of the right LR muscle.
     b. Describes the red image to the left of the white image (the red image is the inner image), there is paralysis of the left MR muscle.

SUGGESTED READING

Walker HK, Hall WD. *Clinical Methods: The History, Physical, and Laboratory Examinations*. 3rd ed. Boston: Butterworths; 1990.

CASE 2.6: EYE CLOSURE AND FACIAL GRIMACING

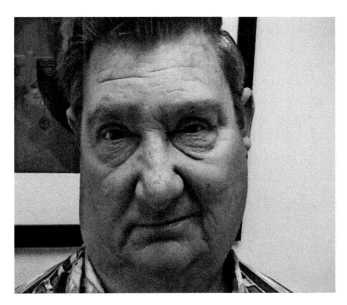

VIDEO 2.6

A 67-year-old man presented with a 5-year history of involuntary bilateral eye closure, facial grimacing, and tongue protrusions. He was initially suspected of having ptosis.

When blepharospasm is the only prominent manifestation of dystonia, it differs from ptosis in that:

1. It responds well to sensory cues.
2. It worsens in the evenings.
3. It causes diplopia.
4. It fluctuates.
5. It is usually reversible.

DIAGNOSIS

- Blepharospasm may be a source of referral to neuromuscular clinics due to confusion with ptosis. Confusion of ptosis with blepharospasm can be dangerous; ptosis may be due to MG where BT is contraindicated.
- Blepharospasm is a forceful involuntary eye closure due to focal dystonia of OO. It is usually bilateral but can be asymmetric.
- In 20% of cases, it starts unilaterally.
- It should be differentiated from ALO, which is due to failure of LPS to contract. Both may coexist.
- Blepharospasm increases under bright light and during time of stress; hence, it may interfere with driving.
- Ptosis may do the same under these conditions. About two-thirds of patients are rendered functionally blind by blepharospasm.
- Blepharospasm may be associated with mandibular and facial dystonia (Meige syndrome).
- The spasms may be transiently alleviated by pulling on the upper eyelid or the eyebrow, pinching the neck, talking, humming, yawning, singing, sleeping, relaxing, reading, concentrating, looking down, and performing other maneuvers or sensory tricks (*geste antagonistique*).
- The cause of blepharospasm may be impairment of the mechanism of blinking. Normally, blinking is reduced by 74% during reading and increased 100% during conversation. Normal individuals blink more frequently during conversation. In blepharospasm, the pattern is reversed.

SUGGESTED READING

Gomez-Wong E, Marti MJ, Tolosa E, Valls-Sole J. Sensory modulation of the blink reflex in patients with blepharospasm. *Arch Neurol.* 1998;55:1233–1237.

CASE 2.7: SYMPTOMS RESOLVED AFTER PRAYER

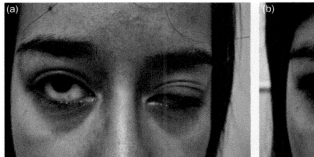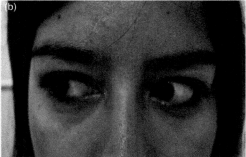

VIDEO 2.7

A 18-year-old woman presented with intermittent left ptosis and fatigable diplopia (Video 2.7A) with positive binding AChR antibodies. She refused treatment, and her symptoms resolved with prayer (Video 2.7B), only to come back 6 months later.

The following is true about resolution of symptoms with prayer:

1. It is due to spontaneous resolution of MG.
2. It is against the diagnosis of MG.
3. MG symptoms are often induced by prayer.
4. It occurs only in seropositive cases.
5. Prayer should be tried first, followed by medication.

DIAGNOSIS

- MG, like other autoimmune diseases, may spontaneously remit temporarily or permanently.
- The natural history of MG was studied in a cohort of 73 patients before the era of disease-modifying agents.
- A total of 22% of patients went into a complete clinical remission, 18% improved considerably, 16% improved moderately, 16% had not changed, 3% deteriorated, and 29% died, including 8 who had thymoma.
- Another study found a remission rate of 10% and a death rate of 35% in 360 patients. Over half of the deaths occurred in the first 3 years. Of the remaining patients, 20% improved, 30% did not change, and 5% got worse.
- Spontaneous remission is more likely as time passes, and complications are more likely during the first 3 years of the diagnosis.
- Remission rate without treatment is 5%, 24%, 33%, and 41% at 1, 3, 5, and 10 years.
- There are no clear factors that are associated with more chances of spontaneous remission.

SUGGESTED READINGS

Beghi E, Antozzi C, Batocchi AP, et al. Prognosis of myasthenia gravis: a multicenter follow up study of 844 patients. *J Neurol Sci.* 1991;106:213–220.

Oosterhuis HJGH. The natural course of myasthenia gravis: a long term follow up study. *J Neurol Neurosurg Psych.* 1989;52:1121–1127.

CASE 2.8: MYASTHENIA WITH DILATED PUPIL

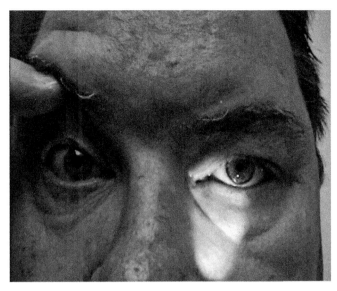

VIDEO 2.8

A 56-year-old man presented with fluctuating right ptosis, which started after recent cataract surgery. He had diplopia due to left MR weakness that started after a right orbital trauma that mandated a major reconstructive surgery several years earlier, but the diplopia had worsened recently. The ptosis was relieved temporarily with an ice pack, and the diplopia resolved when the ptosis was complete. The right pupil was not reactive to light. The AChR Ab titer was positive.

Which of the following argues against the diagnosis of MG?

1. The response of ptosis to the ice pack
2. The resolution of diplopia when the ptosis was complete
3. The appearance of ptosis after surgery
4. The pupillary abnormality
5. None of the above

DIAGNOSIS

- Patients who are referred for neuromuscular evaluation for suspected MG may end up having different diagnoses.
- About 10% of cases referred by neuroophthalmologists to the Nerve and Muscle Center of Texas for confirmation of MG turned out to have an alternative diagnosis, and the misdiagnosis was enhanced by negative brain magnetic resonance imaging (MRI).
- On the other hand, even in serologically proven MG, one may discover irreconcilable findings such as dilated pupil(s). Patients may not be aware of these findings, or they do not give a relevant history because they do not think that it is important.
- This patient had a fixed and dilated right pupil from an old trauma that required orbital surgery, which also changed the anatomy of the orbital muscles. However, the right ptosis is a new finding that prompted a search for MG.
- Resolution of diplopia with complete ptosis is expected, as vision from one eye is not enough to produce diplopia. Monocular diplopia is more likely an image split due to retinal, corneal, or lenticular disease rather than actual diplopia. Very rarely, a central lesion produces monocular diplopia. The double image does not appear when looking through a pinhole.
- The appearance of symptoms of MG after physical or emotional trauma is not unusual. This is the case with all autoimmune diseases.

CASE 2.9: APRAXIA OR PTOSIS?

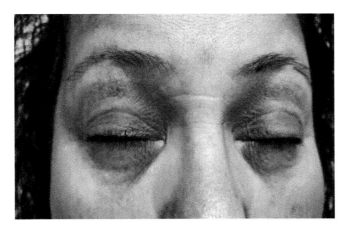

VIDEO 2.9

A 41-year-old woman presented with a 3-month history of diplopia and difficulty opening her eyes. Her examination reveals multidirectional diplopia and weakness of the OO. She also had difficulty opening her eyes once voluntarily closed, suggesting eyelid apraxia. MG serology was positive, and she responded to steroids.

ALO:

1. Can be seen with blepharospasm
2. Can be seen in isolation
3. Can be confused with eyelid myotonia
4. Can be confused with ptosis
5. Never responds to BT

DIAGNOSIS

- Upper eyelid ptosis (drooping) is an important manifestation of MG. It is diagnosed when the upper eyelid covers more than 20% of the cornea.
- ALO is the inability to open the eyes, with preservation of strength and understanding of the command.
- Ptosis may be confused with ALO, but there is usually weakness and fatigability of the LPS and OO.
- ALO is due to abnormality of supranuclear control of eyelid elevation, which requires the activation of the LPS and concurrent inhibition of the OO activity.
- BT injections to the pretarsal muscle may be useful when there is an associated blepharospasm, and it may benefit ALO due to pretarsal motor activity persistence, but not when ALO is due to involuntary LPS inhibition.
- It is crucial that ALO is not confused with ptosis from MG because BT is contraindicated in the latter.

CASE 2.10: MYASTHENIC SYMPTOMS WORSENED WITH STEROIDS

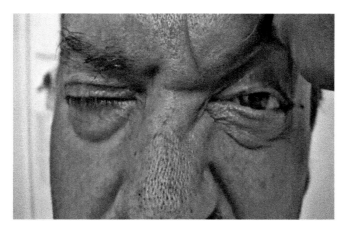

VIDEO 2.10

A 55-year-old man presented with a 6-month history of evening diplopia and dysarthria. Examination is shown in the video. Resting forced vital capacity (FVC) was 50% of normal.

The most specific test for this condition is:

1. AChR Ab titer
2. Repetitive nerve stimulation test
3. Computed tomography (CT) scan of the chest
4. Single-fiber electromyography (SFEMG)
5. Brain MRI

In MG, when respiratory function is compromised, initiation of high-dose steroids:

1. May precipitate respiratory failure
2. Usually improves bulbar symptoms within 24 hours
3. Does not worsen dysphagia
4. Reduces the need for monitoring respiratory functions

DIAGNOSIS

- Examination revealed fluctuating ptosis, diplopia, dysarthria, dysphagia, and weakness of OO, tongue, and multiple extraocular muscles.
- The AChR antibody titer was positive. This is the most specific test for MG.
- Deterioration of myasthenic symptoms after initiation of steroid therapy occurs in 20%–40% of patients and is severe, to a degree that intubation may be necessary, in 8% of cases.
- Worsening of dysphagia would interfere with the ability to take oral prednisone and cholinesterase inhibitors, and that may worsen the situation further.
- Patients with bulbar dysfunction should be watched carefully after steroid initiation; if they do not live close to a medical facility or if they are not able to understand directions well, steroid initiation may be done better under direct supervision in a hospital environment. Pretreatment with plasma exchange (PLEX) or intravenous immunoglobulin (IVIG) is advocated by some experts to counter any early deterioration.
- Gradual initiation of steroids reduces the risk of such deterioration significantly, but it increases the time of total exposure to high-dose steroids, as it will take a few weeks before the maximum dose is reached.
- Worsening usually occurs within two weeks of steroid initiation.
- It is very important that patients are informed of the risk of deterioration and are urged to call the treating physician if they experience dyspnea, dysphagia, or dyspnea.

SUGGESTED READING

Pascuzzi R, Coslett HB, Johns TR. Long term corticosteroids treatment of MG: report of 116 patients. *Ann Neurol.* 1984;15:291–298.

CASE 2.11: IATROGENIC PTOSIS

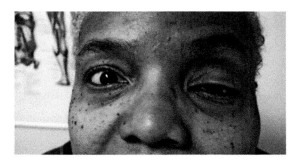

VIDEO 2.11

A 54-year-old woman had left hemifacial spasms treated with BT injection every 3 months. Three days after the last session, she developed blurring of vision.

The shown findings are:

1. Consistent with BT side effects
2. Strongly suggestive of MG
3. Suggestive of botulism
4. Consistent with congenital ptosis
5. None of the above

BT:

1. Blocks ACh receptors
2. Prevents release of ACh
3. Neutralizes ACh
4. Blocks sodium channels
5. None of the above

DIAGNOSIS

- Her examination showed multidirectional diplopia and fatigable left ptosis.
- As the cosmetic use of BT has dramatically increased over the last few years, more patients are referred to neuromuscular clinics to evaluate its complications, especially muscle weakness.
- Transient weakness of the injected muscles is common and intended. More severe weakness of the injected muscles and weakness of muscles that are away from the injection sites may occur and can be alarming and disabling.
- Diplopia occurs in 13% and ptosis in 7% of recipients of BT for hemifacial spasms.
  - Other complications include dysphagia, fatigue, and decreased ability to read emotions due to dampening of emotional signals from face to the brain.
- Sometimes patients who have received cosmetic injections are not aware that diplopia could be related to the injections and therefore do not volunteer their history with the cosmetic procedure.
- BT works by proteolysis of SNAP-25, which is needed for fusion of the vesicle, which is essential for the release of ACh.
- Fortunately, these side effects almost always resolve within a few weeks. Adjustment of future doses of BT and sites of injections is necessary to minimize these complications.

SUGGESTED READINGS

Hayas DA, Glenberg AM, Gutowski KA, Lucarelli MJ, Davidson RJ. Cosmetic use of botulinum toxin-A affects processing of emotional language. *Psych Sci*. 2010 Sep;21(7):895–900.

Yoshimura DM, Aminoff MJ, Tami TA, Scott AB. Treatment of hemifacial spasm with botulinum toxin. *Musc Nerve*. 1992;15(9):1045–1049.

CASE 2.12: FIXED PTOSIS

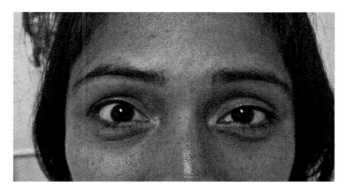

VIDEO 2.12

A 30-year-old woman presented with fixed, painless, nonprogressive left ptosis, which she noticed initially after wearing new contact lenses. Examination revealed normal strength of the OO and LPS and elevated eyelid crease of the ptotic eye.

Levator dehiscence is associated with:

1. Weak OO
2. Morning worsening of the ptosis
3. Trauma to the levator
4. Diplopia
5. None of the above

DIAGNOSIS

- Levator dehiscence is the most common cause of ptosis. In the elderly, it is usually bilateral. In the young population, it is more likely to be unilateral and caused by trauma. Contact lenses may be the source of trauma to the LPS.
- The most characteristic finding is elevation of the eyelid skin crease, which is normally formed by insertion of the tendon of the LPS to the pretarsal plate. Dehiscence is caused by disinsertion of the tendon to the pretarsal plate.
- The levator function is otherwise preserved. The skin above the tarsal plate is thin and may appear semitransparent (especially in the elderly). The pupil and the ocular motility are normal unless they are affected by trauma.
- Oculoplasty is a simple and effective procedure for disabling cases, but usually the condition is not progressive or impairing.

CASE 2.13: FAMILIAL PTOSIS

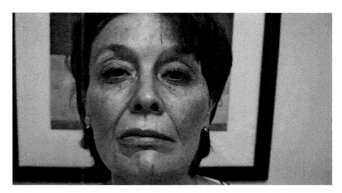

VIDEO 2.13

A 57-year-old woman from Louisiana presented with ptosis, noticed 10 years earlier. The ptosis did not vary during the day. Her father had bilateral ptosis. She had six siblings: a brother and two sisters had ptosis; one had oculoplasty, and the other had cricopharyngeotomy for dysphagia. There was no clinical or electromyographic myotonia.

The most appropriate first test to be performed is:

1. Fundoscopic examination
2. Checking serum lactate and pyruvate levels
3. Repetitive nerve stimulation testing
4. Muscle biopsy
5. Mutation analysis of the *PABPN1* gene

OPMD:

1. Is an autosomal-dominant (AD) disease
2. Is a mitochondrial disorder
3. Has characteristic electron microscopy (EM) findings
4. Is associated with heart block
5. Is associated with retinitis pigmentosa

DIAGNOSIS

- She tested positive for polyadenylate-binding nuclear protein 1 (PABPN1) mutation.
- OPMD is an AD disease that usually presents in the fourth to sixth decade of life with ptosis.
- The ptosis is bilateral and can be asymmetric.
- Ophthalmoplegia occurs in 50% of cases, but diplopia is rare due to chronicity and suppression of one image by the brain. Other causes of peripheral ophthalmoplegia, such as CPEO and CMS, should be considered.
- One-fourth of cases present with dysphagia.
- Facial weakness occurs in some patients.
- Proximal weakness in the arms and legs occur later.
- Temporal wasting and frontal baldness may cause diagnostic confusion with myotonic dystrophy.
- There is a variant where distal muscles are affected (distal OPMD).
- Creatine kinase level is normal or mildly elevated.
- Muscle biopsy is not necessary for the diagnosis, but if obtained, it would show chronic myopathic features and red-rimmed vacuoles similar to the ones seen in inclusion body myositis (IBM).
- Intranuclear tubulofilamentous inclusions measuring 8.5 nm arranged in tangles and palisades are seen in at least 9% of fibers, and they are characteristic.
- Unlike mitochondrial ophthalmopathy, no significant numbers of ragged red fibers are seen for age.
- The pathogenic mutation consists of expansion of GCG repeats within the *PABN1* gene on chromosome 14q11.1.
- Repeats of 8–13 are pathogenic but mitotically stable, unlike myotonic dystrophy. Therefore, anticipation is not observed in OPMD. The expanded repeats lead to formation of misfolded protein that cannot be degraded and cleared so that it forms neurotoxic inclusion bodies.
- There is no cure. Oculoplasty for ptosis and cricopharyngeotomy for dysphagia are helpful if appropriately timed. Patients have normal survival rates.

CASE 2.14: RESPIRATORY FAILURE INDUCED BY STEROIDS

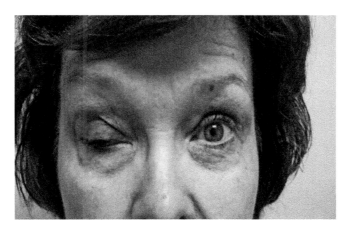

VIDEO 2.14

A 57-year-old woman presented with an 8-week history of drooping right eyelid that was much worse in the evening. She started having frequent coughs during meals 6 weeks later. The AChR antibody titer was 31 nmol/L. She was treated with oral prednisone, 80 mg/day. She was admitted to the hospital 4 days later for severe dysphagia, dysarthria, and dyspnea.

The observed worsening of the bulbar function is most likely due to:

1. Brain stem stroke
2. Wrong diagnosis
3. Nothing in particular; the patient would have worsened anyway
4. Steroid initiation
5. Thymoma

DIAGNOSIS

- Worsening of myasthenic symptoms occurs in 25%–50% of cases, and it is severe in 7% of cases. Patients with bulbar dysfunction should be closely monitored after initiation of steroids. If bulbar function is remarkably compromised, initiation of steroids is safer under observation in the hospital or preceded by IVIG or plasmapheresis.
- The cause of such worsening is not clear. Steroids are known to worsen certain neuromuscular conditions, and therefore they are contraindicated in Guillain-Barré syndrome (GBS) and multifocal motor neuropathy with conduction block.
- Elevation of the eyebrows on the ptotic side is a normal compensatory mechanism. Depression of the eyebrow would suggest a functional (psychogenic) etiology.
- Ptosis in myasthenia can happen without diplopia or bulbar dysfunction. Diagnosis can be difficult to make, especially given that serology and RNS are negative in 40% of cases. Tensilon testing can be helpful in these cases. SFEMG on the weak LPS or OO is more helpful to rule out the disease (if negative), but a positive test is not specific.
- Fluctuation is an important sign in MG, but in chronic cases, muscles may become fixed by fibrosis. A therapeutic steroid trial may be needed to settle the diagnosis.
- The risk of thymoma is the same; therefore, CT scan of the chest should be ordered, even in MG cases that present with ptosis only.

CASE 2.15: WATCH OUT FOR STEROID COMPLICATIONS

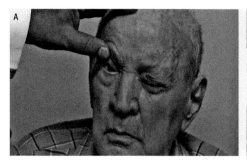 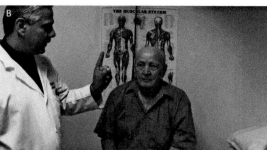

VIDEO 2.15

A 92-year-old man presented with a 2-month history of subacute bilateral ptosis and diplopia. The AChR Ab titer was elevated (Video 2.15A). CT scan of the chest was negative. He did not respond to pyridostigmine 60 mg TID, but 4 weeks after oral prednisone, 60 mg a day, his symptoms resolved.

The most appropriate next step in management of this case is:

1. Add a steroid sparing agent such as azathioprine.
2. Change pyridostigmine to 120 mg five times a day.
3. Continue the same dose of prednisone for a year.
4. Start tapering prednisone to the lowest most effective maintenance dose.
5. Thymectomy.

The prednisone was tapered to 15 mg every other day. A year and a half later, he fell and fractured a femur, which was complicated by deep vein thrombosis (DVT).

Long-term complications of steroids include all of the following except:

1. Cataract
2. Osteoporosis
3. Proximal weakness
4. Hypertension
5. Neuropathy

DIAGNOSIS

- While high-dose oral prednisone is effective in 90% of cases of MG, complications are common, and close monitoring is required, especially in the elderly.
- A total of 25% of patients develop the following complications, which are dose and duration dependent:
  - Osteoporosis: the most serious long-term complication. Menopausal, smoking women are at the highest risk. The risk of femoral fracture after a minor fall is high, and the outcome can be devastating. Weight-bearing exercises such as walking are to be encouraged. A diet rich in calcium, protein, and vitamin D is recommended. An annual bone density scan and supplementation with calcium, 1,000 mg a day, Vitamin D3 1,000 units a day, and etidronate 5 mg a day are recommended.
  - Diabetes mellitus (DM): dietary control and periodic measurement of fasting blood sugar (FBS) or hemoglobin A1c (HbA1c) are advised.
  - Easy bruisability and muscle weakness.
  - Glaucoma and cataract.
  - Gastric erosion and indigestion.
  - Fluid retention.
  - Mood changes, depression, and insomnia.
  - Weight gain.
  - Infection, including thrush.
  - Hypertension.
  - Hypertrichosis.
  - Acne.
- Monitoring of body weight, blood pressure, serum glucose, skin integrity, muscle strength, dietary measures, yearly bone density scan, treatment of insomnia and anxiety, and avoidance of mixing with sick children, are several useful preventive measures.
- Very often, patients ask if they can take influenza vaccination. Influenza vaccination is not contraindicated in MG. Immunosupression or recent treatment with plasmapheresis or intravenous (IV) gammaglobulin may reduce the effectiveness of vaccinations.

CASE 2.16: DROOPY EYELID AND ANISOCORIA

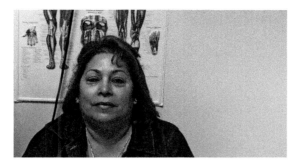

VIDEO 2.16

She had no history of smoking, cough, or migraine. MRI of the brain, including cavernous sinuses and orbits, was normal. Sedimentation rate and antinuclear antibody (ANA) test were negative. Apraclonidine (Lopidine) test result is shown in Figure 2.16.1. Amphetamine drops did not cause a reaction in smaller.

This syndrome is most likely:

1. Horner's syndrome, first-order neuron injury
2. Horner's syndrome, second-order neuron injury

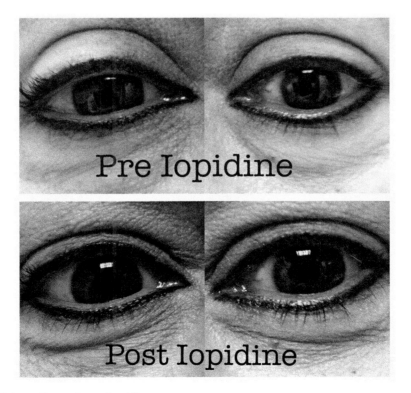

FIGURE 2.16.1 pupils reaction to Lopidine

3. Horner's syndrome, third-order neuron injury
4. Third cranial nerve palsy
5. Adie pupil syndrome

All the following can cause postganglionic Horner's syndrome except:

1. Syringomyelia
2. Carotid artery dissection
3. Cavernous sinus disease
4. Raeder syndrome
5. Cluster headache

DIAGNOSIS

- Right miosis and partial ptosis are characteristic of Horner's syndrome. Also, there was a mild enophthalmos. Elevation of the lower eyelid and injection of the conjunctiva are also typical. Myasthenia does not cause miosis, and oculomotor palsy causes complete ptosis and mydriasis.
- Apraclonidine is an alpha 1 agonist. The denervated right pupil is compensated by increasing alpha 1 receptor density, so it overreacts to apraclonidine drops, leading to reversal of the miosis (the affected pupil becomes bigger than the normal pupil, which reacts normally to the agent). Such a reversal is typical for Horner's syndrome.
- Amphetamine does not elicit pupillary reaction in postganglionic (third-order neuron) Horner's because there are no epinephrine vesicles to be released, as opposed to the normal pupil or preganglionic lesions (first- and second-order neurons).
- This is postganglionic Horner's syndrome. It is usually related to sympathetic pathway lesions in the neck, cavernous sinus, or orbit, as opposed to the brain and cervical cord lesions in preganglionic Horner's. Most postganglionic lesions are benign, as opposed to preganglionic lesions.
- The patient has no history of migraine, and the deficit is fixed, which argues against migraine and Raeder syndrome.
- There is no pain in the right side of the neck to suggest dissection of the carotid artery.
- The relationship to the mentioned surgery is not clear.
- There is no indication of disturbance of the rest of the sympathetic and parasympathetic nervous systems.

CASE 2.17: A WIDE EYE

A 63-year-old man presented with 8 weeks' history of fatigable right ptosis and diplopia, and the exam showed restricted movement of several extraocular muscles and fatigable right ptosis. The AChR antibody titer was negative. RST of the left nasalis showed 20% decrement. He responded to steroids.

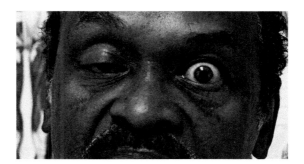

VIDEO 2.17

The left eye shows findings most likely due to:

1. Hyperthyroidism
2. Anxiety
3. MG
4. Hydrocephalus
5. Periodic paralysis

DIAGNOSIS

- This is a 63 YOM with 8 weeks history of fatigable right ptosis and diplopia and the exam showed restricted movement of several EOMs and fatigable right ptosis. AChR antibody titer was negative. RST of the left Nasalis showed 20% decrement. He responded to steroids.
- Eyelid retraction applies when the margin of one of the upper eyelids is elevated above the limbus so that a band of sclera is readily visible in the neutral gaze.
- Eyelid retraction can be associated with thyroid eye disease, familial periodic paralysis, Cushing syndrome, midbrain disease, and hydrocephalus. Unilateral lid retraction is often compensatory to contralateral ptosis and is seen in MG.

CASE 2.18: CHRONIC BILATERAL PTOSIS

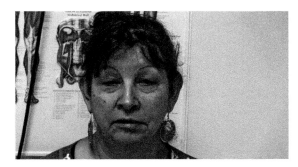

VIDEO 2.18

A 62-year-old woman with 8 years' history of fixed bilateral ptosis (had surgical eyelid lifting) and 4 years' history of dysphagia. Examination revealed normal extraocular movement (EOM) and bilateral fixed ptosis. There were no proximal or axial muscle weakness, reflex, or sensory abnormalities or facial weakness. There was no history of visual or cardiac problems. Creatine phosphokinase (CPK) level was 650 IU/L. No information about her parents or two siblings was available.

This picture is typically seen in:

1. CMS
2. OPMD
3. CPEO
4. PSP
5. Congenital ptosis

DIAGNOSIS

- Genetic testing revealed short triplet repeat expansion (GCG) in the polyadenylation binding protein 2 (*PABP2*) gene in chromosome 14q11, confirming OPMD.
- CMS causes symptoms earlier in life, and they usually are fatigable. Speech abnormalities are common.
- CPEO does not cause such a severe dysphagia.
- PSP causes ophthalmoplegia of upper motor neuron (UMN) type with no ptosis.
- Congenital ptosis appears earlier and does not cause dysphagia.
- OPMD is an AD muscular dystrophy that appears usually in the fifth or sixth decades and presents with progressive ptosis, dysphagia, and proximal weakness.
  - Targeted gene sequencing guided by the typical clinical picture is the best testing strategy.
  - Muscle biopsy is not indicated, except in suspected patients who turn out to have normal *PABP2* alleles.
  - Positive family history, as well as the presence of ptosis and dysphagia, are required for the diagnosis, while ophthalmoplegia is not; it is missing in a significant number of patients.
  - Surgical correction of ptosis and cricopharyngeal myotomy are the only available remedies.
  - Life expectancy is not affected. No cardiac/respiratory involvement is expected.
  - Autosomal recessive (AR) disease is caused by a double dose of the affected allele.

SUGGESTED READING

Brais, B, Rouleau GA, Bouchard J-P, Fardeau M, Tomé FMS. Oculopharyngeal muscular dystrophy. *Sem Neurol.* 1999; 19(1): 59–66.

CASE 2.19: CHRONIC PTOSIS AND HEART BLOCK

A 27-year-old man presented with 10 years' history of progressive, painless, bilateral ptosis and ophthalmoplegia, with no proximal weakness or dysphagia and with normal pupils.

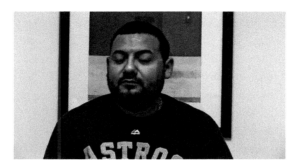

VIDEO 2.19

Electrocardiography (ECG) showed second-degree heart block. Retinal examination was normal. A paternal uncle had EOM abnormality, and he was diagnosed with carotid cavernous fistula. No more information is available.

The history and findings suggest:

1. PSP
2. CMS
3. OPMD
4. CPEO
5. Refractory MG

DIAGNOSIS

- A 27-year-old gentleman with 10 years history of progressive painless bilateral ptosis and ophthalmoplegia with no proximal weakness or dysphagia and with normal pupils.
- This is CPEO.
  - Reported EKG abnormalities may be due to heart block. That suggests Kearns-Sayre syndrome (KSS), which is caused by a large mitochondrial DNA (mtDNA) deletion.
  - Lack of retinitis pigmentosa is not exclusionary. Beside external ophthalmoplegia and onset below 20 years, diagnosis requires one of the following three abnormalities: heart block, retinitis pigmentosa, or CSF protein higher than 100 mg/dl.
  - Chronicity and lack of fluctuation argue against MG.
  - There is no dysphagia to suggest OPMD; age of onset is too early for OPMD.
  - Genetic study on muscle biopsy of this patient confirmed KSS. Mutations are not usually detectable in the blood.
  - This is usually sporadic, and the risk of inheritance is very low.
  - Muscle tissue is needed for mitochondrial deletion studies, as peripheral blood is not sensitive due to heteroplasmy (differential aggregation of mutated mitochondria in different tissue).

SUGGESTED READING

McClelland C. Progressive external ophthalmoplegia. *Curr Neurol Neurosci Rep*. Jun 2016;16(6):53.

DIPLOPIA

CASE 3.1: WEAK LATERAL RECTUS (LR)

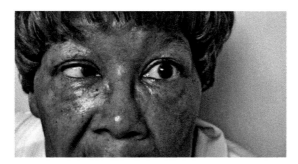

VIDEO 3.1

A 72-year-old African-American woman presented with fluctuating diplopia to lateral gaze bilaterally and elevated acetylcholine (ACh) receptors antibody titer. She had incidental left Bell's palsy 2 years earlier.

Bilateral weakness of the lateral rectus (LR) muscle is a feature of:

1. Amyotrophic lateral sclerosis (ALS)
2. Myasthenia gravis (MG)
3. Benign intracranial hypertension
4. Answers 1 and 2
5. Answers 2 and 3

DIAGNOSIS

- Video 3.1 shows bilateral weakness of the LR.
- About 50% of cases of MG present with ocular symptoms such as ptosis and diplopia.
- A total of 50% of these cases will generalize. Generalization mostly occurs in the first 2 years after the diagnosis and only rarely occurs later.
- Most patients with generalized MG have ocular involvement.
- The cause for preferential involvement of extraocular movement (EOM) is not clear.
  - EOMs are smaller, contract faster than extremity muscles, and have fewer muscle fibers per motor neuron. Such a delicate and fast contraction ability predisposes them to fatigue.
  - It has been proposed that the types of antibodies that attack EOM are different from the ones that affect extremity muscles.
  - The function of EOM is delicate, and even minor weakness can cause symptoms due to misalignment of the EOM, which leads to diplopia.
- EOM involvement in MG is so variable that several diseases can be mimicked, and the diagnosis thus may be delayed, especially when the weakness is limited to the EOMs.
- EOM involvement is usually bilateral but asymmetrical.
- The most common patterns are:
  - Weakness of the superior oblique (SO) and inferior rectus (65%). This leads to vertical diplopia that occurs with sustained upward gaze.
  - Single EOM involvement occurs in 12% of cases.
  - SO weakness causes diagnostic confusion with fourth cranial nerve palsy.
  - LR weakness may mimic sixth cranial nerve palsy.
  - Medial rectus (MR) weakness mimics third cranial nerve palsy.
  - Inferior rectus weakness.
  - Bilateral MR involvement can mimic internuclear ophthalmoplegia.
  - Rarely, bilateral LR weakness may happen, leading to diagnostic confusion with chronic intracranial hypertension, such as seen in benign intracranial hypertension.
  - Benign intracranial hypertension does not cause ptosis.
  - Third cranial nerve palsy causes complete ptosis, but the weakness in this case affected only the LR, and none of the muscles innervated by the third cranial nerve.
  - Diplopia is not a feature of ALS.

CASE 3.2: MEDIAL RECTUS (MR) WEAKNESS

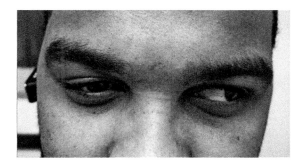

VIDEO 3.2

A 25-year-old man presented with ocular MG controlled with oral steroids. When the steroids were discontinued, he developed weakness of the MRs without ptosis.

Isolated weakness of the MRs can be caused by:

1. MG
2. Bilateral third cranial nerve palsy
3. Multiple sclerosis (MS)
4. Clivus meningeoma
5. Benign intracranial hypertension

DIAGNOSIS

- The medical recti are susceptible to fatigue in MG, and they can be the presenting feature of the disease.
- Lateral gaze may reveal weakness of the MR of the adducted eye and nystagmus of the abducted eye that get coarser with more fatigue of the ipsilateral LR. This is called *pseudo-internuclear ophthalmoplegia.*
- Sustained lateral gaze for 30–45 seconds is usually enough to produce weakness of MR in MG.
- Holding a visual target too close to the patient may produce failure of convergence, which may not be an abnormal sign.
- Moving the visual target away would resolve the produced diplopia if it was due to convergence failure; it would worsen if it was due to MG.
- Associated weakness of the orbicularis oculi (OO) strongly favors myasthenia as a cause of MR weakness.
- In most instances, ptosis, fatigable dysarthria, dysphagia, and weakness of mastication muscles make it easy to diagnose MG, but difficulties arise when the weakness is limited to EOM muscles and when fluctuation is not prominent and abnormal serology is absent.
- Single-fiber electromyography (SFEMG) is useful, especially if a weak facial muscle (frontalis, OO) is tested. Testing EOMs themselves with SFEMG is not an option in clinical practice.
- Clivus meningeoma and benign intracranial hypertension do not cause bilateral MR weakness.

CASE 3.3: POSITIVE EDROPHONIUM TEST

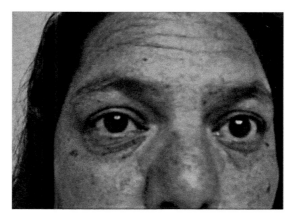

VIDEO 3.3

A 63-year-old woman presented with fatigable, painless, binocular diplopia on left lateral gaze only with reported right ptosis, with a partial response to edrophonium and negative MG serology. Initial brain magnetic resonance imaging (MRI) was normal. She developed nystagmus 3 months later, and a repeat brain MRI was abnormal (Figure 3.3.1).

Edrophonium testing:

1. Is 90% specific for MG
2. If negative, excludes MG
3. Is always negative in brain stem glioma
4. Can be positive in pseudoptosis

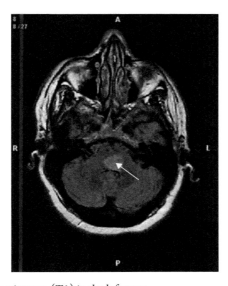

FIGURE 3.3.1 Brain MRI: Hyperintense (T1) in the left pons.

DIAGNOSIS

- This patient was found to have a brain stem glioma.
- Edrophonium inhibits acetylcholinesterase (AChE) and thus prolongs the availability of ACh at the neuromuscular junction, which in turn results in enhanced muscle strength.
- Onset of the action is within 30 seconds, and duration of the action is up to 5 minutes.
- A dose of 2 mg of edrophonium is injected intravenously, and if there is no unwanted reaction such as bradycardia, the remaining 8 mg is injected.
- Facial muscle twitching, lacrimation, salivation, sweating, and flushing are indicators of action.
- Pyridostigmine should be stopped for 24 hours before the procedure.
- Atropine should always be available to reverse severe muscarinic side effects. It will not affect nicotinic side effects.
- A placebo arm is advocated, but its impact on the outcome of the test is questionable.
- It is imperative that a measurable weak muscle is monitored for action such as ptosis or weak EOM.
- A nonspecific response, such as improvement of fatigue, is not essentially a positive response.
- It is 70% sensitive and very nonspecific. False positive response can happen with ALS, brain tumors, and pseudoptosis.
- The use of this test has dramatically declined over the years due to its poor contribution to the diagnosis of equivocal cases and the availability of SFEMG.

CASE 3.4: MYASTHENIA GRAVIS MIMICKER

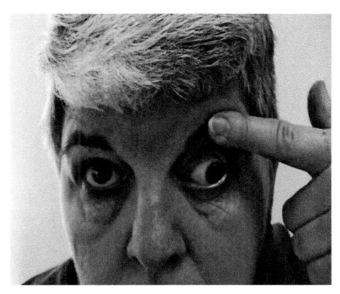

VIDEO 3.4

A 65-year-old woman presented with progressive left ptosis and MR weakness. She had negative MG serology, brain MRI, and magnetic resonance angiogram (MRA) of the brain. She responded partially to pyridostigmine. She developed headaches and left mydriasis 3 months later. Repeat brain MRI and MRA showed a left cavernous sinus lesion. A cerebral arteriogram revealed carotid cavernous sinus fistula (Figures 3.4.1. She improved after embolization.

The following findings are not typical for MG:

1. Severe headache
2. Frontal numbness
3. Nystagmus
4. Morning diplopia
5. All of the above

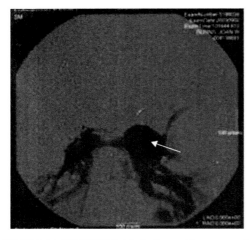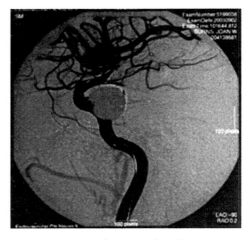

FIGURE 3.4.1 AND FIGURE 3.4.2 Left carotid cavernous fistula (CCF) before (3.4.1) and after (3.4.2) embolization.

DIAGNOSIS

- Carotid cavernous fistula is formed by abnormal communication between the carotid artery and the cavernous sinus. It is more common in young age groups and is mostly traumatic.
- If the cavernous sinus connects to the intracavernous carotid artery, the flow in the fistula would be high. If the cavernous sinus connects to branches of the carotid system within the adjacent dura, the flow would be low (cavernous dural fistula). This is more common in elderly women and is usually spontaneous and idiopathic. Genetic connective tissue disease and hypertension are risk factors. The cavernous sinus contains cranial nerves 3, 4, 5, and 6. Only V1 and V2 of the trigeminal nerve pass through the cavernous sinus. These nerves are affected in the following fashion:
  - Diplopia is the presenting feature in 85% of cases.
  - Cranial nerve 6 is involved in 50%–85% of cases.
  - Cranial nerve 3 is involved in 67% of cases.
  - Cranial nerve 4 is involved in 49% of cases.
- Headache occurs in 53%–75% of cases, and retro-orbital pain occurs in 35% of cases; this argues against MG, which is usually painless. Mild frontal pain may occur in MG, however, due to compensatory activity of the frontalis.
- Proptosis and facial sensory symptoms are common.
- Loss of vision occurs in 33% of cases due to orbital venous congestion and vitreous bleeding.
- After successful closure, cranial nerve dysfunction usually improves over a period of months and persists in a minority of cases.
- While atypical, morning diplopia and nystagmus of a weak MR muscle can be seen in MG.

SUGGESTED READING

Kim MS, Han DH, Kwon OK, Oh CW, Han MH. Clinical characteristics of dural arteriovenous fistula. *J Clin Neurosci.* 2002;9(2):147.

CASE 3.5: UNIFYING DIAGNOSIS
IS NOT ALWAYS POSSIBLE

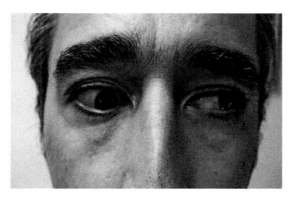

VIDEO 3.5

A 44-year-old man presented with a 6-year history of partially steroid responsive proximal weakness, recurrent steroid responsive oligoarthritis, painless fatigable vertical diplopia, and dysphagia. Creatine kinase (CK) was 450 IU/L, and muscle biopsy revealed endomysial inflammation. The rheumatoid factor was positive. The brain MRI is shown in Figure 3.5.1.

Facioscapulohumeral muscular dystrophy (FSHD) is suggested by the examination and confirmed by mutation analysis, but it does not explain:

1. Diplopia
2. Pectoralis atrophy
3. Oligopolyarthritis
4. Inflammation in muscle biopsy
5. Horizontal clavicles

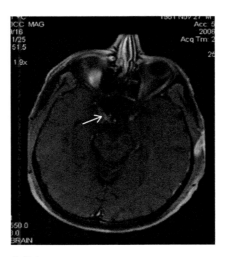

FIGURE 3.5.1 Brain MRI with gadolinium.

DIAGNOSIS

- While the primary diagnostic strategy in neurology is to find a unifying diagnosis to multiple findings, it is sometimes difficult to find one explanation or disease process for all clinical and laboratory data. In such situations, the neuromuscular specialist should be aware of atypical presentations and of exclusive findings of certain diseases.
- This patient has three disorders:
  - FSHD: Pectoralis atrophy, deltoid hypertrophy, horizontal clavicles, and proximal weakness suggested this. The diagnosis is genetically confirmed. Diplopia is not expected, as FSHD does not involve EOMs. Endomysial inflammation is typically seen in these patients.
  - Rheumatoid arthritis: This is suggested by consistently steroid responsive oligoarthritis and very high rheumatoid factors. Endomysial inflammation is also seen in some cases.
  - Apical cavernous meningioma: Diplopia and dysphagia raised the possibility of MG. Initial brain MRI was negative, but the repeat MRI a few months later was abnormal. It showed asymmetry and possible mass in the right cavernous sinus consistent with meningioma. Meningioma may compress the third, fourth, or sixth cranial nerves, depending upon its location and size. Retro-oribital pain, ocular redness, and proptosis are seen if the tumor attains a certain size. Meningeoma was confirmed and treated with radiation.

CASE 3.6: PENALTY FOR CORRECTION OF WRINKLES

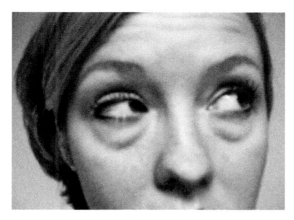

VIDEO 3.6

A 32-year-old female presented with blurring of vision 3 days after receiving botulinum toxin (BT) injections in the face for cosmetic reasons.

BT mechanism of action:

1. Blocks the postsynaptic acetylcholine receptors (AChRs)
2. Blocks acetylcholinesterase (AChE) in the neuromuscular junction
3. Inhibits the release of ACh from the presynaptic terminal
4. Inhibits sodium channels on muscle membrane
5. Answers 1 and 3

DIAGNOSIS

- Video 3.6 showed bilateral ptosis and multidirectional diplopia.
- Cosmetic injection has become the most common application of BT in medicine over the last decade.
- BT is also used to treat focal dystonia (e.g., blepharospasm, cervical dystonia, spasmodic dysphonia), hemifacial spasm, spasticity, and migraine.
- BT inhibits ACh release from presynaptic nerve terminals and therefore prevents the contraction of the related muscles.
- Complications of BT can be functionally and cosmetically significant.
- Diplopia and ptosis are more common the closer the injection is to the eyes. Low frontalis injections may cause ptosis due to involvement of the levator muscle. BT affects the surrounding muscles by diffusion, and it does not have to be injected into them to cause weakness.
- Doses of different BT preparations are not interchangeable, and the use of the wrong conversion factor may lead to overdose.
- Side effects, like good effects, appear within a week and last for 2–3 months. It is important to explain the temporary nature of these potential side effects to the patients.
- Most patients who are referred to neuromuscular centers do not volunteer information about cosmetic use of BT because they are not aware of a relationship between their symptoms and these injections, or they are embarrassed or afraid that they will be thought to be vain.
- Patients with neuromuscular transmission disorders should be warned against any form of BT and should be told about the possibility of precipitating additional weakness or myasthenic crisis.
- Neuromuscular complications of BT are due to weakness of the affected muscles and may include:
  - Diplopia and ptosis from periorbital injections
  - Facial weakness from injection of facial muscles for hemifacial spasm or for cosmetic reasons
  - Dysphagia from cervical injections, mostly for dystonia
  - Jaw ptosis from injections of the masseter and pterygoid, and sometimes lower facial muscles
  - Weakness of finger flexors and extensors from injections for tremors and focal dystonia
  - Foot drop from injections for spasticity and focal foot dystonia

CASE 3.7: OBLIQUE DIPLOPIA

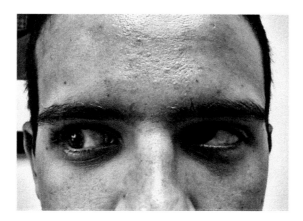

VIDEO 3.7

A 17-year-old man presented with a 1-year history of nonfatigable oblique diplopia. Examination is shown in the video. MG serology and brain MRI were normal.

These findings are typical of:

1. Abducent palsy (sixth cranial nerve)
2. MG
3. Oculomotor palsy (third cranial nerve)
4. Trochlear nerve palsy (TNP; fourth cranial nerve)
5. Convergence spasm

DIAGNOSIS

- TNP may result from lesions anywhere along the course of the nerve from its nucleus in the midbrain to the SO muscle.
- It has the longest intracranial course and is the only nerve with a dorsal exit from the brainstem.
- It passes through the cavernous sinus and enters the SO muscle via the superior orbital fissure.
- The primary action of the SO is intorsion of the globe (to move the eye down and in), and the secondary action is to depress the globe maximally on medial gaze.
- Vertical diplopia that resolves with head tilt to the other side is typical, and patients assume a chronic head tilt to avoid diplopia. Looking downward, such as when going downstairs, may lead to falls due to diplopia.
- On examination, the affected eye is tilted upward (ipsilateral hypertropia), with extorsion. The deviation is greater with the maximum action of the affected muscle (left SO weakness appears with right gaze) and when the head is tilted ipsilaterally.
- Clinical diagnosis of unilateral fourth cranial nerve palsy is performed by three steps:
  1. Determination of the hypertrophic eye: If the left eye is hypertrophic, the weakness may be in the left SO, or IR, or right SR, or IO.
  2. Production of diplopia: If diplopia occurs with right gaze in a left hypermetropic eye, the weakness is then either left SO or IR.
  3. Head tilt: If diplopia worsens with head deviation to the same side of the hypertrophic eye, then the weakness is in that side SO.
- Causes: congenital (40%), traumatic (30%), and idiopathic (30%). The long intracranial course of the nerve carries a long risk for involvement by tumors and increased intracranial pressure (ICP).
- Important causes of fourth cranial nerve palsy seen in neuromuscular clinics include:
  - Cavernous sinus pathology: Other nerves are usually affected (third, fifth, sixth).
  - Retro-orbital pathology: There is usually proptosis and conjunctival congestion.
- Important neuromuscular differential diagnoses of fourth cranial nerve palsy include:
  - MG: SO weakness can be the only manifestation of MG. Usually, other EOMs are affected at some point, especially MR. Weakness of facial muscles and ptosis are common. Fluctuation of diplopia is an important clue.
  - Thyroid ophthalmopathy.

CASE 3.8: OPHTHALMOPLEGIA
WITH ELEVATED CREATINE KINASE (CK)

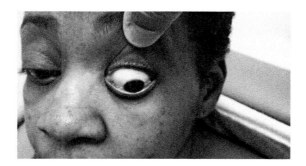

VIDEO 3.8

A 41-year-old woman presented with a 4-week history of diplopia, ptosis, dysphagia, dysarthria, dyspnea, chewing fatigability, skin rash, proximal weakness, and weight loss. Chest X-ray revealed a ground glass appearance, and the CPK level was 1,560 U/L. Electromyography (EMG) revealed paraspinal and proximal fibrillations and myopathic units. Muscle biopsy revealed inflammatory myopathy. The AChR antibodies titer was elevated. CT scan of chest showed no mediastinal abnormalities. She remitted with prednisone and azathioprine.

MG with elevated CK to more than 10 times normal occurs in:

1. Giant cell myositis
2. Musk MG
3. Brachiocervical inflammatory myopathy
4. Paraneoplastic syndrome
5. Answers 1 and 3

DIAGNOSIS

- Mild elevation of CK (less than 500) occurs in 10% of MG patients.
- More severe elevation is not common and should raise the possibility of an associated myopathy, especially if there is severe proximal weakness and myopathic EMG (both can happen in MG, but not typically).
- The most important two neuromuscular syndromes that cause high CK and MG are:
  - Giant cell myositis (granulomatous myopathy, thymoma, and MG)
  - Brachiocervical inflammatory myopathy (BCIM)
- BCIM:
  - Inflammatory myopathy that affects proximal arm more than leg muscles and is associated with ptosis and ophthalmoplegia in 30% of cases and increased AChR Ab in 30% of cases.
  - Weakness of posterior neck muscles, dysphagia, respiratory failure, myalgia, skin rash, and weight loss are characteristic features.
  - Associated mixed connective tissue disease, Sjogren syndrome, rheumatoid arthritis (RA), and scleroderma are common.
  - Irritative myopathy is seen in EMG, and CK may be up to 15 times normal.
  - Muscle pathology shows evidence of primary inflammatory myopathy. Perivascular and perimysial mononuclear infiltration, mycobacteria avium complex (MAC) deposition, and B-cell predominance, along with skin rash and interstitial lung disease, suggest a similar disease to dermatomyositis (DM).
  - The more severe involvement of bulbar, cervical, and upper extremities more than lower extremities and the associated ptosis and ophthalmoplegia are not typical for DM and warrant recognition of a different entity. However, the associated MG can explain all these findings. These could be two autoimmune disorders affecting the same patient.
  - Steroid therapy is usually effective.

SUGGESTED READING

Pestronk A, Kos K, Lopate G, Al-Lozi MT. Brachio-cervical inflammatory myopathies: clinical, immune, and myopathologic features. *Arth Rheum.* 2006 May;54(5):1687–1696.

CASE 3.9: WHICH EXTRAOCULAR MOVEMENT (EOM) IS FIRST AFFECTED IN MYASTHENIA GRAVIS (MG)?

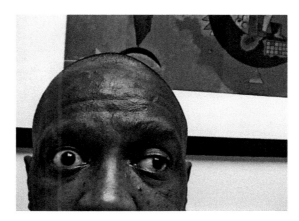

VIDEO 3.9

A 43-year-old man presented with subacute diplopia and ptosis that developed over a few weeks. Examination revealed more involvement of the MRs than LRs, and the triceps than the biceps muscles.

In MG, the following patterns of muscle fatigability are commonly seen:

1. Neck extensors more than flexors
2. MRs more than LRs
3. Triceps more than biceps
4. Ankle extensors more than ankle flexors
5. All of the above

DIAGNOSIS

- More than 50% of patients with MG present with ptosis and diplopia, and half of those generalize within 2 years.
- A total of 15% of patients present with bulbar dysfunction such as dysarthria, dysphagia, and fatigability of muscles of mastication.
- Less than 5% of patients present with proximal limb weakness.
- Less common presentations include:
  - Neck extensor weakness
  - Isolated respiratory muscle weakness
  - Distal extensor muscle weakness
- Extensors are more affected than flexors in MG. Neck extensors are more affected due to their continuous activity to hold the head up.
- From my and other neuromuscular specialists' experiences, triceps muscles are more severely affected in African Americans.
- Myasthenia Gravis may present with painless wrist drop or foot drop, with normal sensation and normal reflexes. This presentation may lead to confusion with ALS or mononeuritis multiplex, especially when coupled with respiratory insufficiency.

CASE 3.10: DIPLOPIA AND WEIGHT LOSS

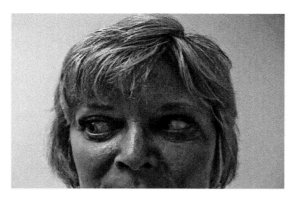

VIDEO 3.10

A 62-year-old woman presented with a 6-month history of diplopia and weight loss. She also developed dysphagia, palpitation, dyspnea, heat intolerance, diffuse headache, and difficulty climbing stairs. She later developed diarrhea and profuse sweating. Examination revealed lid retraction, exophthalmus, and diplopia. She had proximal weakness. Myasthenia serology was negative.

These symptoms are suggestive of:

1. Generalized MG
2. Retro-orbital tumor
3. Thyroid ophthalmopathy
4. Tolosa-Hunt syndrome (THS)
5. Intracranial hypertension

DIAGNOSIS

- Thyroid eye disease is one of the most common differential diagnosis of ocular MG.
- Lid lag due to hyperactive levator palpebrae superioris (LPS) from hyperthyroidism may give a false impression of exophthalmos.
- Unlike MG, thyroid ophthalmopathy (TO) is associated with lid lag instead of ptosis most of the time. However, when exophthalmos is severe, and once hyperthyroidism is treated and lid lag improves, ptosis may develop due to levator dehiscence from protrusion pressure. Ptosis in these cases is nonfluctuating, and the crease line is elevated.
- Infiltration of orbital tissue and EOM with inflammatory cells is the pathological hallmark of TO. The primary antigen is thyroid-stimulating hormone (TSH) receptors, against which antibodies are formed and can be measured commercially.
- TO is the presenting feature of Graves' disease in 20% of cases, and it appears during the disease in 40% of cases, and after the disease in 20%. TO may occur in Hashimoto's thyroiditis and is sometimes isolated.
- TO and MG may coexist, leading to more orbital complications and diagnostic delay.
- Enlargement of EOM is the radiological hallmark of TO. Computed tomography (CT) or MRI scan of the orbits can easily demonstrate this.
- TO may worsen after treatment of Graves' disease, and it may threaten vision.
- Steroid treatment usually helps. Local radiotherapy and decompressive surgery may be needed in refractory cases to save vision.
- Retro-orbital masses and EOM myositis are important differentials for TO, as well as MG.

CASE 3.11: DIPLOPIA AND RETRO-ORBITAL PAIN

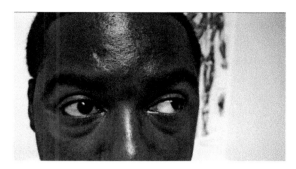

VIDEO 3.11

A 33-year-old man presented with a 2-month history of acute right retro-orbital pain and photophobia, followed by binocular multidirectional diplopia and right forehead numbness.

The most appropriate test is:

1. Repetitive nerve stimulation test
2. MRI of the brain and orbits
3. AChR antibody level
4. CT scan of the chest
5. Lumbar puncture

DIAGNOSIS

- Analysis of 100 cases referred by neuro-ophthalmologists to our clinic for suspicion of myasthenia revealed 10 patients with alternative diagnoses. These patients had normal initial brain MRIs. One of these cases was a patient with THS.
- It is a rare disorder due to granulomatous inflammation in one of the cavernous sinuses, which leads to unilateral retro-orbital pain, and involvement of cranial nerves 3, 4, 5, and 6, resulting in diplopia and facial numbness. Other symptoms may include fever, fatigue, and proptosis.
- MRI of the brain with and without gadolinium and MRA of the brain are essential for the diagnosis, and they can be negative early in the course of the disease (Figure 3.11.1).
- Severe retro-orbital pain and impaired sensation in the forehead (V1 distribution) are not features of MG and should raise the possibility of cavernous sinus pathology.
- The pain of THS usually responds dramatically to oral steroids. Sometimes steroid-sparing agents are needed for long-term remission. A total of 40% of cases relapse after the steroids are tapered.
- A steroid-sparing agent such as azathioprine and methotrexate is usually used in recurrent cases.

Brain MRI with contrast, Coronal section showing enhancing lesion in the right cavernous sinus.

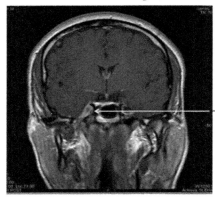

Enhancing lesion in the wall of the right cavernous sinus on the brain MRI scan with contrast. The diagnosis was consistent with Tolosa-Hunt Syndrome. Treatment with prednisone revealed dramatic clinical response. Symptoms recurred after discontinuing of prednisone. The patient was restarted on corticosteroids.

FIGURE 3.11.1 Brian MRI with gadolinium.

CHAPTER 4

OPHTHALMOPLEGIA

CASE 4.1: DIPLOPIA AND BRISK REFLEXES

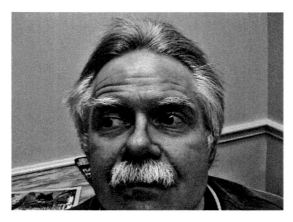

VIDEO 4.1

A 40 year-old man presented with recurrent episodes of transverse myelitis and optic neuritis who gradually developed diplopia to lateral gaze bilaterally, which was not fatigable. Deep tendon reflexes (DTRs), including jaw jerk, were brisk.

Which of the following is incorrect regarding the video findings?

1. Internuclear ophthalmoplegia (INO)
2. The side of the INO is named after the adducted eye.
3. Bilateral lesion of medial longitudinal fasciculus (MLF)
4. Not Pathognomonic of multiple sclerosis (MS)
5. A complication of treatment of MS

DIAGNOSIS

- INO is one of the most localizing signs in neurology. It is due to a lesion of MLF, which connects the nuclei of the sixth and third cranial nerves and is located in the dorsal part of the pons and midbrain.
- The most common cause of INO is cerebrovascular disease, followed by MS. Other causes include tumors, infections, and trauma.
- INO presents with horizontal diplopia, and examination reveals weakness of the ipsilateral adducted eye and nystagmus of the contralateral abducted eye.
- The cause of nystagmus is not clear. It may be an adaptive response to weakness of the adducted eye.
- Myasthenia may mimic INO. MR weakness is common in myasthenia gravis (MG), and adaptive response of the fatigable contralateral lateral rectus (LR) sometimes induces abnormal movement that mimics nystagmus.
  - In the presence of other manifestations of MS and MG, diagnosis is not difficult.
  - However, when these symptoms occur in isolation, the most important differentiating sign is sparing of convergence response in INO due to the preserved integrity of the convergence center.
  - In peripheral medial rectus (MR) weakness, however (third cranial nerve palsy, MG, etc.), such a response is affected.
- INO is named after the side of the adducted eye (MR).

CASE 4.2: FLOPPY BABY WITH OPHTHALMOPLEGIA

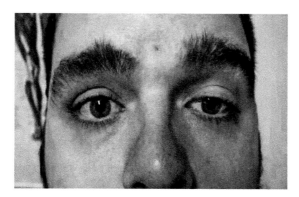

VIDEO 4.2

A 27 year-old man who was born as a floppy baby presented with ophthalmoplegia. Gradually, he was able to walk, but proximal weakness, ophthalmoplegia, and ptosis continued. Repetitive spinal accessory nerve stimulation (RNS) produced a decremental response of the ipsilateral trapezius. He responded to pyridostigmine well.

The following deficits are reported in keep the word postpostsynaptic congenital myasthenic syndrome (CMS):

1. Choline acetyltransferase deficiency
2. Dok-7 mutation
3. Acetylcholine (ACh) esterase deficiency
4. Epsilon mutation
5. Sodium channelopathy

DIAGNOSIS

- CMS is a rare group of disorders that can be confused with seronegative MG, especially when encountered in adult population. They do not respond to immunomodulation or suppression.
- Fatigable weakness of ocular, bulbar, and limb muscles is present since infancy or early childhood.
- Some may improve but exacerbate by infection, medications, and other sources of stress.
- All types of CMS decrement with 2–3-Hz stimulation, but presynaptic forms increment with high-frequency stimulation.
- Some muscles may be spared; therefore, testing multiple muscles is important.
- The presence of family history is helpful, but its absence is not exclusive. Most of these syndromes are autosomal recessive (AR).
- Postsynaptic CMS is the most common type, and the most common of this type is primary deficiency of AChR or primary kinetic defect of these receptors. Rapsyn, epsilon, and Dok-7 mutations are the next most common (the answer is options 2 and 4).
- Quinidine is contraindicated in all CMS instances except slow channel syndrome.
- Pyridostigmine is helpful in most cases, but it should be avoided in endplate acetylcholinesterase deficiency, where ephedrine and albuterol are usually beneficial.
- In most cases except slow channel syndrome, 3,4-diaminopyridine is useful.
- In an adult with fatigable weakness, the following findings would support CMS:
    1. Onset of symptoms at or shortly after birth
    2. Decremental electromyogram (EMG) response to 3-Hz stimulation
    3. Negative double-MG serology
    4. Lack of clinical improvement with immunosuppression
    5. Presence of family history of the similar symptoms.

SUGGESTED READING

Abicht A, et al. Congenital myasthenic syndrome. *GeneRev*. July 14, 2016. https://www.ncbi.nlm.nih.gov/books/NBK1168/

CASE 4.3: BULGY EYES AND HEAT INTOLERANCE

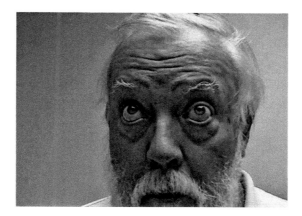

VIDEO 4.3

A 60-year-old man presented with progressive weight loss, diplopia, and heat intolerance. His examination is shown in the video.

Thyroid ophthalmopathy causes diplopia by:

1. Fatty infiltration of the retro-orbital tissue
2. Slowing neuromuscular transmission
3. Enlargement of the extraocular muscles
4. Paralyzing oculomotor nerves
5. Cavernous sinus pathology

DIAGNOSIS

- Examination showed mild restriction of eye movements, exophthalmos, swelling of the eyelids, and congestion of conjunctiva.
- Diplopia and ophthalmoparesis that are produced by thyroid ophthalmopathy (TO) are often confused with MG symptoms.
- The volume of extraocular muscles and retro-orbital tissue is increased due to accumulation of glycosaminoglycans, mostly hyaluronic acid. This leads to accumulation of fluid and bulging of the eyes, which interferes with the function of the extraocular muscles and venous drainage of the orbits.
- Extraocular muscles are enlarged and distorted by inflammatory infiltration and edema. Auto-antibodies to different parts of retro-orbital tissue, including extraocular muscles, are detected in the serum of these patients.
- The activation of T-cells is mostly initiated by thyroid-stimulating hormone (TSH) receptor antigens. This notion is supported by the recovery of TSH receptors' messenger RNA (mRNA) in the orbital tissue.
- There is a correlation between the severity of the ophthalmopathy and the serum level of TSH receptor antibodies.
- TO is more common in women, but it tends to be more aggressive in men.
- Family history, presence of other autoimmune diseases, and smoking are risk factors for TO.

CASE 4.4: HOW LONG SHOULD MYASTHENIA GRAVIS (MG) BE TREATED?

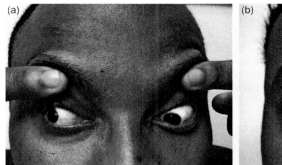 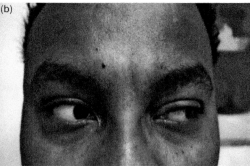

VIDEO 4.4

A 35-year-old man presented with fatigable horizontal diplopia that improved with rest. The AChR antibody titer was elevated. He responded to pyridostigmine for a year, and then he had to increase the dose to 540 mg/day, with minimal benefit. He refused steroids. After a year, he could not drive anymore due to complete ptosis at night. The ophthalmoplegia and ptosis resolved 3 months after steroid therapy (Video 4.4B).

Evidence from clinical trials supports a safe discontinuation of prednisone after a remission for:

1. 2 years
2. 4 years
3. 1 year
4. 5 years
5. No evidence

DIAGNOSIS

- Video 4.4A showed ophthalmoplegia and severe bilateral ptosis.
- There are no guidelines or evidence-based medicine regarding the duration of treatment of MG.
- Most experts try to wean off medications after 2 years of remission.
- A total of 25% of patients may remain in remission after discontinuation of immunosuppression after 2 years.
- Thymectomy improved clinical outcomes over a 3-year period. The utility of thymectomy in purely ocular MG is still not clear.

SUGGESTED READING

Calhoun RF, Ritter JH, Guthrie TJ, et al. Results of transcervical thymectomy for myasthenia gravis in 100 consecutive patients. *Ann Surg*. 1999 Oct;(4):55.

CASE 4.5: OPHTHALMOPLEGIA AND RESPIRATORY FAILURE

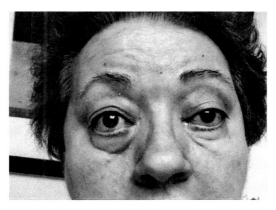

VIDEO 4.5

A 61-year-old woman presented with blurring of vision and leg weakness that had started 2 years earlier. AChR and MuSK antibody testing was negative. Repetitive nerve stimulation showed no significant decrement. A diagnosis of seronegative generalized MG was considered, and she was treated with corticosteroids and thymectomy. Only subjective response to therapy was noted. She developed respiratory failure 1 year later, and she was found to have the demonstrated abnormalities. Serum lactate and pyruvate levels were five times greater than normal, and a left biceps muscle biopsy was abnormal (Figures 4.5.1 and 4.5.2). Mutation analysis of muscle tissue revealed several pathogenic mitochondrial mutations. She died from respiratory failure.

Which of the following features is(are)more consistent with chronic progressive external ophthalmoplegia (CPEO) than with MG?

1. Subacute onset
2. Increased levels of serum lactate and pyruvate
3. Response to steroids
4. Ragged red fibers in muscle biopsy
5. Age of the patient

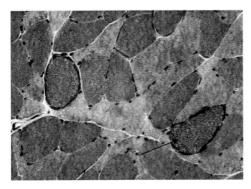

FIGURE 4.5.1 Modified Gomori trichrome stain (100X).

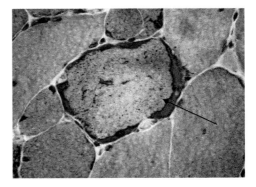

FIGURE 4.5.2 Modified Gomori trichrome stain (400X).

DIAGNOSIS

- The muscle biopsy pictures demonstrated ragged red fibers.
- Although this patient was initially thought to have MG, she ultimately was diagnosed with CPEO. Both MG and mitochondrial disease may present with ophthalmoplegia and ptosis. CPEO is associated with myopathy; however, mild myopathic features also sometimes may be seen in needle EMGs of patients with myasthenia. Patient with mitochondrial disease may report periodic worsening and subjective improvement with steroids. These features can make telling between the two disorders challenging.
- Although diffuse chronic weakness of extraocular muscles does not typically cause diplopia, periodic worsening triggered by external or internal factors may lead to it.
- CPEO may be confused with MG, congenital myasthenic syndrome (CMS), oculopharyngeal muscular dystrophy (OPMD), and progressive supranuclear palsy (PSP). The presence of multisystemic manifestations such as deafness, seizures, strokes, cardiac conduction defects, retinal pigmentary changes, and neuropathy should favor the diagnosis of mitochondrial disorders.
- CPEO usually presents with ophthalmoplegia and ptosis, with or without proximal weakness.
  - Onset usually occurs in the fourth decade, but it can occur at any age.
- Kearns-Sayre syndrome (KSS) is similar to CPEO, but the onset is usually before age 20 years, and there are cardiac conduction defects and retinal pigmentary changes. It is more progressive.
- CPEO is a heterogeneous group of disorders: it can be sporadic; maternally inherited (deletion of the large mitochondrial gene), which constitutes 50% of cases; or autosomal dominant (AD) or AR (nuclear mutations).
- Mild creatine kinase (CK) elevation is common but not required for the diagnosis. EMG is either normal or shows mild myopathic changes.
- Serum resting lactate and pyruvate are increased in 60% of cases.
- Cerebrospinal fluid (CSF) lactate and pyruvate are more sensitive but not specific, as they can be increased in strokes and seizures.
- Muscle tissue is still ideal for the diagnosis of mitochondrial mutations due to segregation of mutated mitochondria in muscle. However, if nuclear mitochondrial mutations are suspected [autosomal polymerase gamma (POLG) mutations, mitochondrial neurogastrointestinal encephalopathy (MNGIE), etc.], peripheral blood may be as good as muscle tissue.
- Muscle biopsy usually shows ragged red fibers, the pathological hallmark of mitochondrial disorders.

CASE 4.6: DEMYELINATING NEUROPATHY WITH OPHTHALMOPLEGIA

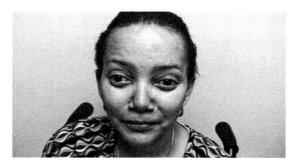

VIDEO 4.6

A 25 year-old woman presented with progressive generalized weakness and loss of balance. She was found to have ophthalmoplegia, ataxia, and areflexia. CSF protein was slightly increased, and motor nerve conduction velocities were moderately decreased. She was diagnosed with Miller Fisher syndrome (MFS). Past medical history was remarkable for chronic abdominal distension and childhood seizures. Also, as a child, she became deaf after being treated with neomycin for a urinary tract infection. The brain MRI is shown in Figure 4.6.1.

Muscle biopsy is expected to show:

1. Myopathic changes
2. Polyglucosan bodies
3. Ragged red fibers
4. Red-rimmed vacuoles
5. Cytoplasmic inclusion bodies

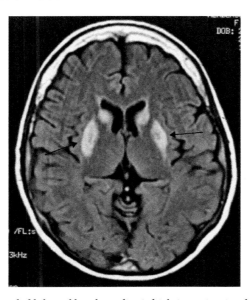

FIGURE 4.6.1 Brain MRI: revealed bilateral basal ganglionic high-intensity signals.

DIAGNOSIS

- Video 4.6 shows ophthalmoplegia, deafness, areflexia, and proximal weakness. This, along with seizures, neuropathy, and MRI findings, raised the possibility of mitochondrial disorder.
- Mitochondrial diseases have a high predilection for organs with a high metabolic rate such as muscle, brain, and nerves.
- Although peripheral neuropathy occurs in more than 50% of cases, it is rarely the presenting symptom.
- Most of the time, the polyneuropathy is axonal, but a demyelinating variant similar to Charcot-Marie-Tooth (CMT) disease and chronic inflammatory demyelinating neuropathy is reported.
- MNGIE syndrome has an associated polyneuropathy in 30% of cases; however, less than 5% of cases are demyelinating.
- In this case, the subacute deterioration, areflexia, and moderate asymmetrical demyelinating neuropathy with ophthalmoplegia and ataxia led to an erroneous diagnosis of MFS.
- Deafness and seizures suggested mitochondrial disease. Gastrointestinal (GI) disturbances with demyelinating neuropathy raised the possibility of MINGIE.
- Subacute deterioration of mitochondrial disorders may be induced by medication, infection, or stress.
- Plasma thymidine phosphorylase elevation is important but not required for the diagnosis of MINGIE.
- Cases of mitochondrial disease erroneously diagnosed as CMT disease are reported. Hereditary neuropathies with negative genetic testing and history of hearing impairment or seizures should be considered for mitochondrial disorders, especially MINGIE, neuropathy, ataxia, and retinitis pigmentosa (NARP), and *POLG1* and *RRM2B* mutations.
- Muscle biopsy revealed myopathic changes and many ragged red fibers.
- This case had MINGIE caused by *RRM2B* mutation.

SUGGESTED READING

Shaibani A, Shchelochkov OA, Zhang S, et al. Mitochondrial neurogastrointestinal encephalopathy due to mutations in RRM2B. *Arch Neuro*. 2009 Aug;66(8):1028–1032.

CASE 4.7: OPHTHALMOPLEGIA AND HEART BLOCK

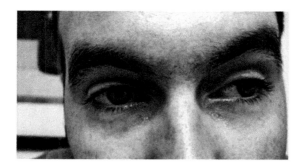

VIDEO 4.7

A 29-year-old man presented with a 3-year history of blurring of vision. There was no visual decline, dysphagia, dyspnea, or leg weakness. There was no family history. Retinal exam was normal and electrocardiogram (ECG) revealed second-degree heart block. MG serology was negative.

The most likely diagnosis is:

1. MG
2. CPEO
3. OPMD
4. CMS
5. PSP

The most likely findings will be:

1. Hyperphosphorylated tau protein accumulation
2. Multiple small mitochondrial deletions
3. Epsilon mutation
4. A single, large mitochondrial deletion
5. Nuclear inclusions

DIAGNOSIS

- Video 4.7 showed partial ophthalmoplegia and ptosis with normal facial strength.
- The onset of KSS typically occurs before age 20 years, and death may occur in the fourth decade.
- KSS is a multisystemic disease with variable tissue involvement due to heteroplasmy.
- The following clinical features may be present:
    - Progressive external ophthalmoplegia and ptosis.
    - Pigmentary degeneration of retina: Visual loss is mild and occurs in 50% of cases.
    - Heart block: This usually occurs years after the development of ophthalmoplegia and leads to syncope and even sudden death.
    - Dysphagia (50%).
    - Mitochondrial myopathy (90%).
    - Sensorimotor neuropathy (10%).
    - Deafness (95%).
    - Ataxia (cerebellar or sensory) (90%).
    - Encephalopathy (seizures, strokes, dementia).
    - Endocrinopathy: impaired glucose tolerance, hypothyroidism, hypoparathyroidism.
- Laboratory and imaging findings:
    - Lactic acidosis due to anaerobic metabolism.
    - Mild CK elevation, myopathic EMG.
    - Brain MRI: white matter changes in the basal ganglia and thalamus.
    - Ragged red fibers in muscle pathology in 98% of cases. Mitochondrial DNA (mtDNA) mutation is detected in muscle.
    - High CSF protein.
- Genetics: 80% of cases are due to a single, large mtDNA mutation. Most cases are sporadic.
- Treatment: There is no cure. Monitoring of ECG and early pacemaker placement and screening for and treatment of diabetes mellitus (DM), hypothyroidism, and oculoplasty are examples of medical interventions that are needed in some of these patients.

CASE 4.8: PTOSIS AND ANISOCORIA

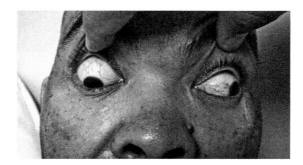

VIDEO 4.8

A 63-year-old man presented with droopy eyelids and diplopia. Examination is shown in the video. The AChR antibody titer was remarkably high.

Pupillary abnormalities in patients with MG could be due to all of the following except:

1. Physiologic anisocoria
2. MG itself
3. Prior ocular trauma
4. An independent optic neuropathy
5. A tonic pupil

DIAGNOSIS

- Video 4.8 showed weakness of MR bilaterally, moderate left ptosis, and anisocoria. The right pupil is slightly larger and less reactive than the left one.
- Unlike presynaptic neuromuscular disorders such as botulism and Lambert-Eaton myasthenic syndrome (LEMS), dysautonomia is not a feature of MG. Therefore, pupillary changes are not expected and should strongly argue against the diagnosis of MG.
- However, some patients have unrelated pupillary abnormalities that may cloud the diagnosis of MG.
  - The most common are physiological anisocoria, tonic pupils, and traumatic pupillary abnormalities.
  - These abnormalities are not associated with other features of dysautonomia, such as xerostomia, areflexia, diarrhea, hypotension, bradycardia, urinary retention, and erectile dysfunction.
- Having a tonic pupil is common among an otherwise normal population and is usually caused by damage to the ciliary ganglia by viral infection. The tonic pupil reacts slowly to light and better to accommodation. Sometimes it is associated with loss of ankle reflexes and other DTRs due to involvement of dorsal root ganglia. Unlike normal pupils, tonic pupils react to pilocarpine due to denervation hypersensitivity.
- Light response of pupils in physiological anisocoria are normal (direct, indirect, and accommodation response).
- Patients do not usually volunteer information about old trauma to the eye, and the clinician must have a high index of suspicion.
- Mydriasis and isolated MR weakness were concerning for oculomotor nerve palsy. In contrast, involvement of both MRs and LRs, fluctuating ptosis, and normal level of consciousness could be explained by a unifying diagnosis of MG.

CASE 4.9: FLUCTUATING EOM WEAKNESS WITHOUT DIPLOPIA

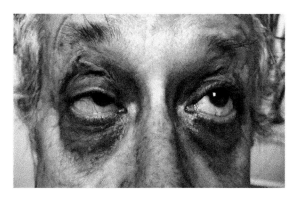

VIDEO 4.9

A 70 year-old man presented with a 1-year history of variable right ptosis. His family noticed divergent eyes when he was tired, but he did not have diplopia. He had dysphagia and dysarthria. AChR antibody testing was positive.

In MG, the lack of diplopia despite fatigable extraocular muscles occurs in the following circumstances:

1. Complete ptosis
2. Negative serology
3. Monocular blindness (macular degeneration)
4. Negative repetitive nerve stimulation (RNS)
5. Thymoma

DIAGNOSIS

- Examination of the patient confirmed the presence of fatigable right ptosis and superior rectus weakness without diplopia.
- Chronic diffuse ophthalmoplegia, such as CPEO and OPMD, is not typically associated with diplopia. The chronicity and gradual progression of these disorders allow the brain to suppress one image and thus avoid diplopia.
- Fluctuating binocular diplopia is an important feature of MG and results from fatigable weakness of one or more extraocular muscles. The diplopia can be horizontal, vertical, or oblique, depending on the affected muscles.
- However, diplopia is not reported by the patient if one eye does not produce an image due to complete ptosis, monocular blindness, long-standing strabismus, or other conditions.

CASE 4.10: OPHTHALMOPLEGIA WITH FREQUENT FALLS

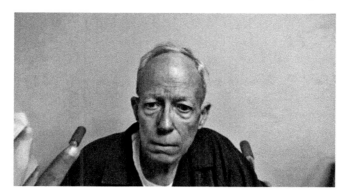

VIDEO 4.10

A 73-year-old man presented with frequent falls.
The likely cause of the falls in this case is:

1. Neuropathy
2. Parkinson disease
3. PSP
4. MG
5. OPMD

DIAGNOSIS

- *Ophthalmoplegia* means paralysis of one or more extraocular muscles.
- There are several ways of classifying ophthalmoplegia:
  - Acute or chronic:
    - Acute ophthalmoplegia is usually associated with diplopia, unlike chronic ones.
  - External or internal:
    - Pupillary dilatation (internal ophthalmoplegia) is not a feature of MG but may be seen in compressive oculomotor palsy and in presynaptic neuromuscular disorders.
    - External ophthalmoplegia is usually a feature of muscle disease (CPEO, OPMD), myasthenia, or noncompressive oculomotor palsy (diabetic third cranial nerve palsy).
  - Supranuclear or infranuclear:
    - Supranuclear, as in PSP
    - Infranuclear, such as myopathies and neuromuscular junction disorders
- Doll's eye movement is preserved in the supranuclear type.
- This case showed the patient looking to the right as a reflex to the speaker's voice (seen at 00:16 of the recording). He could not do the same movement on command. This pattern is typically seen in supranuclear ophthalmoplegia.
- PSP: neurodegenerative disease of the central nervous system (CNS) characterized by:
  - Impairment of vertical gaze (later becoming global gaze palsy) and axial rigidity, leading to frequent falls.
  - Dysarthria, dysphagia, dementia, and emotional incontinence are common.
  - Rare blinking and facial dystonia.
  - Tau-positive filamentous inclusions intracellularly in specific anatomic areas are characteristic.
  - Other features of multisystem atrophy (MSA) may be evident, such as extrapyramidal symptoms.
- Diagnosis remains clinical, and prognosis is poor.

CASE 4.11: DIPLOPIA AND TRICEPS FATIGABILITY

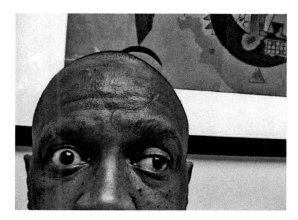

VIDEO 4.11

A 43-year-old man reported diplopia triggered by facing bright lights while driving. Sunglasses and prisms helped temporarily, but symptoms returned after a few months. He then developed difficulty doing bench presses. Examination is shown in the video.

The most likely diagnosis is:

1. INO
2. CMS
3. CPEO
4. MG
5. OPMD

DIAGNOSIS

- Video 4.11 showed fatigable ptosis and weakness of multiple extraocular muscles and fatigable triceps.
- The triceps muscle is commonly involved in MG, especially in African Americans, and it rarely can be the presenting feature of the disease. Biceps are much less affected.
- Patients tend to modify their activities to avoid using the triceps for months or years before other muscles become affected and medical advice is sought.
- The triceps muscles may be strong in the beginning of resistance but fatigue easily; therefore, in every suspected myasthenic, triceps muscles should be tested for fatigue.
- None of the mentioned options causes fatigue of triceps, other than MG and CMS.
- Triceps weakness and fatigability may persist despite improvement of other muscles.

SUGGESTED READING

Abraham A, Kassardjian CD, Katzberg HD, Bril V, Breiner A. Selective predominant triceps muscle weakness in African American patients with MG. *Neuromuscul. Disord.* 2017 Jul:27(7):646–649.

CASE 4.12: DROOPY EYELIDS AND FAINTING

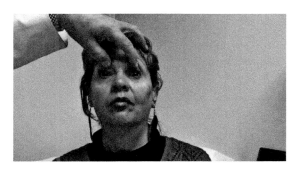

VIDEO 4.12

A 53-year-old woman presented with symptoms since age 23, consisting of droopy eyelids and impairment of night vision. She fainted one time and was taken to the emergency room. She was discharged from the hospital with a pacemaker. She had seven children who were all healthy. Myasthenia serology was negative, but she thought that pyridostigmine was helpful.

The most likely diagnosis is:

1. OPMD
2. CMS
3. MG
4. KSS
5. Myotonic dystrophy (MD)

DIAGNOSIS

- Video 4.12 showed fixed ophthalmoplegia and bilateral ptosis. Night vision loss suggested retinitis pigmentosa, which was confirmed by fundoscopic examination. Syncope was due to heart block, which was not a feature of MG.
- The diagnosis of KSS was made based on mitochondrial analysis of muscle tissue.
- Positive response to pyridostigmine is not specific.
- Cardiac conduction abnormalities are common in mitochondrial disorders and predict high mortality and morbidity.
- Early detection by regular monitoring is important to reduce the chance of sudden death, as progression to high-grade atrioventricular (AV) block is not predictable.
- Cardiac conduction abnormalities occur in 85% of patients with KSS and 10% of other mitochondrial disorders, mostly *m.3243>G* and *m.8344A>G* mutations.
- Other cardiac conduction defects, such as supraventricular arrhythmias, prolonged QT interval, and preexcitation syndromes, are all reported more in patients with mitochondrial disorders than in the general population.
- Different kinds of cardiomyopathies are reported in 40% of mitochondrial disorders.
- Cases of predominant cardiac involvement with minimal additional manifestations are reported in some mitochondrial mutations.

SUGGESTED READING

Bates MG, Bourke JP, Giordano C, d'Amati G, Turnbull DM, Taylor RW. Cardiac involvement in mitochondrial DNA disease: clinical spectrum, diagnosis, and management. *Eur. Heart J.* 2012;33:3023–3033.

CASE 4.13: PTOSIS SINCE CHILDHOOD

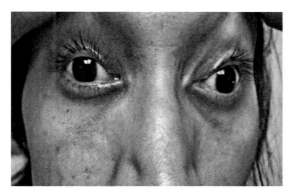

VIDEO 4.13

A 36-year-old man presented with bilateral fixed ptosis that he has had since 10 years of age. Over the previous 10 years, he developed mild dysphagia and proximal leg weakness. Examination revealed no sensory abnormalities, cardiac conduction problems, deafness, or visual impairment. Serum resting lactate and pyruvate were normal. Brain MRI was normal. EMG revealed mild myopathic features in the proximal leg muscles. RNS test was negative. CK level was normal. MG serology was negative. Muscle biopsy showed many ragged red fibers.

The next most useful diagnostic step is to send muscle tissue for:

1. Mitochondrial mutations
2. Muscle end plate analysis
3. Polyadenylate binding protein nuclear 1 (*PABPN1*) mutation
4. Muscle microarray
5. Chromosomal analysis (karyotype)

DIAGNOSIS

- Video 4.13 showed fixed and severe bilateral ptosis and ophthalmoplegia.
- Mitochondrial disorders are commonly seen in neuromuscular clinics, as well as other subspecialty clinics, due to their protean manifestations and the wide range of affected age groups.
- Mitochondria are bacteria that insinuated into the living human cell a billion years ago and have lived in it symbiotically, therefore losing their full independence.
- mtDNA contains only 37 genes, and encodes 13 of the 80 proteins that compose the respiratory chain. Nuclear DNA (nDNA) controls the remaining 99% of mitochondrial proteins.
- Phenotypic variation depends on the proportion of pathogenic mitochondria in the tissue. Heteroplasmy implies the presence of pathogenic and healthy mitochondria side by side in the same host. In a neuromuscular patient, the presence of multisystemic involvement such as seizures, deafness, neuropathy, myopathy, ophthalmoplegia, cardiomyopathy, and other symptoms should raise the possibility of mitochondrial disorders.
- The phenotype may change as the patient ages, due to mitotic segregation of pathogenic mitochondria during cell division.
- mtDNA mutations are maternally inherited, which prevents male to male transmission. Pedigree analysis can be very helpful.

Neuromuscular mitochondrial disorders:

- mtDNA mutations:
  - mtDNA deletions:
    - KSS
    - CPEO
  - Point mutations:
    - Myoclonic epilepsy, lactic acidosis, and strokes (MELAS)
    - Myoclonic epilepsy and ragged red fibers (MERRF)
    - NARP
    - Mitochondrial myopathies: exercise intolerance, rhabdomyolysis, and myalgia
- nDNA mutations:
  - MNGIE
  - *ANT1* mutations
  - POLG mutations:
    - AD or AR CPEO
    - Sensory ataxia neuropathy dysarthria and ophthalmoplegia (SANDO)
    - Mitochondrial encephalopathy with lactic acidosis and stroke (MELAS)
  - Twinkle mutations

CASE 4.14: MUSCLE STIFFNESS AND WEIGHT LOSS

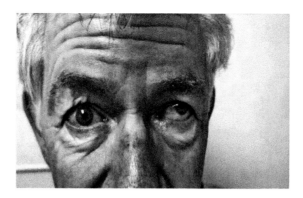

VIDEO 4.14

A 62-year-old man developed severe intermittent stiffness of the back and leg muscles (triggered by cold), diplopia, progressive hearing loss, and intermittent severe vertigo. He also developed photophobia, headache, and irritability. He had nasopharyngeal carcinoma treated with radiation 3 years earlier. Symptoms responded well to diazepam. EMG showed no myotonia or spontaneous motor unit discharges. RNS was normal. The AChR antibody titer was negative. Sodium channel (SC4A) mutation was negative. The glutamate acid decarboxylase (GAD) antibody titer was more than 30 nU/ml.

The most likely diagnosis is:

1. Progressive encephalomyelitis rigidity and myoclonus (PERM)
2. Neuromyotonia
3. Paramyotonia congenita (PMC)
4. MG
5. None of the above

DIAGNOSIS

- Paraneoplastic neuromuscular syndromes may present individually or in combination.
- Some of these syndromes are not difficult to diagnose, such as progressive cerebellar ataxia in a patient with small cell lung cancer or lymphoma.
- Diagnostic difficulties arise when the cancer is not diagnosed or when the symptoms are vague and diffuse, as in this case.
- Cold-sensitive muscle stiffness is typically seen in PMC, which is not a paraneoplastic syndrome. However, the age of the patient and EOM abnormality were atypical for this disorder.
- Stiff person syndrome (SPS) was a strong possibility. Axial stiffness is not as prominent in paraneoplastic stiff person syndrome compared to the idiopathic syndrome.
- The patient responded well to diazepam, which supported the diagnosis of SPS.
- The displayed ophthalmoplegia was difficult to reconcile with a typical case of SPS.
- LEMS, which may occur on a paraneoplastic basis, can have abnormality of extraocular motility. However, eye findings are typically less prominent than in MG, and LEMS patients more typically present with proximal weakness and autonomic symptoms, and their examination shows facilitation of strength and reflexes with exercise. In this case, voltage-gated calcium channel antibodies were negative, RNS was normal, and there was no facilitation of compound muscle action potential (CMAP) amplitudes with exercise.
- The constellation of vertigo, deafness, headache, photophobia, and rapid progression in a patient with cancer suggested paraneoplastic brain stem encephalitis. Elevated CSF protein supported that conclusion. The negative brain MRI may be due to the subtle nature of the inflammation.
- SPS with encephalitis is reported with some malignancies and is associated with increased antibodies to anti-amphiphysin.
- PERM:
  - A variant of SPS that is associated with ophthalmoplegia, nystagmus, myoclonus, hearing loss, vertigo, and dysautonomia.
  - Reported with lymphoma.
  - Death within 4 years is common in most cases.

SUGGESTED READING

Wessig C, Klein R, Schneider MF, Toyka KV, Naumann M, Sommer C. Neuropathology and binding studies in anti-amphiphysin-associated stiff-person syndrome. *Neurol.* 2003;61(2):195.

CASE 4.15: FAMILIAL PTOSIS

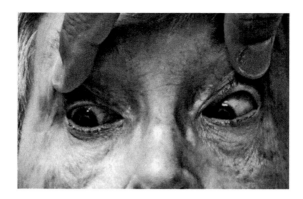

VIDEO 4.15

A 77-year-old woman presented with a 20-year history of droopy eyelids and dysphagia. She had a brother and a sister with the same. She had mild proximal weakness. CK level was 200 U/L and EMG was myopathic.

This disorder is due to a mutation of:

1. *PABPN1*
2. mtDNA
3. The rapsyn gene
4. The Na channel gene
5. The Ca channel gene

DIAGNOSIS

- OPMD is an AD myopathy with complete penetrance.
- A single founder chromosome in the French Canadian population is responsible.
- Incidence in French Canadians is as high as 1:8,000.
- It is due to GCG repeat expansion of the *PABPN1* gene on chromosome 14q11.2-q13.
- *PABPN1* is localized to the nucleus, where it regulates mRNA polyadenylation.
- The expanded allele ranges between 8 and 13 repeats.
- The mutation codes for a protein with a long polyalanin tract, which causes the PABPN1 protein to form clumps within muscle cells that cannot be degraded (intranuclear inclusions); muscle death ensues, though the pathophysiology remains unclear.
- Muscle pathology shows red-rimmed vacuoles and 8.5-nm tubulofilamentous nuclear inclusions.
- Muscle biopsy is no longer necessary since DNA extracted from white blood cells is adequate for the identification of mutation.
- Muscle biopsy is indicated if the genetic testing is negative or if there are atypical features, such as a CK more than 10 times normal, multisystemic features suggestive of mitochondrial disorder, or extreme fatigability suggestive of a neuromuscular junction disorder.
- The trinucleotide expansion is short and stable; therefore, anticipation is *not* a feature.
- Testing other family members for molecular diagnosis can be problematic since symptoms usually start after age 45 years.

CASE 4.16: OPHTHALMOPLEGIA WITH CEREBELLAR ATAXIA AND DEMYELINATING NEUROPATHY

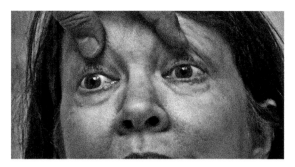

VIDEO 4.16

A 63-year-old woman presented with a 10-year history of droopy eyelids and falls. Examination is demonstrated. Nerve conduction study (NCS) showed demyelinating neuropathy. Brain MRI was normal. A maternal aunt was diagnosed with MS. CSF was normal.

The most likely diagnosis is:

1. Multisystem atrophy
2. Spinocerebellar ataxia (SCA)
3. Mitochondrial disorder
4. Chronic inflammatory demyelinating polyneuropathy (CIDP)
5. Paraneoplastic syndrome

DIAGNOSIS

- Examination showed proximal weakness, distal sensory loss, hyporeflexia, cerebellar ataxia, optic atrophy, ptosis, and ophthalmoplegia.
- While SCA 28 and 30 can cause chronic ophthalmoplegia and ptosis, demyelinating neuropathy and the resulting areflexia are well reported in mitochondrial disorders, but not in hereditary SCAs, where DTRs are usually brisk and the neuropathy, if it exists, is axonal.
- Mitochondrial disorders involve multiple systems, including brain, nerves, muscles, and heart. CNS features, such as seizures and MRI T2 signal abnormalities in the basal ganglia and thalami, are important.
- In this case, POLG pathogenic mutation was identified, which explained this syndrome of mitochondrial SCA.
- These clinical and genetic findings are reported in cases of mitochondrial spinocerebellar ataxia and epilepsy (MSCAE), although epilepsy occurs in only 63% of cases.
- DNA polymerase Gamma (pol G) is the enzyme that replicates and repairs mtDNA. More than 120 pathogenic mutations have been reported in the gene encoding POLG, such as:
  - AD and AR PEO, MSCAE, Alper syndrome, Parkinsonism, encephalopathies, and myopathies.
- MSCAE is a recessive disorder that appears at age 2–24 years, mostly as balance loss and seizures; 89% of patients develop neuropathy with areflexia. Epilepsy occurs in 63% of cases.
- Median survival is 20 years. Treatment is supportive.

SUGGESTED READING

Tzoulis C, Bindoff LA. The syndrome of mitochondrial spinocerebellar ataxia and epilepsy caused by POLG mutations. *ACNR*. 2009;9(3).

CASE 4.17: RECURRENT PTOSIS SINCE CHILDHOOD

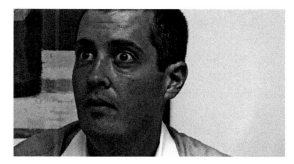

VIDEO 4.17

A 32-year-old man presented with ptosis since childhood and visual impairment since the age of 29. Examination is shown in the video. He also had mild proximal weakness. Ophthalmological examination revealed pigmentary changes in the retinas. ECG revealed prolonged PR interval. CK level was 334 U/L. EMG revealed proximal myopathic changes. A left biceps muscle biopsy is shown in Figure 4.17.1.

The most appropriate next step is to look for:

1. A large mitochondrial deletion in muscle tissue
2. A large mitochondrial deletion in the white blood cells
3. A deletion in nuclear mitochondrial genes, such as POLG
4. A point mutation in the mitochondrial genome
5. Twinkle gene mutations in ocular muscles

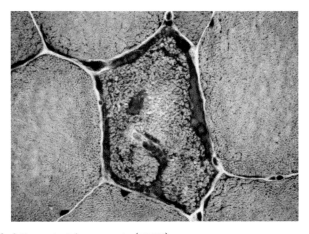

FIGURE 4.17.1 Modified Gomori trichrome stain (400X).

DIAGNOSIS

- Examination revealed fixed ophthalmoplegia and bilateral ptosis. The muscle biopsy picture showed a ragged red fiber. The age of onset, the chronicity of symptoms, the cardiac conduction abnormalities, and retinal pigmentary changes were all consistent with KSS.
- KSS is a multisystemic disease mainly affecting the muscles, eyes, and heart. It is usually caused by spontaneous mutation. In some cases, it can be inherited via mitochondrial, AD, or AR modes.
- Symptoms usually appear before the age of 20 years.
- KSS is an important cause of progressive ophthalmoplegia without pupillary involvement, nonfluctuating ptosis, progressive loss of vision due to retinitis pigmentosa, cardiac conduction defect, and sometimes ataxia. The CSF protein level is usually elevated.
- Proximal weakness, facial weakness, deafness, dementia, seizures, and DM also occur in some patients, which emphasize the widespread nature of this mitochondrial disease.
- Prevalence is 2:100,000 individuals.
- A single, large deletion ranging from 1,000 to 10,000 nucleotides is usually detected.
- KSS is a progressive disorder. Heart block can cause death in 20% of cases. Early pacemaker implantation prolongs life expectancy.
- Gomori trichrome stain of skeletal muscle usually shows a higher concentration of mutated mitochondria in some fibers that accumulates in the periphery of the muscle fibers (ragged red fibers).
- No treatment is available. Blepharoplasty is indicated for severe ptosis.

CASE 4.18: OPHTHALMOPLEGIA AFTER SINUS INFECTION

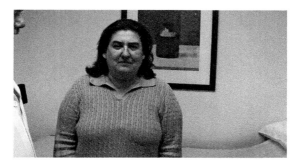

VIDEO 4.18

A 56-year-old woman with acute external ophthalmoplegia that was preceded by upper respiratory tract infection. Myasthenia serology was negative. CSF examination performed 2 days after the symptoms started was normal. Brain MRI was normal. The GQ1B antibody titre was elevated.

The most likely cause of this postinfectious ophthalmoplegia is:

1. MG
2. Partial MFS
3. Brainstem pathology
4. OPMD
5. CPEO

DIAGNOSIS

- This a case of partial MFS. 10% of patients with MFS do not develop ataxia or areflexia (acute ophthalmoparesis without ataxia).
- The normal CSF exam could be attributed to the short interval between the appearance of the symptoms and the spinal tap.
- Ocular MG may rarely present acutely. Negative serology does not exclude this possibility, of course, but a positive GBQ1 antibody titer confirmed MFS.
- Brainstem pathology and cavernous sinus pathology was ruled out by normal mental status and normal imaging.
- The symptoms resolved within 6 weeks.
- MFS typically presents with a triad of ophthalmoplegia, ataxia, and areflexia.
  - Onset is usually triggered by upper respiratory tract infection (RTI) or GI infection.
  - Anti-GQ1B antibodies are positive in 90% of cases.
  - The clinical course of MFS is self-limiting, and neurological deficits resolve in weeks to months, starting as early as 2 weeks following the onset of symptoms.
  - The rapid onset of ophthalmoplegia can help distinguish MFS from conditions that progress chronically, such as mitochondrial myopathies, oculopharyngeal dystrophy, myotonic dystrophy, thyroid eye disease, and some cases of ocular MG.
  - In a review of 31 patients with acute onset of complete bilateral external ophthalmoplegia, MFS was found to be the underlying etiology in the majority of cases.

SUGGESTED READINGS

Anthony SA, Thurtell MJ, Leigh RJ. Miller Fisher syndrome mimicking ocular myasthenia gravis. *Optom Vis Sci.* 2012 Dec;89(12):e118–e123.

Lee S, Lim G-H, Kim LS, et al. Acute ophthalmoplegia (without ataxia) associated with anti-GQ1b antibody. *Neurol.* 2008;71:426–429.

CASE 4.19: CAN'T MOVE EYES OR OPEN THEM WIDE

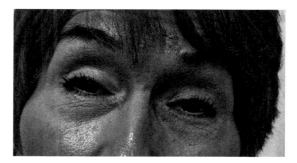

VIDEO 4.19

A 64-year-old French-Canadian woman with chronic, bilateral, nonfatigable ptosis and mild ophthalmoplegia who developed slowly progressive proximal weakness of the arms and legs over the last several years. Besides the demonstrated findings, the CK level was persistently and mildly elevated and her EMG was myopathic.

Al of the following are true of the demonstrated disorder except:

1. It can be AD.
2. It can be AR.
3. It can be X-linked.
4. It is caused by a triplet repeat expansion.
5. Anticipation is not a feature.

DIAGNOSIS

- Family history of the same in her father and his sister and multiple cousins suggest an AD inheritance.
- This clinical picture is very typical for OPMD.
    - This disease is not expected to affect the heart, cognition, or pulmonary function.
    - It is mostly an AD muscle disease that appears in early middle age, with 50% chance of passing the gene to the offspring.
    - It is caused by mutation of the *PABPN1* gene on chromosome 14q, which contains a GCG trinucleotide repeat. Expansion of this repeat from the normal 6 copies to 8–13 copies is the genetic hallmark of the disease.
    - Although a triplet repeat expansion, anticipation is not typical (the appearance of more severe and earlier disease in subsequent generations). The pathogenesis is not understood.
    - The vast majority of cases are AD. Rare AR cases appear earlier in age and are more severe.
    - Familial ptosis and dysphagia are typical. Complete ophthalmoplegia is uncommon (unlike CPEO and CMS).
    - Prevalence among the French-Canadian population is 1:1000. The overall prevalence is 1:10:000.
    - Dysphagia may lead to recurrent pneumonia later in the course of the disease.
    - Proximal weakness and mild facial weakness may also occur later.
    - Genetic test is positive in 99% of cases, and therefore muscle biopsy is not indicated.

CHAPTER 5

FACIAL WEAKNESS

CASE 5.1: MUSCLE STIFFNESS AND SYNCOPE

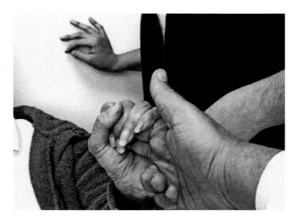

VIDEO 5.1

A 65-year-old woman presented to the emergency room twice during a year due to syncope. She was found to have complete heart block and had a pacemaker. Her creatine kinase (CK) level was 800 U/L with normal echocardiogram and thallium stress test results. She had no family history of muscle disease. Her father had cataract surgery at age 50 years.

The history and examination provide findings typically seen in:

1. Myotonia congenita (MC)
2. Myotonic dystrophy
3. Paramyotonia congenita (PMC)
4. Schwartz-Jampel syndrome
5. Anderson-Tawil syndrome

DIAGNOSIS

The slow relaxation phase that improves with repeated testing (warming-up phenomenon) is typically seen in myotonia. The frontal baldness and facial weakness suggest myotonic dystrophy. Cataracts in her father, with minimal muscular symptoms and more severe symptoms in the patient, suggests anticipation. Syncope due to heart block is common in myotonic dystrophy.

- Myotonic dystrophy:
  - Myotonic dystrophy is the most common inherited neuromuscular disorder (13.5/100,000 live births).
  - It is an autosomal-dominant (AD) disease due to mutation of the dystrophia myotonic protein kinase (*DMPK*) gene located in the noncoding region of the gene.
  - Severity correlates with the cytosine-thymine-guanine (CTG) repeat number:
    - 50–150 repeats: mild disease
    - 100–1,000 repeats: moderate disease
    - More than 1,000 repeats: severe
  - Earlier and more severe symptoms in successive generations are characteristic of the disease, and this is called *anticipation*.
    - Anticipation is explained by successive prolongation of the CTG repeat expansion due to instability of the gene.
    - The number of repeats varies from one tissue to another.
    - Loss of DMPK function is associated with altered Ca^{++} homeostasis. The exact molecular mechanism by which the genotype produces the phenotype is not clear.
- Clinical features:
  - Myotonia: correlates with CTG repeats
  - Ptosis and facial weakness
    - No ophthalmoplegia
  - Proximal and distal weakness
  - Apathy and mental retardation
  - Hypersomnia
  - Hypogonadism, hypothyroidism, and diabetes mellitus (DM)
  - Cardiac abnormalities
  - Tachyarrhythmia
  - Atrial flutter and fibrillation
  - Sudden death
  - Cardiomyopathy
    - Annual electrocardiography (EKG) is indicated, and cardiac intervention is needed if there is a progressive prolongation of the PR interval or QRS duration.
  - Dysphagia and megacolon
  - Medications to be avoided: tricyclic antidepressants, beta blockers, and anti-arrhythmics

CASE 5.2: FACIAL WEAKNESS AND ELEVATED CEREBROSPINAL FLUID (CSF) PROTEIN

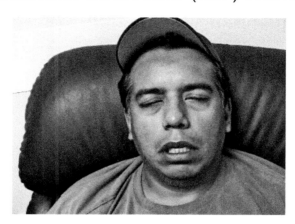

VIDEO 5.2

A 30-year-old man presented with a 2-week history of acute tingling of the feet and hands, difficulty raising his arms, and a 1-week history of slurring of speech and dryness of the eyes. He had no preceding fever. The cerebrospinal fluid (CSF) protein level was 280 mg/ml, and the nerve conduction study (NCS) revealed prolonged F responses and distal latencies, with motor slowing of several nerves in all extremities.

Bilateral facial palsy, defined as a simultaneous or sequential weakness of both sides of the face, is a feature of:

1. Guillain-Barré syndrome (GBS)
2. Sarcoidosis
3. Lyme disease
4. Bilateral Bell's palsy
5. All of the above

DIAGNOSIS

- Bilateral facial nerve palsy complicates 0.3%–2% of facial paralysis.
- Facial onset GBS is one of several clinical variants of the syndrome.
  - It is symmetric and occurs early, along with weakness in the extremities. It should be noted that asymmetric facial diplegia may occur later in the disease, while other motor symptoms are stable or improving.
  - A total of 86% of cases are preceded by upper respiratory tract infection (URTI) by 2–4 weeks.
  - Age range: 23–65 years.
  - Facial diplegia progresses over 4 weeks. It is important to close the eyes with eye patches or Scotch tape at bedtime to avoid exposure keratitis.
  - Foot numbness
  - Mild or no weakness
  - Areflexia
  - CSF albumino-cytologic dissociation
  - Demyelination noted in NCS in 64% of patients.
- Causes of facial diplegia:
  - GBS
  - HIV infection: may occur before seroconversion
  - Sarcoidosis
  - Melkersson syndrome
  - Hereditary: Möbius syndrome and congenital facial paresis
  - Leprosy
  - An-α-lipoproteinemia (Tangier)
  - Lyme disease
  - Other peripheral causes:
    - Motor neuron disorders such as Kennedy disease
    - Myasthenia gravis (MG)
    - Myopathies: myotonic dystrophy, facioscapulohumeral muscular dystrophy (FSHD), inclusion body myositis (IBM)
- Other regional variants of GBS:
  - Miller Fisher syndrome (MFS)
  - Pharyngeal-cervical-brachial variants
  - Paraparetic variant
  - Acute sensory polyneuropathy
  - Acute autonomic neuropathy

SUGGESTED READING

Susuki K, Koga M, Hirata K, Isogai E, Yuki N. A Guillain-Barré syndrome variant with prominent facial diplegia. *J Neurol.* 2009 Nov;256(11):1899–1905. doi:10.1007/s00415-009-5254-8. Epub 2009 Jul 25.

CASE 5.3: RESOLUTION OF FACIAL WEAKNESS

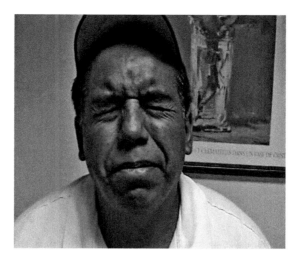

VIDEO 5.3

The patient was treated with intravenous immunoglobulin (IVIG) 1 gm/kg of body weight every day for two days. This examination was done a month later.

Which of the following treatments are proved to be effective first-line therapies in GBS?

1. Intravenous (IV) gammaglobulin
2. IV steroids
3. Plasmapheresis
4. Rituximab
5. Azathioprine

DIAGNOSIS

- IV steroids did not outperform a placebo in the treatment of GBS; in fact, some treated patients became worse. Adding IV steroids to IVIG did not offer any benefit in clinical trials.
- IVIG and therapeutic plasma exchange (TPE) are equally effective and have comparable side effect profiles.
  - The main IVIG complications are headache, myalgia, renal impairment, and deep vein thrombosis (DVT).
  - The main side effects of TPE are hypotension, hypocalcemia, and vascular access–related complications such as infection, obstruction, and bleeding.
- TPE after IVIG does not make sense, and IVIG after TPE does not offer benefits.
- Patients with congestive cardiac failure (CCF) are more suitable for TPE, while patients with infection are more suitable for IVIG.
- TPE onset is shorter than IVIG, but vascular access is inhibitory.
- With the introduction of smaller machines and outpatient availability and the ease of vascular access, TPE is being used more widely than before.
- Subcutaneous immunoglobulin (SCIg) is emerging as an alternative to IVIG, but clinical trials are lacking so far.
- While all GBS patients need to be monitored closely to detect bulbar involvement early, not every GBS patient has to be treated. Treatment is indicated in:
  - Patients with ambulation problems
  - Patients seen within 6 weeks of the onset of symptoms
- Milder cases and cases seen later in the disease course are not generally treated.
- Dosage:
  - TPE: 250 ml/kg/bwt over 10–14 days. It usually translates to 5–6 (one plasma volume per session) exchanges over 2 weeks.
  - IVIG 2 gm/kg/bwt over 2–5 days.
- Improvement is noted in 1–3 weeks after treatment.
- Chronic inflammatory demyelinating polyneuropathy (CIDP) may present acutely and therefore can be confused with GBS. A total of 10% of treated GBS patients relapse within weeks. In these cases, CIDP should be considered.

CASE 5.4: CARPOPEDAL SPASMS

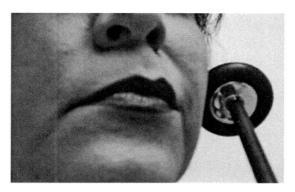

VIDEO 5.4

A 27-year-old woman had developed tingling of the hands and feet with intermittent spontaneous painful spasms of the fingers and toes, facial twitching, and nervousness over the preceding 6 months. Electromyography (EMG) revealed many doublets.

These symptoms and signs suggest:

1. Hypercalcemia
2. Hypocalcemia
3. Tetanus
4. Myokymia
5. Neuromyotonia

DIAGNOSIS

- A low ionized calcium level leads to hyperexcitability of peripheral nerves, which can be tested by tapping the facial nerve at the angle of the jaw to produce twitching of the ipsilateral facial muscles (Chvostek sign). A more sensitive sign is produced by inflating the blood pressure cuff pressure above systolic for 2–3 minutes, which leads to carpal spasms at the metacarpophalangeal joint (MPJ) (obstetrician hand). This is called the *Trousseau sign*.
- Hypocalcemia may be produced by:
  - Hypovitaminosis D
  - Hypoparathyroidism
  - Pseudohypoparathyroidism
- Hypomagnesemia (alcoholism, malabsorption, or diuresis) may produce a similar picture. It is imperative that the magnesium level is checked when the calcium level is normal in patients with paroxysmal nocturnal hemoglobinuria (PNH) disorders.
- Hyperventilation leads to peripheral nerve hyperexcitability by shifting calcium from free to albumin bound (alkalosis makes albumin more acidic). In this case, total calcium remains normal.
- Doublets and triplets [single motor unit action potentials (MUAPs)] repeated, firing rapidly in succession with interdischarge intervals between 2 and 20 ms) are typical EMG findings in hypocalcemia and they can be brought up by asking patients to hyperventilate. Fasciculations may also be observed, along with perioral and acral paraesthesias.
- True hypocalcemia, unlike hyperventilation, is usually associated with proximal weakness, and more reports linking vitamin D deficiency with myopathy have been published recently.
- Recent literature sheds light on the following additional risk factors of vitamin D deficiency:
  - Extensive use of sunscreen that blocks 95% of ultraviolet (UV) light from penetrating skin
  - Wearing a burka or other heavy, sun-blocking clothes
  - Obesity: low bioavailability of vitamin D
  - Dark skin: because melanin blocks UV

CASE 5.5: UNILATERAL FACIAL WEAKNESS

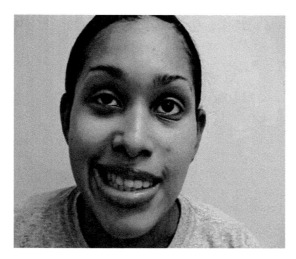

VIDEO 5.5

A 17-year-old woman developed sudden left retroauricular pain, followed by facial asymmetry and impairment of hearing and taste. Examination is shown in the video.

The cause of impairment of taste and hearing is:

1. Damage to the chorda tympani
2. Damage to the medullary nucleus
3. Damage to the nerve to the stapedius
4. Damage to the trigeminal nerve
5. A central lesion

DIAGNOSIS

- Examination showed weakness of the left side of the face that involved both volitional and emotional components and involving the upper and lower parts of the face.
- Facial palsy is a common presentation to neuromuscular clinics.
- The facial muscles are supplied by the facial nerves, which emerge from the pontomedullary junction and enter the face through the parotid glands.
- The chorda tympani carries taste sensation to the anterior two-thirds of the tongue and joins the facial nerve later in the course. It also carries parasympathetic supply to the lacrimal and salivary glands except for the parotids. The smallest muscle in the body (the stapedius) is supplied by a branch of a facial nerve, and it tenses and relaxes the tympanic membrane during transmission of air vibrations to produce clear distinction of sound.
- Facial nerve may be affected by myopathies (FSHD, IBM, etc.), polyneuropathies (CIDP, Familial amyloid neuropathy [FAN]), mononeuropathies (Bell's palsy, sarcoidosis), MG, brain stem pathology (ischemic, glioma), and cerebral pathology (infarction).
- The face is bilaterally innervated, and therefore central facial weakness saves the upper part of the face, while peripheral facial palsy (as in Bell's palsy) leads to the loss of upper and lower facial strength.
- Bell's palsy is an acute peripheral facial paralysis due to viral invasion of the nerve at the stylomastoid canal. HSV1 is the most common proven infection, followed by herpeszoster activation, cytomegalovirus (CMV), and Epstein-Barr virus (EBV).
- Acute retroauricular pain is followed by facial palsy, loss of taste of the anterior two-thirds of the tongue, hyperacusis, and dry eyes.
- Onset occurs over 1–2 days, maximum weakness in 3 weeks, and recovery in 6 months.
- Recurrence occurs in 7% of cases, and a second recurrence in 2%.
- Prednisone (60–80 mg a day for a week) is shown to reduce the risk of unfavorable outcome if given early in the course of the disease.
- Antiviral therapy is not routinely indicated, as double-blind clinical trials did not favor them.

CASE 5.6: FACIAL WEAKNESS AFTER DIVORCE

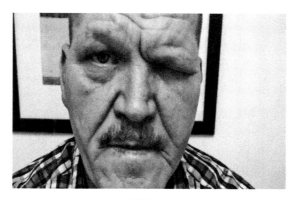

VIDEO 5.6

A 55-year-old man presented with a history of metastatic prostate cancer and a recent divorce and loss of his job. He suddenly could not open his left eye and developed frontal headache with no sensory symptoms. Examination that took place a month later is shown in the video. The symptoms resolved with an intramuscular, normal saline injection in the face.

The features that suggest nonorganic weakness in this case are:

1. Preservation of the nasolabial fold (NLF)
2. Lack of facial weakness
3. Exaggerated wrinkles and facial folds in the affected side
4. Concurrent stress
5. All of the above

DIAGNOSIS

- His examination showed exaggeration of the upper facial folds and no objective facial weakness. There was no atrophy of the NLF.
- Facial weakness is often a manifestation of functional disorders and malingering since it can be easily mimicked. However, it is not difficult for a neurologist to recognize functional facial weakness.
- The elevation of the ipsilateral eyebrow and the closure of the ipsilateral eye are very suggestive of a functional overlay.
- Exaggeration of forehead wrinkles and preservation of the NLF are also suggestive of a non-organic cause. In Bell's palsy, it is hard to close the affected eye, and the NLF becomes flat within a few days.
- Underlying stress may not be easy to figure out.
- Despite chronicity, atrophy does not occur, and symptoms improve with distraction.
- Many patients respond to treatment with a placebo.

CASE 5.7: FACIAL ASYMMETRY AFTER
A HURRICANE

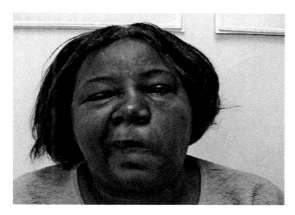

VIDEO 5.7

A 65-year-old woman relocated to Houston after losing her house and job because of Hurricane Katrina. She developed frequent, sustained, and painful right facial muscle spasms every time she saw her friends who lived in the same area. The condition always resolved with prayer.

The following facts support functional rather than organic hemifacial spasms:

1. They are sustained.
2. They are painful.
3. They are associated with profound speech abnormality.
4. They are worsened by stress.
5. They are improved by prayer.

DIAGNOSIS

- There was no facial weakness, but her voice changed during the spasms. The Chvostek sign was negative.
- Stress may be associated with a wide spectrum of clinical manifestations; some of them are difficult to differentiate from their organic counterparts.
- Rarely is the source of stress apparent, but when it is, the diagnosis is facilitated.
- Symptoms are usually not typical for any recognized neurological presentation.
- It is important to differentiate between:
  - Conversion: Stress is converted into acute somatic symptoms such as weakness or numbness, usually in young females.
  - Somatization: Stress is converted into chronic multiple somatic symptoms, usually in middle-aged females.
  - Factitious disorder: Symptoms are induced by the administration of pharmacologically active substances, such as insulin injections to produce hypoglycemia.
  - Malingering: Fabrication of symptoms.
    - The first three are involuntary, and the fourth is a conscious falsification.
- While psychogenic symptoms typically improve with prayer and get worse with stress, this does not exclude organicity, as many organic symptoms improve with these measures, too.

CASE 5.8: COULD NEVER BLOW UP A BALLOON

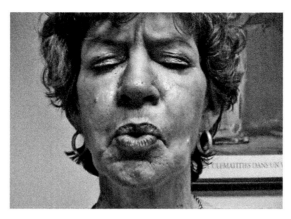

VIDEO 5.8

A 63-year-old woman presented with a 20-year history of inability to stand on her heels and a 10-year history of inability to stand up from a deep chair and difficulty raising her arms. She could never blow up a balloon. Her examination is shown in the video. The combination of facial weakness, foot drop, and scapular winging that evolves over years is very typical of FSHD.

What do the identified structures in Figure 5.8.1 (marked by arrows) represent?

1. Scapulae
2. Hypertrophied trapezius
3. Levator scapulae
4. Fat pad
5. Sternocleidomastoid

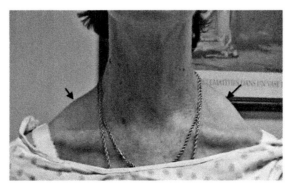

FIGURE 5.8.1 A patient with FSHD.

DIAGNOSIS

- Facial weakness is frequently the first sign of FSHD, although it is not usually noticed by patients, but rather by their friends and family.
- Retrospectively, many patients give a history of difficulty with blowing up balloons, using straws, and whistling for years before the diagnosis. Patients cannot pucker their lips during the exam. Labial dysarthria may occur. A transverse smile is common.
- Inability to close eyes completely during sleep may cause exposure keratitis. Patching the eyes during sleep may be necessary.
- Facial involvement occurs in 95% of cases. In the remaining 5%, the face is spared.
- These are usually of late onset and are associated with small deletions.
- In 7% of cases, facial involvement is predominant, and scapuloperoneal weakness is found only in the examination.
- Facial weakness is common in IBM and myotonic dystrophy. Dysphagia and true proximal weakness are rare in FSHD.
- The inability to abduct arms is not due to weakness of the arm abductor muscles, but rather due to instability of the scapulae, which ascend and rotate during arm abduction, forming the arrowed prominences.

CASE 5.9: A PENALTY FOR FACIAL LIFT

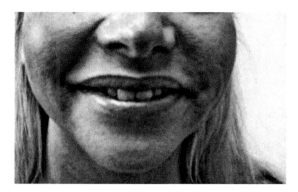

VIDEO 5.9

A 45-year-old woman had a bilateral transoral cheek implantation, facelift, and rhinoplasty 3 months earlier. She could not pucker her upper lip or whistle since surgery. There was no weakness in the rest of the face, and her facial sensation was normal. EMG revealed denervation of the upper lip only.

The abovementioned findings suggest an injury to the following branches of the facial nerve:

1. Main trunk
2. Marginal branches
3. Buccal branches
4. Frontal branches
5. Cervical branches

DIAGNOSIS

- Rhytidectomy (facelift) is the sixth-most-common plastic surgery in the United States, and each facelift costs $10,000 on average.
- Nerve injury is one of the most common complications. The facial and greater auricular nerves are the most commonly affected.
- Many cases recover spontaneously within a few months.
- Permanent motor nerve paralysis occurs at a rate of 0.5%–2.6% of cases.
  - The marginal branch is most commonly injured, followed by the frontal and buccal branches. In this case, the buccal branches were severed.
- Pseudoparalysis of the marginal mandibular nerve due to cervical branch injury can be distinguished from true marginal mandibular injury by the fact that the patient is able to evert the lower lip because of a functioning mentalis muscle.
- The prevalence of cervical branch injury in facelifts is reported at 1.7%.
- Sensory nerve injuries are more common, with great auricular nerve injury reported in up to 7% of cases.

CASE 5.10: WEAKNESS OF FACE AND FINGERS

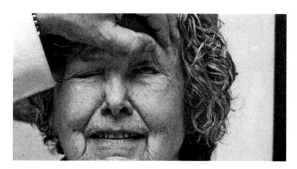

VIDEO 5.10

A 77-year-old woman reported a 5-year history of difficulty climbing stairs and dysphagia. The CK level was 190 IU/L, and the EMG revealed many short-duration polyphasic units in the proximal leg muscles and finger flexors.

Muscle biopsy in this disease is not expected to show:

1. Endomysial inflammation
2. Cytoplasmic inclusion bodies
3. Red-rimmed vacuoles
4. Denervated fibers
5. Perifascicular atrophy

DIAGNOSIS

- Video 5.10 revealed facial weakness, finger flexor weakness, and proximal leg weakness.
- IBM is the most common myopathy after age 50 years. It is more common in males.
- While a typical picture is that of chronic progressive weakness of the quadriceps (more than the iliopsoas), finger flexors, and biceps (more than the deltoids) and dysphagia, phenotypic variations are well reported.
- In this case, the quadriceps muscles were not clinically affected.
- Dysphagia occurs in two-thirds of cases.
- Unlike polymyositis and dermatomyositis, facial weakness occurs in one-third of cases, although it is often discovered during examination and the patient does not complain about it. It can be so severe that eyes cannot be kept closed during sleep, which may lead to exposure keratitis.
- Typical pathological findings include:
  - Chronic myopathic changes (variation of fiber size and shape, necrotic and phagocytic fibers, split fibers, patchy loss of oxidative activity, increased connective tissue, etc.).
  - Endomysial inflammation with invasion of nonnecrotic fibers by mononuclear inflammatory cells.
  - Red-rimmed vacuoles and eosinophilic cytoplasmic inclusion bodies.
  - Nuclear inclusion bodies seen under electron microscopy (EM).
  - Congophilic material usually adjacent to the vacuoles.
  - Denervated fibers.
    - Perifascicular atrophy is not a feature of IBM. It is typically seen in dermatomyositis.

CASE 5.11: NASAL SPEECH

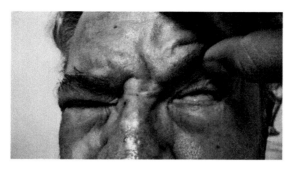

VIDEO 5.11

A 65-year-old man presented with a 3-month history of nasal speech and regurgitation of water through the nose.

Facial weakness and nasal speech are typically seen in:

1. MG
2. Lambert-Eaton myasthenic syndrome (LEMS)
3. IBM
4. FSMD
5. CIDP

DIAGNOSIS

- Video 5.11 revealed facial weakness and nasal speech.
- Facial weakness is common in MG and several myopathies like IBM and myotonic dystrophy.
- LEMS usually presents with proximal weakness mimicking myopathy. Facial weakness is rare.
- GBS may lead to facial diplegia.
- Palate weakness, causing nasal speech and regurgitation of food through the nose, is not commonly seen in any of the mentioned possibilities except MG.
- The most common causes of nasal speech are local factors such as adenoids, deviated septum, and allergic rhinitis. Neurologic causes are rare and include MG, poliomyelitis, and diphtheria.

CASE 5.12: FACIAL TWITCHING

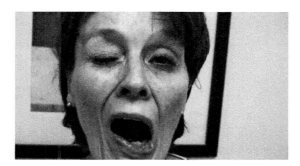

VIDEO 5.12

A 48-year-old woman had right Bell's palsy 2 years earlier, from which she recovered, except for the finding shown in Video 5.12.

The eye blinking is:

1. Due to viral reactivation
2. Due to synkinesis of facial nerves
3. Is not related to Bell's palsy
4. Is reversible most of the time

DIAGNOSIS

- Facial synkinesis is a common complication of Bell's palsy.
- During nerve regeneration, nerve misdirected wiring may occur, leading to the misconnection of different nerve fibers that are intended for different functions.
- It is more likely to happen in severe cases.
- Synkinesis is manifested during the recovery process, usually months after the initial insult.
- The most common symptoms of facial synkinesis are:
  - Eye closure, with volitional contraction of mouth muscles
    - This patient demonstrated an involuntary blinking of the right eye whenever she opened her mouth.
  - Facial movements with volitional eye closure
  - Neck tightness (platysmal contraction) with volitional smiling
  - Hyperlacrimation (also called *crocodile tears*)
    - A case where eating or just thinking of food provokes excessive lacrimation: This has been attributed to neural synkinesis between branches to the salivary glands and the lacrimal glands.
    - The condition is chronic and may be helped by botulinum toxin (BT) injections to the lacrimal glands.

CASE 5.13: INABILITY TO SING AND KISS

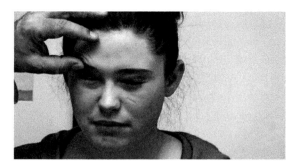

VIDEO 5.13

A 17-year-old girl presented with a 1-year history of inability to sing in church because her voice faded soon after she began singing. The binding acetylcholine receptor (AChR) antibody titer was 403 nmol/L.

Such a very high AChR antibody titer:

1. Indicates a poor prognosis
2. Indicates severe disease
3. Is associated with a high risk of generalization of MG
4. Is associated with thymoma
5. Confirms the diagnosis of MG

DIAGNOSIS

- Video 5.13 showed upper and lower facial weakness.
- Absolute titer of AChR-binding antibodies does not correlate with the severity of MG in the general population, although in individual patients, improvement is often seen with reduction in titer by more than 50%.
  - These antibodies are positive in 80%–90% of generalized MG, and 50%–70% of ocular MG.
  - False positives rarely occur in:
    - LEMS
    - Graft vs. host disease (GVHD)
    - Autoimmune hepatitis
    - Healthy relatives of patients with myasthenia
    - Patients with thymoma
    - Lung cancer
    - Motor neuron disease
    - Snake venom poisoning
- There is no difference in phenotype or responsiveness to treatment between seronegative and seropositive individuals (regardless of the titer).
- Antibodies may not even decline with treatment, despite good clinical response.
- Seroconversion occurs in 20% of cases within a year; therefore, repeating the test in negative cases is advised.
- Anti-ACh receptor blocking and modulating antibodies are reported in 5% of AChR-binding antibody cases. They may be useful if the binding antibodies are negative. This test is reported on a percentage basis and should be considered significant only when present at a high percentile. Minimally positive test results in normal patients are not uncommon.
- Anti-ACh blocking antibodies are highly specific. False positives are reported in LEMS only rarely, and in patients exposed to curarelike drugs. These are essentially never present in isolation. Accordingly, these are not used as a screening test for MG, and their only practical role is to aid in the identification of a potentially false-positive result.
- Other than confirming the diagnosis, the AChR antibody titer does not have a prognostic value, correlates with severity, or predicts thymoma.

CASE 5.14: CROOKED SMILE SINCE CHILDHOOD

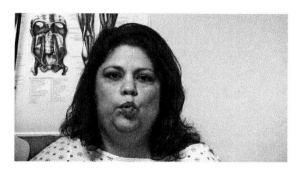

VIDEO 5.14

A 42-year-old woman presented with a history of DM and hypertension; she was noticed to have a crooked smile since the age of 12 years. Gradually, she noticed difficulty raising her arms and pain in the upper back. She had normal deep tendon reflexes (DTRs), sensation, foot extensors, hearing, and vision. Physical findings are shown in the video. She had one child and four siblings. There was no family history of a neurological illness.

The most likely cause of facial weakness in this case is:

1. Facial nerve palsy
2. FSHD
3. Scapuloperoneal syndrome
4. Congenital facial weakness
5. Demyelinating neuropathy

DIAGNOSIS

- Asymmetrical facial weakness, scapular winging, inverted axillary folds, and proximal leg weakness since age 12 are very suggestive of FSHD. Mutation analysis confirmed deletion of D4Z4 at 4q35.
- It is the second-most-prevalent form of muscular dystrophy (MD) after Duchenne muscular dystrophy (DMD), with a prevalence of 5/100,000.
- Asymmetry in FSHD is so striking that some patients are diagnosed with facial nerve palsy. Asymmetrical foot drop is common.
- It is an autosomal-dominant (AD) disease, but 30% of cases are caused by de novo mutation.
- The genotype-phenotype relationship is far from being understood. Interestingly, a toxic gain of function of the *DUX4* gene is found to play a role. This is the first time where "junk DNA" is found to reanimate and cause disease.
- Life span is normal. A total of 20% of patients eventually require a wheelchair and 1% artificial ventilation.

SUGGESTED READING

Lemmers RJ, van der Vliet PJ, Klooster R, et al. A unifying genetic model for facioscapulohumeral muscular dystrophy. *Science*. 2010 Sep 24;1650–1653.

CASE 5.15: CHRONIC FACIAL WEAKNESS AND DEAFNESS

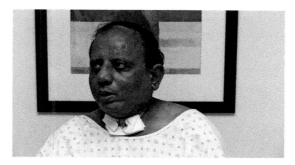

VIDEO 5.15

A 66-year-old Indian man who reports bilateral facial weakness that started when he was 15–20 years old and affected both the upper and lower parts of the face. He had 2 healthy brothers and 1 son. His parents did not have evidence of a neuromuscular problem. He developed hoarseness 2–3 years later and was found to have bilateral vocal cord paralysis, which required tracheostomy several years later. He denies swallowing or chewing difficulty, diplopia, or sensory symptoms. He denies headache or weakness in the arms, legs, or bowel, or bladder disturbances. He denies muscle cramps or twitching or weakness in the arms or legs. Magnetic resonance imaging (MRI) of the brain, cervical spine, thoracic spine, repeat CSF exam, and investigation for sarcoidosis were all negative. EMG/NCS revealed no evidence of neuropathy. The tongue was denervated. Chronic slowly progressive course of findings shown in Video 5.15 were associated with hearing impairment.

The most likely diagnosis is:

1. Bulbar onset amyotrophic lateral sclerosis (ALS)
2. Spinal muscular atrophy (SMA)
3. Madras motor neuron disease
4. Brown-Violette-Van Laere syndrome (BVVLS)
5. Facial onset sensorimotor neuropathy (FOSMN)

DIAGNOSIS

Madras motor neuron disease:

- Blink reflex testing confirmed bilateral facial palsy. Brainstem-evoked responses suggested central interruption of the auditory pathway.
- Chronic slowly progressive cranial polyneuropathy, including facial nerves, vestibulo-cochlear nerves, hypoglossal nerves, and vagus nerves, the lack of sensory symptoms, and normal MRI of the brainstem suggested that the lesion was at the level of the motor neurons.
- He had mild proximal weakness in the arms and legs and generalized areflexia with normal sural responses, which also supported the notion of lower motor neuron (LMN) disease.
- There was no evidence of upper motor neuron (UMN) involvement, and the long duration strongly argued against ALS.
- He had no family history to suggest spinal muscular atrophy.
- He had no gynecomastia to suggest Kennedy disease.
- Degenerative pathology was much more likely than autoimmune disease because of chronicity and the normal CSF exam and the lack of response to steroids.
- FOSMN is a consideration, but the lack of sensory symptoms is atypical.
- The Madras variant of motor neuron disease (MND) is reported in South India (where he is from) and is most likely the cause. Degeneration of cranial nerve nuclei 7, 9, and 10 and progressive hearing loss are typical. The cause is not clear.
- BVVLS in the Western literature seems to be the equivalent of this, except that the former is not associated with riboflavin receptor mutation (it tested negative in this case).

SUGGESTED READING

Gourie-Devi, M, Nalini A. Madras motor neuron disease variant, clinical features of seven patients. *J Neurol Sci.* 2003 May 15;209(1–2):13–17.

CASE 5.16: ANARTHRIA AND FACIAL WEAKNESS

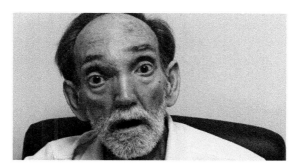

VIDEO 5.16

A 70-year-old healthy man with 8 months' history of progressive dysarthria (which progressed to anarthria), dysphagia, drooling, and weight loss. Examination showed atrophy and fasciculations of the tongue. Forced vital capacity (FVC) was 800 ml, creatine phosphokinase (CPK) was normal, and EMG showed denervation of the tongue.

Regarding facial weakness in MND, the following is true except:

1. Common in early ALS
2. Is noted in advanced cases of ALS
3. Is a common feature of FOSMN
4. Not against the diagnosis of ALS
5. Is common in Madras MND disease

DIAGNOSIS

This is a case of advance bulbar onset ALS. Frank facial weakness is not common early in the disease, except in some variants like Madras disease and FOSMN. As the disease progresses, facial weakness becomes noticeable. Special care should be taken to prevent exposure keratitis in these cases.

CASE 5.17: FACIAL WEAKNESS AND INFLAMMATORY MYOPATHY

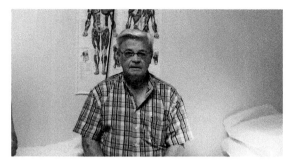

VIDEO 5.17

A 78-year-old man presented with the clinical findings shown in Video 5.17. The CPK level was 460 IU/L. EMG revealed irritative myopathy of the quadriceps and hip flexors. A muscle biopsy is shown in Figure 5.17.1. To confirm the diagnosis of IBM, the most diagnostically helpful antibodies are:

1. NT5C1A
2. HMGCR
3. SRP
4. Jo1
5. Mi

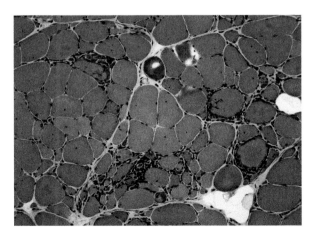

FIGURE 5.17.1 H&E stain of left biceps muscle tissue.(100X)

DIAGNOSIS

- Frequent falls is the most common presentation of IBM due to knee extensor weakness.
- Weakness of the facial muscles and finger flexors and more weakness of biceps than deltoids, and quadriceps than iliopsoas, are typical.
- Muscle biopsy revealed inflammatory myopathy with no red-rimmed vacuoles, cytoplasmic inclusion bodies, or congophilia. Rimmed vacuoles and cytoplasmic inclusion bodies are not seen in 20% of cases, especially early in the disease.
- NT5C1A antibody titer is positive in 51%–75% of cases and helps confirm atypical cases. However, it is false positive in 30% of cases. [4%–20% of PM and DM and 20% of systemic lupus erythematosus (SLE) and Sjogren syndrome cases.]
  - Preliminary data suggest that cases associated with NT5C1A antibodies have more severe facial and bulbar involvement.

SUGGESTED READING

Goyal NA, Cash TM, Alam U, et al. Seropositive for NT5c1A antibody in IBM predicts more severe motor, bulbar and respiratory involvement. *J Neurol Neurosurg Psych*. 2016 Apr;87(4):373–378.

CHAPTER 6

TONGUE SIGNS

CASE 6.1: SLURRED SPEECH AND TROUBLE SWALLOWING

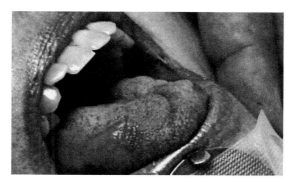

VIDEO 6.1

A 53-year-old woman presented with a 3-month history of slurring of speech and excessive drooling. She was suspected of having a stroke. Brain magnetic resonance imaging (MRI) was normal. She developed dysphagia a month later. Examination demonstrated key physical and neurophysiological findings. She had no weakness in the extremities.

The following are bad prognostic signs in this disease:

1. Onset in the legs
2. Bulbar onset
3. Spasticity
4. Old age
5. Female gender

DIAGNOSIS

- Examination showed atrophy and fasciculations of the tongue with jaw hyperreflexia, and tongue electromyography (EMG) revealed fast-firing motor units in the background.
- A third of amyotrophic lateral sclerosis (ALS) patients present with dysarthria and, to a lesser extent, dysphagia. The appearance of dysphagia before dysarthria is not typical of ALS.
- Early in the course of the disease, and when clinical findings are confined to the bulbar muscles, diagnosis of ALS may be difficult, particularly if upper motor neuron (UMN) symptoms are predominant.
- Tongue fasciculation and jaw hyperreflexia are important clues to bulbar ALS, but when the lesion is confined to the UMN (PLS picture), confirmation of the diagnosis remains difficult.
- Bulbar onset occurs more in females, and it carries a worse prognosis than extremities onset ALS.
- Hypersialosis is common and may further disturb swallowing. If anticholinergic drugs fail, botulinum toxin (BT) injection to the salivary glands can be effective.
- Pseudobulbar affect (a tendency to laugh or cry with minimal provocation and with no emotional component) is common in bulbar ALS and is attributed to a UMN lesion; it may respond well to tricyclic antidepressants or dextromethorphan/quinidine.
- Trials of riluzole showed that this medicine works better in bulbar onset ALS.
- Intravenous (IV) edaravone (Radicava) was just approved by the U.S. Food and Drug Administration (FDA) for the treatment of ALS. The active group declined less at week 24 compared to the placebo group in a 6-month clinical trial. The mechanism of action is not known.
- The main differential diagnosis of bulbar palsy is myasthenia gravis (MG), particularly Musk Ab–associated MG. Therefore, acetylcholine receptor (AChR) antibody titer should be checked and, if negative, Musk Ab titer.
- It is important to monitor pulmonary function tests (PFTs) because early institution of biphasic positive airway pressure (BIPAP) is shown to improve quality of life and may prolong survival.
- Monitoring of swallowing is essential, and early percutaneous endoscopic gastrostomy (PEG) improves morbidity.
- Chronic lower motor neuron (LMN) bulbar palsy should raise the possibility of Kennedy disease, and one needs to examine the breasts for gynecomastia and obtain mutation analysis for androgen receptors.
- Ptosis and ophthalmoplegia do not occur in bulbar ALS.
- Bulbar onset and old age are bad prognostic signs in ALS.

SUGGESTED READING

Tanaka M, Sakata T, Palumbo J, Akimoto M. A 24-week, Phase III, double-blind, parallel-group study of edaravone (MCI-186) for treatment of amyotrophic lateral sclerosis (ALS). *Neurol* 86(16):Suppl P3.189.

CASE 6.2: CHOKING WITH SALIVA

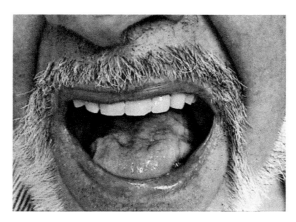

VIDEO 6.2

A 65-year-old man presented with a 6-month history of difficulty lifting his head for a long time. He developed slurring of speech, especially at night, and excessive salivation and choking 2 months later. He lost 10 pounds. In addition to what is shown in Video 6.2, there was hyperreflexia of the jaw jerk and deep tendon reflexes (DTRs) in the upper and lower extremities. EMG revealed denervation of the tongue, neck extensors, and upper extremities, proximally and distally. The thoracic paraspinal muscles and leg muscles were not denervated.

This patient qualifies for which diagnosis, according to modified El Escorial criteria (EEC)?

1. Clinically definite ALS
2. Clinically probable ALS
3. Clinically probable, lab-supported ALS
4. Possible ALS
5. No ALS

DIAGNOSIS

- Video 6.2 revealed weak neck extensors, atrophy, and fasciculation of the tongue and dysarthria.
- There are several sets of ALS diagnostic criteria.
- In 1990, the World Federation of Neurology met in El Escorial in Spain and set diagnostic criteria for ALS that were mainly intended for research purposes. These criteria were modified 8 years later in order to allow more subjects to be enrolled in clinical trials. EEC are the gold standard of ALS diagnosis, but the lack of sensitivity continues to encourage experts to modify them.
- It is estimated that 25% of patients with progressive UMN and LMN lesions proven at autopsy never met EEC.
- EEC do not capture those restricted variants such as primary lateral sclerosis (PLS), progressive muscular atrophy (PMA), and pseudobulbar palsy (PBP) that may never generalize.
- The following are the modified EEC for the diagnosis of ALS. All require progressive course and exclusion of other causes by appropriate imaging and neurophysiological tests:
  - Clinically definite ALS: clinical evidence of UMN and LMN lesion in three regions
  - Clinically probable ALS: clinical evidence of UMN and LMN lesion in two regions and some UMN rostral to the LMN signs
  - Clinically probable, lab-supported ALS: clinical evidence of UMN and LMN lesions in one region, or clinical UMN signs in one region and EMG evidence of LMN in at least two limbs
  - Possible ALS: signs of UMN and LMN lesions in one region only, or UMN signs in two or more regions
- The regions in question are bulbar, cervical, thoracic, and lumbar.
- LMN evidence of denervation, according to EEC, is only fibrillations. (Awaji criteria allow for fasciculation.)
- This case qualified as clinically probable ALS. There was evidence of UMN and LMN signs in the bulbar and cervical regions only.

CASE 6.3: JUST A LISP

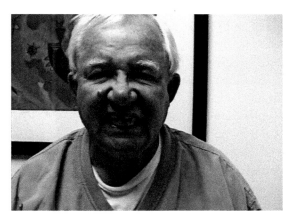

VIDEO 6.3

A 70-year-old man presented with a 6-month history of a lisp, noted by his friends, that became worse the more he spoke. There was no diplopia, ptosis, dysphagia, muscle wasting, or extremities weakness. Since he was stressed, it was considered psychogenic. The AChR antibody titer was high, and the lingual dysarthria responded to steroids.

Lingual dysarthria can be a feature of:

1. MG
2. ALS
3. Hypoglossal neuropathy
4. Hysteria
5. Lambert-Eaton myasthenic syndrome (LEMS)

DIAGNOSIS

- The tongue consists of four pairs of extrinsic and four pairs of intrinsic muscles. Tongue movement is served by the hypoglossal nerve.
- Tongue weakness is a feature of several neuromuscular disorders. It may present as dysarthria or inability to move food in the mouth properly.
- These disorders include:
  - Muscle disease (polymyositis)
  - Nerve disease [Guillain-Barré syndrome (GBS)]
  - Neuromuscular junction (NMJ) disorders (MG, LEMS, botulism)
  - Motor neuron disease (MND) (ALS, Kennedy disease), and
  - Mitochondrial disorders like sensory ataxia, neuropathy dysarthria, ophthalmoplegia (SANDO).
- Bulbar weakness without prominent ocular symptoms is not unusual in MG. As a matter of fact, it is a common manifestation of MuSK antibodies associated with MG, where atrophy of the tongue and face may lead to diagnostic confusion with bulbar onset ALS. Even tongue fasciculations are reported in MuSK antibody–associated MG.
- Fatigability of dysarthria (worsening with speech) is more typically seen in MG.
- In MG, the tip of the tongue is often affected early, leading to a lisp; in ALS, the bulk of the tongue is affected, leading to a "heavy tongue," like the tongue of an intoxicated person.
- Cerebellar dysarthria is irregular. The patient cannot count fast with regular intervals and consistent volume.

CASE 6.4: TONGUE PROTRUSIONS

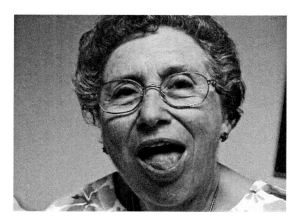

VIDEO 6.4

A 73-year-old woman presented with a 2-year history of abnormal tongue movement. There was no family history of a similar disorder. She had chronic nausea treated with metoclopramide for several months before these symptoms started.

The following drugs can cause this syndrome:

1. Metoclopramide
2. Hydrochlorothiazide
3. Promethazine
4. Tetracycline
5. Steroids

DIAGNOSIS

- Video 6.4 showed involuntary, painless, repetitive protrusion of the tongue, which was alleviated as the patient touched her face with her hand. There was no abnormal movement of the other facial muscles.
- Patients with oromandibular dystonia (OMD) are sometimes referred to neuromuscular clinics due to lingual dysarthria, dysphagia, choking, and weight loss that lead to suspicion of a neuromuscular disorder such as ALS or MG.
- Involuntary tongue protrusion in dystonia is usually associated with mouth opening and contraction of cervical muscles.
- The tongue in this syndrome is not weak or atrophied, and it is not fatigable.
- Oculogyric crisis, if it happens, can be easily differentiated from the weak extraocular muscles that occur with MG.
- OMD is usually alleviated with sensory tricks such as touching the face.
- Like tardive dyskinesia, tardive dystonia can be produced by prolonged administration of drugs that block dopamine, such as phenothiazine and metoclopramide.
- OMD can also be produced by neurodegenerative disorders, but it is usually idiopathic.
- BT injection into the genioglossus, which protrudes the tongue, usually works and does not cause swallowing problems.

CASE 6.5: GROOVED TONGUE

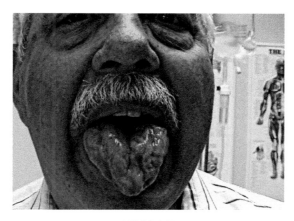

VIDEO 6.5

A 45-year-old diabetic man presented with a 5-year history of intermittent diplopia and foot numbness. Examination is shown in the video. He also had mild sensory impairment in the feet and absent ankle jerks. Nerve conduction study (NCS) revealed mild sensory neuropathy.

The following tongue abnormalities are not uncommonly seen in chronic MG:

1. Weakness
2. Atrophy
3. Grooving
4. Fasciculation
5. All of the above

DIAGNOSIS

- Video 6.5 showed mild fatigable right ptosis and grooved tongue.
- In chronic MG, atrophy of the tongue leads to formation of a triple-furrowed appearance, with grooves paralleling median sulci on each side.
- Tongue atrophy and weakness are commonly seen in MuSK MG.
- Tongue fasciculation is not a feature of MG (there is one questionable case report in the medical literature).

CASE 6.6: FAMILIAL MUSCLE STIFFNESS

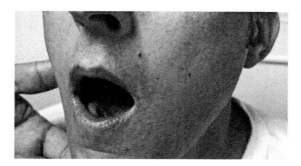

VIDEO 6.6

A 38-year-old man had developed symptoms since age 21 years consisting of muscle stiffness, painful muscle spasms, difficulty chewing, and memory problems. He had several cousins and a sister with the same symptoms. His tongue examination is shown in the video.

This demonstrated reaction of the tongue is due to:

1. Atrophy
2. Myotonia
3. Pain
4. Weakness
5. Reaction to cotton in the Q-tip

DIAGNOSIS

- Video 6.6 showed persistent grooving of the tongue after applying pressure with a Q-tip.
- In patients with a myotonic disorder, myotonia can be:
  - Spontaneous, affecting extremities during walking or running, which leads to falls
  - Induced by:
    - Percussion of selected muscles, such as
      - Thenar eminence: Percussion leads to sustained abduction or opposition of the thumb.
      - Wrist extensors: Percussion leads to sustained wrist extension.
    - Pressure: Application of sustained pressure on the tongue leads to grooving due to sustained poor relaxation of the pressed muscles. Percussion of the tongue may produce the same effect, but it is more technically difficult to perform.
    - Gripping: Grip myotonia leads to difficulty in the relaxation of finger flexors after a forceful handshake.
- When examining for myotonia, it is important to repeat the tapping or pressure in order to examine for the "warming up" phenomenon, which means improvement of relaxation of the affected muscle by repeated challenges. This is typically seen in myotonia. On the other hand, paramyotonia (PMC) worsens with repeated challenges. Cold has the same effect on PMC.
- Myotonia of the tongue explains dysarthria in these patients and cold-induced dysarthria in patients with sodium channelopathy.
- Tongue myotonia is more pronounced than grip myotonia in myotonic dystrophy type 2.
- In our experience, tongue myotonia responds to mexiletine, as well as grip myotonia.

CASE 6.7: TONGUE TWITCHING AFTER RADIOTHERAPY

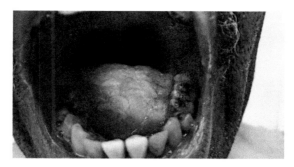

VIDEO 6.7

A 53-year-old male presented with trouble swallowing and excessive drooling. His examination is shown in the video. DTRs were revealed as normal. Clinical findings did not change when he was seen 5 years later.

Tongue fasciculation occurs in all the following conditions except:

1. ALS
2. Kennedy disease
3. After radiotherapy
4. Organophosphorous compound poisoning
5. Snake venom poisoning

DIAGNOSIS

- Video 6.7 showed dysarthria, tongue fasciculation, excessive salivation, and atrophy of the cervical muscles.
- The effect of radiation on the nervous system can be:
  - Acute
  - Subacute
  - Remote
- Remote effects of radiation may appear several years later in the form of motor neuron dysfunction in the irradiated area.
- Painless atrophy, weakness, and fasciculation may lead to diagnostic confusion with ALS.
  - Unlike ALS, DTRs are usually absent in the affected area and the course is not relentless.
- A typical course is that of initial worsening, and then stabilization.
- Myokymia in EMG is a highly characteristic sign.
- While ALS is the most ominous cause of tongue fasciculation, other causes should be born in mind, which include:
  - LMN disease [Kennedy disease, spinal muscular atrophy (SMA), poliomyelitis]
  - Brainstem lesions
  - Base of skull tumor
  - Skull base irradiation
  - Hypoglossal neuropathy
  - Organophosphorus poisoning
  - Snake venom poisoning
- Tongue weakness is an important sign that can precede fasciculation and atrophy in LMN syndromes and NMJ disorders. Strength of the tongue muscles is tested by asking the patient to push the tongue against the cheek and against the examiner's finger from outside.
- Advanced ALS patients may be unable to move their tongues at all. They are usually anarthritic.
- Irradiation of para-aortic lymph nodes for lymphoma or testicular tumors may produce LMN syndrome in the legs years later.
- It is always important to ask about history of irradiation in patients with fasciculation and atrophy because patients do not think of such connections and may not volunteer such information.

CASE 6.8: UNEXPECTED ELECTROMYOGRAPHY (EMG) FINDING

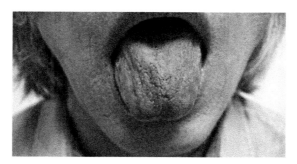

VIDEO .68

A 61-year-old woman presented with bilateral hand pain that prompted an EMG, which revealed widespread spontaneous activity and tongue movements, as shown in Video 6.8. She was referred for confirmation of "ALS." Her examination revealed percussion myotonia of the thenar muscles that worsened with repeated tapping (PMC), and the EMG showed diffuse myotonic discharges. She had abnormal sodium channel (SCNA) mutation consistent with paramyotonia congenita (PMC) that was asymptomatic. The tongue had normal bulk and strength and showed rhythmic contractions that were part of her essential tremor.

Unlike tremor of the tongue, ALS-related fasciculations are:

1. Irregular
2. Frequent
3. Associated with weakness and atrophy
4. Answers 1, 2, and 3
5. Answers 1 and 3

DIAGNOSIS

- Tongue tremor is a common finding and is usually part of essential or physiological tremor.
- It is regular, with a frequency of 6–10 Hz.
- Sometimes tongue tremor is punctuated by "jerks," leading to even more confusion with fasciculation.
- The tongue is not weak and not atrophied. It is important to inspect and examine the strength of the tongue in all cases of abnormal tongue movement to look for atrophy and weakness.
- Normal jaw jerk supports the benign nature of the abnormal tongue movement.
- Needle EMG of the extrinsic tongue muscles revealed rhythmic contractions and motor units with normal configuration and firing frequency.
- Fasciculations of ALS are irregular, infrequent, and associated with atrophy and weakness of the tongue.

CASE 6.9: FACIAL TWITCHING AND LARGE BREASTS

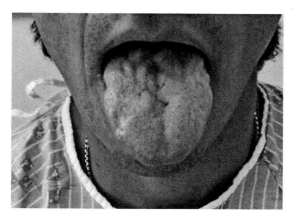

VIDEO 6.9

A 42-year-old man from Mexico had noticed facial twitching whenever he became nervous since age 20 years. A few years later, he also noticed mild slurring of speech. His examination is shown in the video. Genetic testing was diagnostic.

Mutation of which gene is expected in this case?

1. Androgen receptors (ARs)
2. Superoxide dismutase (SOD)
3. Valosin-containing protein
4. TAR DNA-binding protein 43 (TDP-43)
5. Fused in sarcoma (FUS)

DIAGNOSIS

- Video 6.9 showed atrophy and fasciculation of the tongue, abnormal facial movements, and large male breasts (gynecomastia). These findings are very suggestive of Kennedy disease.
- Kennedy disease is an X-linked SMA.
- Mean age of onset of symptoms is 27 years.
- Due to mutation of ARs, affected males display impotence, gynecomastia, testicular atrophy, and infertility.
- The presence of muscle cramps, proximal symmetrical weakness, and elevated creatine kinase (CK) leads to suspicion of a myopathy.
- The presence of foot numbness and areflexia leads to suspicion of neuropathy. NCS usually shows mild sensory neuropathy.
- Dysphagia, dysarthria, and fatigability of chewing muscles and dropped jaw (due to trigeminal palsy) leads to suspicion of MG.
- Any young male with proximal weakness and neurogenic EMG should be examined for Kennedy disease.
- Molecular basis: CAG repeat expansion (40–65 repeats). Androgen plays a role in cell survival and dendritic growth.
- A heterozygous female may show tongue fasciculation and muscle cramps in the seventh decade.
- An autosomal-dominant (AD) clinical variant of Kennedy disease is reported, with no clear identification of the molecular basis yet.

CASE 6.10: RESTLESS TONGUE

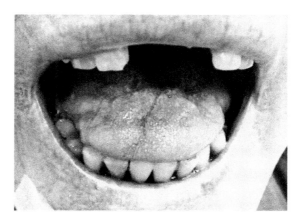

VIDEO 6.10

A 76-year-old man who had had radiotherapy for carcinoma of the tonsils 20 years earlier presented with dysphagia and excessive drooling. Examination showed atrophy and spontaneous movements of the tongue and absent jaw jerk. EMG of the tongue revealed bursts of discharges in a semirhythmic pattern.

The shown in the video activity is reported in all the following conditions except:

1. Delayed, postirradiation MND
2. Bell palsy
3. Episodic ataxia 1
4. Radiation-induced plexopathy
5. Myopathy

DIAGNOSIS

Video 6.10 showed atrophy and myokymia of the tongue, which is confirmed by EMG.
Myokymia is characterized by:

- Has single motor unit action potential (MUAP) firing as bursts of multiplets.
- Has 30–40-Hz discharges in short bursts.
- Bursts occur at 2–10 Hz.
- Burst duration is 100–900 milliseconds.
- Semirhythmic burst pattern.
- Bursts start and stop abruptly.
- Spontaneous.

Causes of myokymia:

- Brainstem glioma
- Multiple sclerosis (MS)
- Neuromyotonia
- Benign fasciculation syndrome
- Traumatic and inflammatory neuropathies such as Bell's palsy
- Postirradiation neuronopathy
- Episodic ataxia

Delayed postirradiation toxicity to motor neurons is well recognized and usually occurs years after
exposure. Myokymia is very characteristic.

CASE 6.11: NECK PAIN AND TONGUE DEVIATION

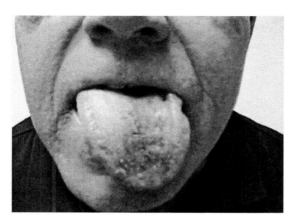

VIDEO 6.11

A 56-year-old man presented with acute left neck pain, followed by dysarthria. A few months later, the examination shown in Video 6.11 was made.

The most likely cause for these findings is:

1. Brainstem tumor
2. Trauma to the tongue
3. Carotid artery dissection
4. Jugular foramen tumor
5. Stroke

DIAGNOSIS

- Video 6.11 showed left tongue deviation.
- The hypoglossal nerves, which are the motor nerves to the tongue, can be affected anywhere in their pathway, from their origin in the medulla oblongata to the tongue muscles.
- Unilateral hypoglossal palsy leads to deviation of the tongue to the weak side (unlike paralyzed palate, where the uvula deviates to the healthy side).
- Important causes of hypoglossal palsy from the neuromuscular standpoint include:
  - Hereditary neuropathy with liability to pressure palsy (HNPP): Usually, there is a history of pressure, such as sleeping with the jaw supported by an arm, leading to pressure on the hypoglossal nerve. There is a history of other self-limiting focal neuropathies in the past.
  - Carotid artery dissection: Usually, this is caused by trauma to the neck. Common findings are acute neck pain and Horner's syndrome due to interruption of the sympathetic fibers to the ipsilateral pupil, which are conveyed via the carotid arteries.
  - As a part of Parsonage-Turner syndrome (hypoglossal nerves are less commonly affected than the anterior interosseus, suprascapular, long thoracic, and phrenic nerves).
  - Glomus tumor: Usually, the hypoglossal nerve is affected along with other lower cranial nerves. Progression is usually slow.
  - Idiopathic (usually acute and self-limiting, similar to Bell's palsy).
- Patients with more diffuse diseases like ALS and Kennedy disease may present with slight tongue asymmetry resulting from tongue atrophy, but unilateral tongue weakness is not a feature.

CASE 6.12: MUSCLE STIFFNESS AND WINTER WEAKNESS

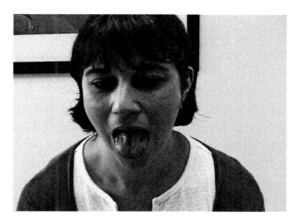

VIDEO 6.12

A 40-year-old woman developed painful muscle stiffness, especially during winter, and episodic generalized weakness, usually after heavy meals. There was no family history of significance. Examination of the tongue is shown in the video. She had a positive genetic testing.

The expected mutation affects the gene of the following channels:

1. Sodium
2. Calcium
3. Potassium
4. Chloride
5. None of the above

DIAGNOSIS

- Video 6.12 showed percussion myotonia of the tongue. Her EMG revealed generalized myotonic discharge.
- Myotonia is characterized by the persistence of strong contraction of muscle after stimulation has ceased. The contraction can be initiated voluntarily, mechanically, or electrically.
- Percussion of the tongue leads to localized constriction (napkin ring sign).
- Tongue myotonia is not specific to any myotonic disorder.
- Worsening of myotonia with repeated testing and cold suggests PMC.
- Periodic weakness suggests hyperkalemic periodic paralysis, which is allelic to PMC. It usually starts in adolescence, and each episode lasts less than 2 hours.
- PMC is caused by a sodium channel (SCN4A) mutation.
- Prolonged decrease of compound muscle action potential (CMAP) amplitude with long exercise testing is typical.
- Mexiletine at 150–1,000 mg a day is effective by blocking sodium channels.
- Hyperkalemic periodic paralysis usually responds to hydrochlorothiazide or acetazolamide therapy.

CASE 6.13: EAR PAIN AND TONGUE DEVIATION

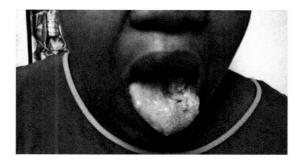

VIDEO 6.13

A 41-year-old woman presented with a 1-year history of tinnitus and left otalgia, followed by the mentioned symptoms and demonstrated signs.

The most likely cause of the left tongue atrophy in this case is:

1. Carotid dissection
2. Parsonage-Turner syndrome
3. Cavernous sinus pathology
4. Retro-orbital pathology
5. Glomus jugulare

DIAGNOSIS

- Hearing impairment, vocal cord paralysis, tongue deviation, and facial pain suggest involvement of the 8th, 10th, 12th, and 5th cranial nerves. Among the mentioned choices, glomus jugulare is the only one that can be that extensive.
- Glomus jugulare is a neuroendocrine neoplasm, 97% of which are benign.
- It originates from paraganglia in chromaffin negative glomus cells that are derived from embryonic neural crest. A total of 75% are sporadic, asymptomatic, or cause painless masses.
- Common sites are the head and neck, and it mostly originates in the middle ear and spreads to the jugular foramen and beyond, leading to multiple compressive cranial neuropathies.
- It is a slowly evolving tumor that appears at age 40–70 years.
- Symptoms usually start with tinnitus, conductive hearing loss, and as it progresses, it leads to vertigo, nystagmus, and facial palsy.
- Jugular foramen pathology symptoms include:
  - 9th and 10th: dysphonia, dysphagia
  - 11th: weak trapezius and sternocleidomastoid muscle
  - 12th: tongue hemiatrophy
- Carotid canal: Horner's syndrome
- Symptoms of the 5th and 6th cranial nerves indicate inoperability.
- Radiation surgery usually leads to a cure or long-term control.
- Carotid dissection may lead to hypoglossal palsy but does not extend to the abducens or trigeminal nerve.
- Cavernous sinus pathology may lead to involvement of the 3rd–5th cranial nerves but does not extend to the hypoglossal nerve.
- Retro-orbital pathology does not go that far either.
- Parsonage-Turner may cause hypoglossal neuropathy but does not affect the rest of the cranial nerves.

DYSARTHRIA

CASE 7.1: CRYING AND LAUGHTER

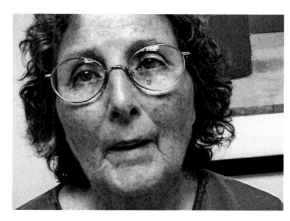

VIDEO 7.1

A 63-year-old woman presented with a 6-month history of speech difficulty and outbursts of laughter and crying that were unprovoked and sometimes socially inappropriate. She developed swallowing difficulty 3 months later. Her examination revealed tongue atrophy and fasciculations and brisk jaw jerk.

The following statements regarding dysarthria in amyotrophic lateral sclerosis (ALS) are true except:

1. It usually precedes dysphagia.
2. It usually follows dysphagia.
3. It is associated with tongue weakness.
4. It is usually of mixed upper motor neuron (UMN) and lower motor neuron (LMN) type.
5. It is associated with a poor prognosis.

DIAGNOSIS

- Dysarthria in ALS occurs in 80% of cases. In only 25% of cases, dysarthria is the first symptom of the disease.
- It is estimated that dysarthria appears after 80% of motor neurons are lost.
- The average time between the onset of dysarthria and the diagnosis of ALS ranges from 33 months before the diagnosis to 60 months after.
- As an initial symptom, dysarthria is eight times more common than dysphagia.
- ALS patients usually have mixed flaccid and spastic dysarthria, but there is no cerebellar element in it; therefore, it is regular.
  - In some cases, flaccid dysarthria predominates (weakness is proportional to atrophy).
  - In other cases, spastic dysarthria is the only presenting symptom, posing a diagnostic challenge. No atrophy or fasciculation of the tongue is noticed, and jaw jerk is brisk. Side-to-side tongue movement is slow.
- Speech in ALS is characterized by being slow and laborious, with imprecise consonant production, hypernasality, emission of air during speech, and hoarseness.
- Other bulbar symptoms like emotional lability and dyspnea coexist.
- Dysarthria eventually progresses to anarthria, imposing serious communication problems and social isolation. Therefore, it is important to adopt new communication strategies before anarthria occurs.
- Tongue weakness is an important cause of dysarthria in ALS patients and it is an independent risk factor for poor survival.
- Speech disturbances in ALS also may be related to concomitant frontotemporal dementia, dysphonia, or breathing problems.

SUGGESTED READING

Tomik B, Guiloff RJ. Dysarthria in amyotrophic lateral sclerosis: a review. *ALS*. 2010;11:4–15.

CASE 7.2: DYSARTHRIA AND FALLS

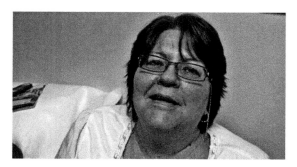

VIDEO 7.2

A 57-year-old woman was referred for a 2-year history of progressive loss of balance, speech difficulty, and hyperreflexia. Magnetic resonance imaging (MRI) of the brain and spinal cord revealed nonspecific white matter lesions in the brainstem and cerebellum. Cerebrospinal fluid (CSF) was positive for oligoclonal bands (OCBs).

Unlike that of ALS, dysarthria of progressive multiple sclerosis (MS) is usually associated with:

1. Jaw hyperreflexia
2. Tongue atrophy
3. Irregular speech rhythm
4. Dyspnea
5. Emotional lability

DIAGNOSIS

- Examination showed scanning speech and dysdiadochokinesia.
- Patients with progressive dysarthria are referred for neuromuscular evaluation due to suspicion of ALS or myasthenia gravis (MG). However, many of them end up having a nonneuromuscular diagnosis such as MS, cerebrovascular disease, movement disorders, or functional etiology. Therefore, a neuromuscular specialist needs to learn about these diseases and the pattern of speech disturbances in them.

Dysarthria in MS is:

- Usually of mixed type: spastic and cerebellar due to vulnerability of the cerebellum and corticobulbar tracts to MS pathology. No LMN signs are expected, such as tongue atrophy or fasciculation.
- Cerebellar elements are suggested by the irregularity of dysarthria and the presence of ataxia, dysmetria, nystagmus, and dysdiadochokinesia.
- It is slowly progressive or relapsing-remitting, depending on the type of MS. In relapsing-remitting MS (RRMS), acute dysarthria and ataxia may be misdiagnosed as a stroke, while in progressive MS, dysarthria may be misdiagnosed as ALS.
- The cerebellar element (if present) facilitates the diagnosis, but difficulty arises when the dysarthria is spastic and progressive. Of course, one will have to find evidence of demyelination in other sites and/or at other times.
- Emotional lability usually exists, and it is different than that of ALS by being more about a decreased crying or laughter threshold than classic, paroxysmal giggling.

SUGGESTED READING

Hartelius L, Runmarker B, Andersen O. Prevalence and characteristics of dysarthria in a multiple-sclerosis incidence cohort: relation to neurological data. *Folia Phoniatr Logop*. 2000 Jul–Aug;52(4):160–177.

CASE 7.3: RELAPSING REMITTING DYSARTHRIA

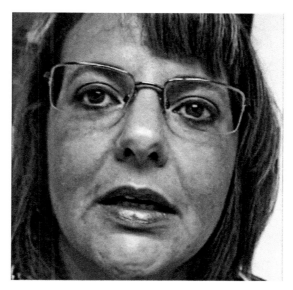

VIDEO 7.3

A 33-year-old woman presented with acute dysarthria and ataxia that responded to steroids. She had multiple white matter lesions in the brainstem and cerebellum and positive OCBs in the CSF. She had multiple relapses in the following few years.

The most likely diagnosis is:

1. ALS
2. MG
3. MS
4. Chronic inflammatory demyelinating polyneuropathy (CIDP)
5. Neuromyelitis optica (NMO)

DIAGNOSIS

- This case illustrates similar findings to Case 7.2, but the symptoms were intermittent.
- Examination demonstrated explosive irregular speech, cerebellar ataxia, impaired heel-to-shin test, dysdiadochokinesia, and hyperreflexia.
- Dysarthria simply means difficulty with articulation.
- Anatomically, it is either flaccid (LMN disorder), spastic (UMN disorder), or cerebellar (irregular).
- In ALS, it is usually of mixed UMN and LMN type. The cerebellar quality should raise a question about the diagnosis of ALS.
- In MS, it is usually of mixed spastic and cerebellar type; any LMN findings should raise a question about the diagnosis.
- Multisystem atrophy also may produce spastic/cerebellar-type dysarthria. The age group tends to be older, and no evidence of demyelination is found on the MRIs.
- Cerebrovascular disease also may produce mixed spastic and cerebellar dysarthria.
- LMN dysarthria may be caused by other forms of motor neuron disease (MND), such as Kennedy disease or postirradiation bulbar palsy. Other clinical features and the time course are important to differentiate.
- MG is the most challenging differential diagnosis, especially MuSK Ab–associated MG, which tends to affect bulbar muscles more than ocular muscles. MuSK MG may cause atrophy of the pharyngeal, lingual, and facial muscles, and there are case reports of tongue fasciculation.
- Repetitive nerve stimulation (RNS) testing is abnormal in 25% of ALS cases, and negative MG serology in seen in 20% of MG cases.
- Mild worsening of symptoms in the evenings is common in ALS.
- Positive single-fiber electromyography (SFEMG) is common in ALS.
- From what has been said, the diagnosis of bulbar ALS or MG may be delayed until other findings appear to make the diagnosis clearer.
- A therapeutic trial of prednisone may help the diagnosis. A negative 6-week trial of prednisone at 1 mg/kg of body weight would strongly argue against MG. Initial worsening of symptoms of MG after initiation of steroids should not be seen as evidence against the diagnosis of MG, as 7%–15% of cases worsen within 2 weeks of initiation. Myasthenic crisis can be induced with steroids, particularly in those with bulbar dysfunction.

CASE 7.4: SPASTIC DYSARTHRIA

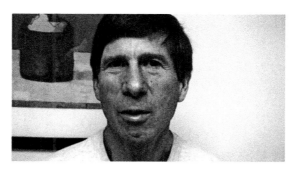

VIDEO 7.4

A 62-year-old man presented with a 1-year history of speech difficulty. His tongue was not atrophied and did not show fasciculation, but it was weak and the jaw jerk was brisk. There was no major dysphagia or diplopia, and there was no weakness of the extremities. Electromyography (EMG) was normal, including the tongue. Brain MRI was normal. Gradually, he became more dysarthric and more spastic in the legs. The acetylcholine receptor (AChR) antibody titer was 0.9 nmol/L.

The most likely diagnosis is:

1. Bulbar MG
2. MuSK MG
3. Bulbar-onset primary lateral sclerosis (PLS)
4. Bulbar-onset ALS
5. Brainstem tumor

DIAGNOSIS

- The examination showed spastic dysarthria and hyperreflexia.
- A variant of ALS in which degeneration is restricted to the UMNs has been recognized for many years and is called PLS.
- It usually affects males around age 50 years, starting in the legs in 87% of cases, which leads to spastic gait.
- Eventually, pseudobulbar symptoms occur in 40% of cases, but rarely are they the presenting features. Asymmetry is noticed in 50% of cases.
- Lower-extremity-onset cases are confused with myelopathies. Neuroimaging excludes compressive etiology, but noncompressive myelopathies can be challenging to sort out. These may include B_{12} and copper deficiency, hereditary spastic paraplegia, MS, and adrenomyeloneuropathy.
- Bulbar-onset PLS remains a diagnosis of exclusion.
- The following tests are usually performed to rule out other causes: MG serology, EMG, brain MRI, CSF examination, hereditary spastic paraplegia mutation analysis, and B_{12} and copper levels.
- A weakly positive AChR antibody titer is reported in ALS and should not lead to erroneous diagnosis of MG and subsequent unnecessary immunosupression. MG does not cause spastic dysarthria.
- The course of PLS is progressive, and in some cases, it becomes full-blown ALS.

CASE 7.5: DYSARTHRIA LONG AFTER RADIOTHERAPY

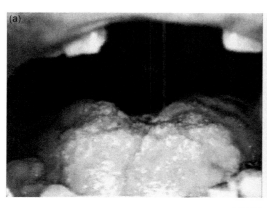

VIDEO 7.5

A 76-year-old man presented with a 2-year history of slurring of speech and swallowing difficulty. His past medical history was remarkable for cancer of the tonsils treated with radiation 20 years earlier. Examination and EMG of the tongue are shown in Videos 7.5A and 7.5B, respectively. He worsened for a year and needed a percutaneous endoscopic gastrostomy (PEG) tube placement, and then he stabilized. This video was taken 10 years later.

The demonstrated EMG discharges are:

1. Fasciculation
2. Complex repetitive discharges
3. Myokymia
4. Myotonic discharges
5. Voluntary activity

The following is correct regarding postirradiation bulbar palsy:

1. It may occur years after exposure to radiation.
2. It follows the same course as ALS.
3. Myokymia is a typical EMG feature.
4. It does not occur with low-dose irradiation.
5. Usually, it resolves spontaneously.

DIAGNOSIS

- Video 7.5A and 7.5B show myokymia of the tongue and restriction of movement of the soft palate.
- It occurs in 10% of patients treated with radiation directed to the neck region. It can happen even with exposure to a small dose of radiation.
- Bulbar palsy is often accompanied by cervical amyotrophy, hypoglossal nerve palsy, and Horner's syndrome.
- Average time of onset after exposure is 5.5 years.
- Symptoms may progress for years before they reach a plateau. Spontaneous resolution does not occur.
- The subacute onset and subsequent stuttering of symptoms support vascular etiology rather than a direct neuronal toxicity.
- A similar picture of MND may evolve in the lumbar region after irradiation of the pelvic area.
- Chronic denervation in the affected areas (and sometimes beyond) is reported. More specifically, myokymia is seen in the vast majority of cases.

SUGGESTED READING

Chew NK, Sim BF, Tan CT, Goh KJ, Ramli N, Umapathi P. Delayed post-irradiation bulbar palsy in nasopharyngeal carcinoma. *Neurol.* 2001; 57(3):529–531.

CASE 7.6: FAMILIAL DYSARTHRIA, SENSORY ATAXIA, AND ELEVATED CREATINE KINASE (CK)

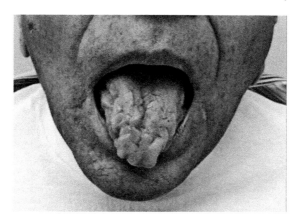

VIDEO 7.6

An 80-year-old man presented with a 10-year history of slurring of speech, weakness and atrophy of the legs and arms, and loss of balance. Examination revealed sensory ataxia, impaired foot sensation to vibration, diffuse areflexia, fasciculation of the face and chest muscles, and weakness of the tongue and face. Speech was nasal. EMG revealed widespread chronic denervation of the legs, arms, and tongue. Creatine phosphokinase (CPK) level was 1,500 U/L. He had a brother with similar symptoms.

Which of the following is the most likely diagnosis?

1. Chronic myopathy
2. Axonal neuropathy
3. Kennedy disease
4. Acid maltase deficiency
5. ALS

DIAGNOSIS

- Video 7.6 showed gynecomastia and nasal speech. Due to the presence of chronic diffuse denervation, bulbar symptoms, and gynecomastia, mutation analysis for androgen receptor (AR) mutation was obtained, and it was positive.
- Kennedy disease is an X-linked recessive disease caused by mutation of the *AR* gene on Xq12.
  - The mutation is in the form of CAG repeat expansion.
  - Most affected people have a repeat number of 40–65 (normal range is 10–36).
  - Cytosine-thymine-guanine (CTG) repeats produce a polyglutamate tail, which leads to abnormal folding of the ARs, resulting in partial proteolysis. Androgen plays a role in cell survival and dendritic growth.
  - Autosomal-dominant (AD) bulbospinal atrophy with gynecomastia is also reported.
- Pathologically, the disease is characterized by degeneration of the motor and sensory neurons. Extraocular muscles are spared.
- Age of onset: 15–60 years.
- Heterozygous females may display tongue fasciculations and muscle cramps in the seventh decade.
- Muscle cramps, fatigue, and leg weakness are common early symptoms.
- Full-blown picture of the disease is characterized by:
  - Proximal weakness, atrophy, and fasciculations
  - Tongue weakness and fasciculations
  - Facial myokymia
  - Dysphagia, dysarthria
  - Diffuse areflexia
  - Reduced sensation in the feet and hands and small sensory nerve action potentials (SNAPs)
  - Action tremor
  - Gynecomastia, testicular atrophy, erectile dysfunction
  - Diabetes mellitus (DM)
- Needle electromyography: chronic diffuse denervation expressed as giant motor unit potentials with fast firing rates.
- Mildly elevated creatine kinase (CK).
- It affects 2:100,000 of the population.
- Every male with muscle cramps, high CK, and neurogenic EMG should be tested for Kennedy disease, especially if there is gynecomastia or bulbar weakness.
- In chronic motor neuron disorders, the presence of high CK and low SNAPs should raise the possibility of Kennedy disease.

CASE 7.7: CEREBELLAR ATAXIA AND TONGUE FASCICULATION

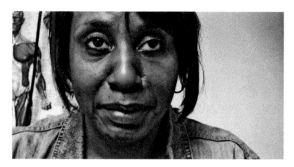

VIDEO 7.7

A 43-year-old woman presented with a 10-year history of twitching of the facial muscles and loss of balance. Brain MRI revealed mild cerebellar atrophy. EMG confirmed fasciculation of the face and tongue, but there was no widespread denervation.

The most likely diagnosis is:

1. Spinocerebellar ataxia (SCA) type 3
2. Kennedy disease
3. SCA-2
4. Familial ALS
5. Friedreich's ataxia

DIAGNOSIS

- Video 7.7 demonstrated dysarthria, dysmetria, dysdiadochokinesia, nystagmus, hyperreflexia, and fasciculation of the tongue and lower facial muscles.
- Patients with spinocerebellar ataxias are sometimes referred to neuromuscular clinics due to gait imbalance, slurring of speech, and associated neuropathy. In this case, the referral was based on facial twitching and ataxia.
- Cerebellar involvement is not a feature of ALS or Kennedy disease. Friedreich's ataxia does not cause fasciculations and hyperreflexia.
- Hereditary ataxias comprise a large group of genetic spinocerebellar degenerations; the pathology of most of them extends beyond the cerebellum.
- Neuromuscular components may include neuropathy, optic atrophy, myopathy, and MND.
- While fasciculations are not unique to a type of SCA, SCA-3, also known as *Machado-Joseph disease (MCD),* is the best-known entity associated with fasciculation.
- MCD is characterized by:
  - Progressive cerebellar ataxia, extrapyramidal rigidity, and peripheral neuropathy.
  - It is an AD disease caused by an unstable CAG repeat expansion on chromosome 14.
  - Mean age of onset is 37 years, but the age of onset and severity correlate with the degree of triplet repeat expansion.
  - The disease displays the phenomenon of anticipation: earlier and more severe in successive generations due to repeat expansion.
  - Some patients develop vocal cord paralysis and dysautonomia.
  - Later in the disease, axonal (mostly sensory) neuropathy appears, accelerating disability.
  - Patients with shorter repeat length may present at a later age with neuropathy and ataxia. This group comprises 30% of patients and is more likely to be seen by a neuromuscular specialist.
  - Progression of neuropathy seems to correlate with the CAG expansion as well.

SUGGESTED READING

França M Jr, D'abreu A, Nucci A, Cendes F, Lopes-Cendes I. Prospective study of peripheral neuropathy in Machado-Joseph disease. *Muscl Nerve.* 2009;40(6):1012–1018.

CASE 7.8: A LISP DURING DIVORCE

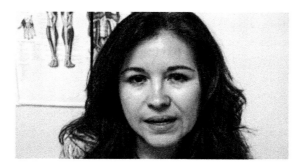

VIDEO 7.8

A 39-year-old woman presented with intermittent speech difficulty that began 7 months earlier. She was going through a divorce. She had no dysphagia. She had normal strength, including in the tongue, and sensation, but her deep tendon reflexes (DTRs) were brisk. Myasthenia serology, RNS testing, and single-fiber EMG were negative.

The following feature would argue the most against MG:

1. Poor response to steroids
2. Concurrent stress
3. Intermittent nature of the symptoms
4. The absence of diplopia
5. Improvement after resolution of stress

DIAGNOSIS

- Weakness of the tongue is a feature of:
  - ◆ Bulbar and pseudobulbar palsy: ALS, Kennedy disease, and other MNDs. The weakness is associated with atrophy and fasciculation except in PLS cases.
  - ◆ NMJ disorders like MG. Atrophy is not a feature except in MuSK MG. Fluctuation of symptoms is typical.
  - ◆ Hypoglossal palsy: brainstem pathology, hypoglossal neuropathy such as neuritis or carotid dissection, and so on. This is usually unilateral and is associated with atrophy.
- Dysarthria is a product of interference with articulation mechanism, and it could be:
  - ◆ Labial
  - ◆ Lingual
  - ◆ Palatal
  - ◆ Facial: Bell's palsy
- Lingual dysarthria is characterized by difficulty pronouncing lingual sounds like *T, L,* and *D.*
- In ALS, tongue weakness is almost always present by the time that dysarthria appears. It is important to examine tongue strength by asking the patient to push the tongue against the cheek and the examiner's finger from outside.
- In MG, the weakness is intermittent and gets worse with repetition. Tongue weakness may not be detected by examination.
- Labial dysarthria usually accompanies lingual dysarthria in MG.
- What makes the diagnosis more difficult is that myasthenia serology and RNS testing is negative in 40% of bulbar MG cases.
- Functional weakness is difficult to exclude, and many cases of MG are considered to be hysterical initially. Precipitation and relief of symptoms in relation to stress are not uncommon in MG.
- Negative response to steroids is seen in only 10% of MG cases and therefore argues the most against the diagnosis of MG.
- Negative SFEMG of a weak muscle argues strongly against MG.
- The speech of this woman returned to normal a few months after her divorce and new marriage.

CASE 7.9: NASAL SPEECH AND HYPERCKEMIA

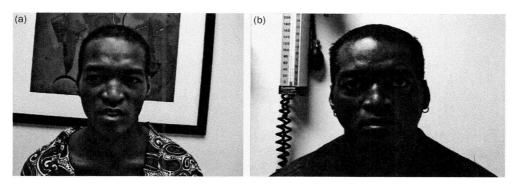

VIDEO 7.9

A 36-year-old man presented with a 4-week history of progressive nasal speech, dysphagia, and proximal and distal weakness of the extremities. He lost 30 pounds. EMG showed the demonstrated activity in the arms, legs, and thoracic paraspinal muscles. Nerve conduction study (NCS) was normal. The CPK level was 2,210 U/L. The erythrocyte sedimentation rate (ESR) was 74 mm/hour. He did not respond to 60 mg/day of prednisone given for 6 weeks. Muscle pathology is shown in Figure 7.9.1. There was also severe endomysial inflammation consisting mainly of CD4 cells.

These pathological findings are typically seen in:

1. Dermatomyositis
2. ALS
3. Spinal muscular atrophy (SMA)
4. Polymyositis
5. Inclusion body myositis (IBM)

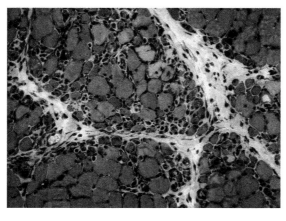

FIGURE 7.9.1 H &E stain, 100x.

DIAGNOSIS

- The pathology picture shows perifascicular atrophy (atrophy of multiple layers on the margin of the fascicles due to ischemia).
- The typical presentation of dermatomyositis is that of subacute, symmetrical, proximal weakness, periorbital swelling, violaceous rash on the knuckles, Gottron's sign, elevated CK, and irritative myopathy in EMG and the normal sensory system. Reflexes are usually normal.
- The typical ALS presentation is that of progressive dysarthria, dysphagia, distal more than proximal weakness and atrophy, hyperreflexia, and a normal sensory system. CK may be mildly elevated, and EMG shows widespread denervation.
- In this case, an alternative diagnosis to ALS was sought due to the following factors:
  - There is a lack of atrophy despite severe weakness.
  - Weight loss in ALS occurs late and is proportional to dysphagia and low dietary intake.
  - Dysphonia and nasal speech are not common in ALS. Instead, dysarthria is typically seen, and it precedes dysphagia.
  - Elevated CK: While hyperCKemia is common in denervated conditions like ALS, the CK level is usually below 1,000 U/L.
  - Elevated ESR (although not specific), along with weight loss, suggested systemic inflammation.
  - Bilateral foot drop occurred, with preservation of the bulk of extensor digitorum brevis (EDB). In ALS, EDB mass is lost due to neurogenic atrophy.
  - Due to these factors, a muscle biopsy was done, which revealed:
    - Endomysial and perivascular mononuclear inflammatory cell infiltration
    - Predominance of CD4 in the inflammatory infiltrate
    - Perifascicular atrophy, as shown in Figure 7.9.1
    - Positive mycobacteria avium complex (MAC) antibody reaction
- Nasal speech is not common in dermatomyositis, and we speculate that inflammation and weakness of the palatine muscles are responsible for this finding.
- Skin rash is not required for the diagnosis of dermatomyositis. Pathological findings are specific and can differentiate it from other inflammatory muscle diseases.
- The patient returned to normal strength after treatment with intravenous (IV) cyclophosphamide (Video 7.9B).

CASE 7.10: THYMECTOMY OR NOT?

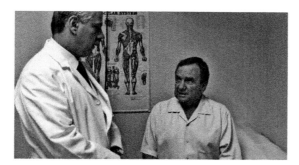

VIDEO 7.10

A 69-year-old man presented with a 2-month history of speech difficulty. The AChR antibody titer was 23 nmol/l. He had a history of a large ascending aortic aneurysm, coronary artery disease, and prostate cancer.

True or false? Thymectomy in this case is advisable.

DIAGNOSIS

- The examination shown in Video 7.10 revealed labial and lingual dysarthria with a nasal component, facial weakness, and fatigability of the proximal leg muscles.
- Thymectomy is indicated for thymoma, which occurs in 5%–15% of myasthenics.
- For nonthymomatous myasthenics, thymectomy is generally advised for all patients with generalized MG of age 18–65 years. In our practice, we advise it for patients up to 70 years old if they are healthy otherwise. This patient has many comorbid conditions beside his borderline age limit; therefore, we did not advise it.
- There is no role for emergency thymectomy since its impact will not appear before a year.
- The thymus gland plays an important role in the pathogenesis of MG mostly due to the presence of myoid cells in the thymus that have molecular similarities with the nicotinic, postsynaptic AChRs.
- Retrospective studies have shown an increased long-term remission rate of MG after thymectomy compared to nonthymectomized patients.
- The practice of thymectomy has been performed for more than 70 years since Blalock published a series of poorly controlled nonthymomatous myasthenics who improved dramatically after thymectomy.
- Thymic hyperplasia is seen in the majority of these patients pathologically.
- In the elderly, the thymus is reduced to a small tag that is difficult to identify, and it is not pathologically active anyway. Therefore, thymectomy is not indicated.
- Transternal thymectomy is more likely to remove any ectopic thymic tissue. It is preferred in patients with thymoma. Transcervical thymectomy has become popular and may be as effective.
- Interestingly, MuSK antibody–associated MG may not be as responsive to thymectomy, and therefore surgery is not indicated.
- A recent randomized trial of thymectomy in nonthymomatous MG confirmed improved outcomes over a 3-year period.

SUGGESTED READINGS

Gil GI, Kaminski HJ, Aban IB, et al. Randomized trial of thymectomy in myasthenia gravis. *NEJM*. 375(6):511–522.

Blalock A. Thymectomy in the treatment of myasthenia gravis, report of 20 cases. *Thoracic Surg*. 1944;13:316–339.

CASE 7.11: MORBIDITY IN ALS: CAN IT BE IMPROVED?

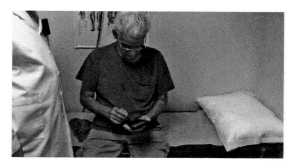

VIDEO 7.11

A 70-year-old man presented with a 6-month history of progressive speech difficulty, cough, orthopnea, weight loss, and excessive salivation. Examination revealed (in addition to what is shown in Video 7.11) atrophy and fasciculation of the tongue, diffuse hyperreflexia, and normal cognition and strength of the extremities. Myasthenia serology was negative. Sensory and motor NCSs were normal. Needle examination of the extremities and thoracic paraspinal muscles was normal, but the tongue was denervated. The CPK level was 450 U/L. Brain MRI was normal.

Which of the following can improve quality of life in bulbar ALS?

1. A PEG tube
2. Biphasic positive airway pressure (BIPAP)
3. Botulinum toxin (BT) for refractory hypersialosis
4. An electronic communication system
5. All of the above

DIAGNOSIS

- Bulbar involvement is a bad prognostic sign in ALS. Serial assessment of bulbar function is recommended in these patients.
- There are certain measures that are shown to reduce morbidity and improve lifestyle in ALS patients with bulbar dysfunction.
  - Dysphagia: Early PEG placement is important to prevent more loss of muscle mass, which may worsen respiratory insufficiency due to its effect on the respiratory muscles. Cough, voice change, and weight loss are early signs of aspiration. Recurrent pneumonia is a late sign. Modified barium swallowing may cause aspiration. The isosmolar contrast agent iotrolan, which has no significant adverse effects even in the case of aspiration, is recommended.
  - Dyspnea: Early institution of BIPAP helps sleep apnea and improves sleep and, secondarily, reduces daytime fatigue and lack of concentration.
  - Dysarthria: Early institution of a communication system is important to reduce incidence of depression and poor healthcare delivery due to lack of communication. Electronic communication devices with a keyboard or a scanner to detect head or eye movements and with a voice output enable patients to use telephones and computers in a very effective way. Patients can be sent for recording of their voice patterns before they develop severe dysarthria so that the communicative device can be programmed with their own voice instead of a robotic sound.
  - Sialorrhea: Anticholinergic drugs, like nortriptyline at 25–75 mg at bedtime or glycopyrrolate at 1–2 mg daily, are usually effective. Refractory cases may benefit from BT injection to the salivary glands. Surprisingly, worsening of dysphagia is not encountered as much as expected.
  - Emotional lability: This is due to involvement of the suprabulbar pathways and may not be associated with depression. Tricyclic antidepressant drugs like nortriptyline usually help. Nuedexta (dextromethorphan/quinidine) is also shown to be effective.

SUGGESTED READING

Kühnlein P, Gdynia HJ, Sperfeld AD, Lindner-Pfleghar B, Ludolph AC, Prosiegel M, Riecker A. Diagnosis and treatment of bulbar symptoms in amyotrophic lateral sclerosis. *Nature Clin Prac Neurol.* 2008;4:366–374.

CASE 7.12A: SELF-MEDICATED MYASTHENIC

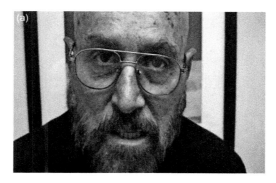

VIDEO 7.12A

A 56-year-old man presented with nasal speech and diplopia. The AChR antibody titer was 24 nmol/L. He responded well to prednisone, but after 3 months, he discontinued it and started taking short courses of the drug only when his symptoms exacerbated.

Poor treatment compliance (PTC) in MG is probably:

1. More common than in CIDP.
2. More common in young female patients.
3. Contributory to poor outcomes.
4. PRN Steroid administration by patients is as effective as chronic steroid administration by a neurologist.
5. Overall side effects of PRN steroids in MG are less than chronic use.

DIAGNOSIS

- PTC in MG accounts for 23% of unsatisfactory outcome rates, which are estimated to be 20%.
- The phenomenon of PTC in MG has not been studied systematically in terms of its characteristics, impact, and solutions; therefore, the following discussion is based on our experience.
- The most common causes and risk factors of PTC in MG are:
  - Side effects of steroids that can be disabling and disfiguring, particularly weight gain.
  - PTC is more common in females, especially young females.
  - The fluctuating nature of the disease enforces the feeling by some patients that they do not need to be treated continuously.
  - The good response of the symptoms to treatment, with reversal to normal function, tempts some patients to change the dosage or to quit medications on their own.
- PTC may take the following forms:
  - Discontinuation of medications altogether.
  - Lowering the dose of prednisone and increasing it when symptoms come back, trying to find the minimal effective dose. Unfortunately, when relapse occurs, the dose of prednisone frequently will have to be increased to the highest level again and then be tapered. A small increment does not usually induce remission.
- Some patients disappear for some time before they appear again with a relapse. Recurrence may not happen immediately after the medications are discontinued, which reinforces the notion that discontinuation of the medications is not the cause of the relapse.
- Some patients do not inform their physicians that they have changed the dosage on their own, and they pretend that they do not know why the symptoms came back.
- Compliance is usually improved after one or two relapses, which make patients more serious about taking the medications.
- PTC is more common in MG than in chronic diseases that do not usually respond completely to treatment, such as CIDP. The residual symptoms act as a reminder that treatment must continue.
- The need for frequent PRN courses of steroids usually leads to severe chronic side effects, compared to an initially high dose followed by tapering to a low maintenance dose.
- It is possible that PRN use of steroids makes the disease less responsive to high-dose steroids when needed for exacerbations.
- Confidence of patients in their physicians may improve compliance.

SUGGESTED READING

Dunand MB, Botez SA, Borruat FX, Roux-Lombard P, Spertini F, Kuntzer T. Unsatisfactory outcomes in myasthenia gravis: influence by care providers. *J Neurol.* 2010;257(3):338–343.

CASE 7.12B: THE PATIENT IN CASE 7.12A AFTER TREATMENT

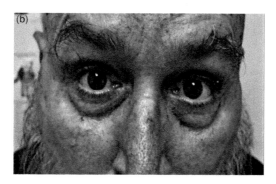

VIDEO 7.12B

The symptoms for the patient in Case 7.12A were reversed after 2 months of steroid therapy. The next step in management is to:

1. Start azathioprine
2. Taper prednisone
3. Start mycophenolate
4. Discuss thymectomy
5. Discontinue pyridostigmine

DIAGNOSIS

- There are different methods of management of MG. The most common way is to start reducing the dose of prednisone after 6 weeks of initiation. The tapering schedule varies greatly, even among experts. The key is to taper over a few months to the lowest effective and safe maintenance dose, which is usually 10–20 mg of prednisone every other day.
- If symptoms return before that dose could be reached, a steroid-sparing agent is added to achieve that goal. Most of the steroid-sparing agents take months to work. Azathioprine may take up to 6 months. Mycophenolate fell out of favor after two clinical trials showed no significant impact compared to a placebo. A recent methotrexate double-blind trial showed negative results.
- Pyridostigmine may still be used during the remission phase, but preferably on a PRN basis.
- Thymectomy pros and cons are to be discussed with the patient after the disease is brought into remission. There is no role for emergency thymectomy in a nonthymomatous patient.

CASE 7.13: TONGUE FASCICULATION
AND POSITIVE MG SEROLOGY

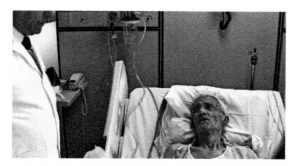

VIDEO 7.13

A 75-year-old man presented with a 6-month history of speech difficulty, dysphagia, and fatigue that was more pronounced in the evenings. There was no diplopia or ptosis. He developed progressive dyspnea and lost 10 pounds over 6 months. RNS of the left spinal accessory nerve revealed 15% decremental response. A binding AChR antibody titer was increased to 0.5 nml/L. He was diagnosed with MG and was transferred to our hospital for plasmaphoresis. Examination is shown in the video. He also had hyperreflexia and mild proximal weakness in the arms.

Mild elevation of AChR Ab in this case:

1. Excluded the diagnosis of ALS
2. Indicated coincidental MG and ALS
3. Was an artifact
4. Along with positive RNS, excluded ALS
5. Is reported in ALS

DIAGNOSIS

- EMG was done in the hospital and revealed denervation of the tongue and upper extremity muscles and thoracic paraspinal muscles.
- The AChR antibody titer is about 90% specific for MG. False positive mild elevation is reported in patients with
  - ◆ Thymoma without MG
  - ◆ Family history of MG
  - ◆ Exposure to snake toxin
  - ◆ ALS
- The patient in this case met the diagnostic criteria of ALS, and the course of the disease was as expected for ALS. The presence of AChR antibodies did not change the prognosis.
- These antibodies suggest NMJ involvement in ALS. Decremental response occurs in 15% of ALS patients due to dysfunction of presynaptic calcium channels.
- Although the antibody titer is usually below 0.5, a titer as high as 50 nmol/L nm is reported in ALS.

SUGGESTED READINGS

Mittag T, Caroscio J. False positive immunoassay for acetylcholine receptor antibody in ALS. *NEJM*. 1980;302:868.

Okuyama Y, Mizuno T, Inoue H, Kimoto K. Amyotrophic lateral sclerosis with anti-acetylcholine receptor antibody. *Intern Med*. 1997;36(4):312–315.

CHAPTER 8

DYSPHONIA

CASE 8.1: FLUCTUATING NASAL SPEECH

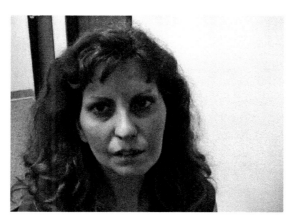

VIDEO 8.1

A 24-year-old woman presented with a 9-month history of gradually increasing and fluctuating nasal speech and regurgitation of water through her nose. Her soft palate was restricted, and tongue and facial muscles were weak. Repetitive nerve stimulation (RNS) testing, Tensilon testing, acetylcholine receptor (AChR) antibody titer, and computed tomography (CT) scan of the chest were noncontributory.

The most specific and appropriate next test is:

1. MuSK antibody titer
2. Single-fiber electromyogram (EMG)
3. Repeat CT of the chest
4. Repeat RNS test
5. None of the above

DIAGNOSIS

- The MuSK antibody test was positive.
- This form of autoimmune MG accounts for 40%–70% of AChR-Ab negative MG (AChR-Ab MG).
- Only rarely do AChR-Ab MG and MuSK-MG coexist.
- MuSK enhances aggregation of acetylcholine (ACh) in the microtubules.
- Mostly present at age 30–50 years.
- A total of 80% of patients are female.
- Onset is usually subacute.
- Dysarthria and dysphonia are universal.
- Dropped head syndrome due to weak neck extensors is common.
- Atrophy of the pharyngeal muscles and tongue is common in chronic cases, leading to diagnostic confusion with amyotrophic lateral sclerosis (ALS). Even tongue fasciculation was reported.
- Respiratory failure is common, and myasthenic crisis is more frequent than AChR Ab MG.
- It rarely starts with extraocular muscle weakness.
- Positive RNS and thymic hyperplasia are uncommon.
- A positive Tensilon test is less likely than with AChR Ab MG.
- Unlike AChR Ab MG, severity of MuSK Ab MG correlates with MuSK-Ab titer.
- Thymectomy may not be effective and is not routinely indicated.
- It is less responsive to pyridostigmine, steroids, and intravenous immunoglobulin (IVIG) and is more responsive to plasmapheresis and rituximab.
- In our experience, rituximab may induce long-term remission in refractory cases.

CASE 8.2: FAMILIAL HOARSENESS AND FOOT DROP

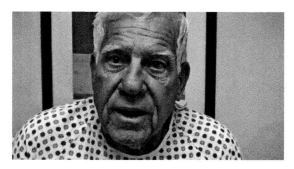

VIDEO 8.2

A 78-year-old man presented with a 7-year history of slowly progressive hoarseness and painless, bilateral foot drop. He had mild proximal leg weakness. There was no dysphagia or ptosis. The creatine kinase (CK) level was 400 U/L, and EMG showed 30% short-duration units in the proximal and distal leg muscles. His twin brother developed similar signs. Muscle biopsy revealed nonspecific myopathic features, with several red-rimmed vacuoles.

The most likely diagnosis is:

1. Oculopharyngeal muscular dystrophy (OPMD)
2. Myotilinopathy
3. Dysferlinopathy
4. Calpainopathy
5. Cavuolinopathy

DIAGNOSIS

- LGMD 1A is an autosomal-dominant (AD) limb girdle muscular dystrophy caused by mutation of myotilin on chromosome 5.
- Myotilin is a sarcolemma protein that is important for the integrity of cell membrane function.
- A total of 50% of cases have no family history.
- Onset is usually at age 40–70 years.
- Weakness, myalgia, and hoarseness are common.
- Wrist flexion weakness and ankle extensor weakness occur with disease progression.
- Dropped head syndrome occurs in some patients, as does facial weakness.
- Dysarthria, dysphonia, and nasal speech occur in 30% of cases.
- Cardiomyopathy occurs in 50% of cases.
- Progression is slow.
- CK is commonly two times higher than normal.
- EMG usually shows irritative myopathy.
- Muscle biopsy usually shows rimmed and autophagic vacuoles.
- Distal weakness with dysphonia is also seen in Charcot-Marie-Tooth (CMT) disease types 2C, 2K, and 4A. EMG and nerve conduction study (NCS) are usually enough to distinguish neuropathic from myopathic syndromes.
- If clinically suspected, mutation analysis of the suspected genes is recommended, and if negative, muscle biopsy would be indicated to look for diagnostic clues. If myotilin histoimmunochemistry or genes are normal, one will have to look for a similar disorder, called *distal myopathy with vocal cord and pharyngeal weakness (MPD2)*.
  - MPD2 is an AD disease that is reported in North America and Bulgaria and is caused by mutation of a nuclear gene called *Martin 3 (MATR 3)* on chromosome 5q31.2.
  - Average age of onset is 46 years, and weakness starts in the distal anterior leg muscle (foot drop) and sometimes spreads to the arms.
  - The voice is affected in 65% of cases and usually occurs after limb weakness.
  - Dysphagia is common.
  - Serum CK: normal to eight times normal.
  - EMG: Chronic myopathic changes.
  - Muscle pathology: nonspecific chronic myopathic changes, rare rimmed vacuoles.
  - *MATR 3:* variable staining of myonuclei.

CASE 8.3: CHRONIC NASAL SPEECH

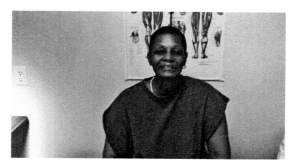

VIDEO 8.3

A 46-year-old woman presented with a 10-year history of speech and swallowing difficulty. Her neck extensors were 4/5, and extraocular movements (EOMs) were full. There was mild tongue weakness. There was no ptosis. Symptoms consistently became worse in the evenings and when she was tired. There were times when her symptoms became very mild. The AChR antibody titer was negative. EMG revealed no proximal myopathic abnormalities. RNS testing and CT scan of the chest were normal. Brain magnetic resonance imaging (MRI) was normal. She did not respond to pyridostigmine.

The most reasonable next step is to test for:

1. MuSK antibody–associated MG
2. Diphtheria
3. Kennedy disease
4. Hypoglossal palsy
5. Brainstem glioma

DIAGNOSIS

- MuSK MG is more common in females and mostly affects the pharyngeal muscles.
- It can go undetected for years due to negative AChR antibodies and the lack of ocular symptoms.
- Atrophy of pharyngeal muscles and even tongue fasciculation are reported, leading to misdiagnosis as ALS.
- Response to pyridostigmine, prednisone, and thymectomy is not as good as in AChR Ab–associated MG.
- Plasmaphoresis and rituximab are reported to be effective when other measures fail.
- Rare cases of ocular MG are reported in association with MuSK antibodies.
- Double-positive serology is also reported.

CASE 8.4: VOCAL CORD PARALYSIS
AND DISTAL WEAKNESS

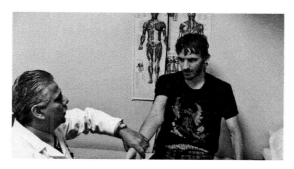

VIDEO 8.4

A 31-year-old man presented with hand and foot numbness since he was 8 years old. Gradually, he developed ataxia, as well as distal arm and leg weakness and loss of reflexes. He also developed hoarseness. Cerebrospinal fluid (CSF) protein was 50 mg/dl with normal cells. NCS revealed the following: peroneal and tibial motor conduction velocities of 34–35 milliseconds and compound muscle action potential (CMAP) amplitudes of 1 millivolt, with distal motor latencies of 8–9 milliseconds and prolonged F responses. Sural responses were absent, and he had bilateral focal ulnar slowing at the elbows. EMG was normal. Ear, nose, and throat (ENT) evaluation revealed vocal cord paralysis. He was treated with IVIG for 8 months with no improvement. His mother had similar symptoms. He had high foot arches. Testing for CMT type 1A was negative.

These associations are typically seen in:

1. Chronic inflammatory demyelinating polyneuropathy (CIDP)
2. CMT 2D
3. CMT 4B
4. CMT 4A
5. CMT 4E

DIAGNOSIS

- A combination of vocal cord paralysis and distal weakness is seen in LGMD 1A (myotilin-opathy) and in CMT 2C, 2K, and 4A.
- CMT 2C: AD axonal neuropathy due to mutation of the *TRPV4* gene on chromosome 12.
- CMT2K is due to GDAP1 protein mutation on chromosome 8 q21.11 and has several phenotypes:
  - Axonal, recessive
  - Axonal, dominant
  - Recessive, intermediate A (CMT RIA)
    - It presents in early childhood with gait imbalance and causes distal loss and proximal and distal weakness. NCS shows mixed demyelinating and axonal features. Nerve pathology shows mixed axonal and demyelinating features.
- CMT 4A: GDAP1 mutation, the same gene as CMT 2K
  - Usually starts before 2 years of age.
  - Progressive, distal weakness, vocal cord paralysis, and absent reflexes.
  - Motor conduction slowing and low CMAP amplitudes.
  - Pathology is mostly demyelinating.
- Ganglioside-induced, differentiation-associated protein 1 in humans is encoded by the *GDAP1* gene.
  - This gene encodes a member of the ganglioside-induced, differentiation-associated protein family, which may play a role in a signal transduction pathway during neuronal development. Mutations in this gene have been associated with various forms of CMT disease.

CASE 8.5: ACUTE HOARSENESS
AND SEVERE ARM PAIN

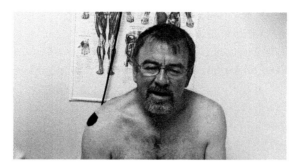

VIDEO 8.5.1

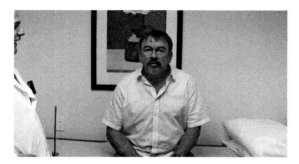

VIDEO 8.5.2

A 56-year-old man with acute vocal cord paralysis, severe right periscapular pain, and proximal right arm weakness, atrophy, and areflexia.

This is most likely a case of:

1. Hereditary neuralgic amyotrophy (HNA)
2. Parsonage-Turner syndrome (PTS)
3. Pancoast tumor
4. Cervical radiculopathy
5. ALS

DIAGNOSIS

- Sudden severe neuropathic pain, followed by muscle weakness and wasting, are typical features of idiopathic neuralgic amyotrophy (INA) (PTS).
- Predisposing factors include infection, exercise, surgery, vaccination, stress, and trauma.
- In 19.4% of patients, nerves outside the brachial plexus are affected; 8.2% for the lumbosacral plexus; 6.6% for the phrenic nerve; 2% for the recurrent laryngeal nerve; and 2.6% for other nerves.
- A total of 70% of cases are unilateral.
- Painless PTS occurs in 3.7% of cases.
- 71.5% of cases involve only one arm, and in 28.5% both arms, typically in an asymmetric fashion (97.1%).
- Surprisingly, recurrences were seen in 26.1% of the INA patients (19.1% two attacks, 4.5% three, 4% four, and 1% five or more attacks). The median time to recurrence was slightly more than 2 years.
- There is no evidence that steroids will affect the natural history of the disease, but if administered early, they may reduce pain and improve tolerance of physical therapy.
- Recovery may take a year or more (Video 8.5.2 shows findings after a year).

SUGGESTED READING

van Alfen N, van Engelen BG. The clinical spectrum of neuralgic amyotrophy in 246 cases. *Brain* 2006;129(2):438–450.

CASE 8.6: DYSARTHRIA AND INCOORDINATION

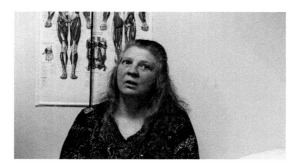

VIDEO 8.6

A 54-year-old woman presented with slurring of speech and loss of balance that she has suffered with since she was 30 years old. She denied weakness, sensory symptoms, memory problems, or visual symptoms. She had a sister with similar symptoms. Brain MRI revealed atrophy of cerebellar hemispheres and nonspecific white matter changes. Genetic testing for hereditary ataxias was negative. She was diagnosed with cerebellar ataxia of unknown type. The patient had three children in their 20s, none of which were symptomatic. Examination is shown in the video.

This picture is consistent with:

1. Paraneoplastic cerebellar degeneration
2. Hereditary spastic paraplegia (HSP)
3. Telangiectasia ataxia syndrome
4. Chronic progressive multiple sclerosis (CPMS)
5. Primary lateral sclerosis (PLS)

Genetic testing revealed homozygous pathogenic mutation of the *SPG7* gene.

DIAGNOSIS

Spastic paraplegia 7 features the following:

- Progressive leg spasticity with mild vibratory impairment in the feet and cerebellar features like nystagmus and dysarthria.
- Onset is usually in adulthood.
- Duration is not consistent with paraneoplastic cerebellar degeneration or PLS.
- The lack of typical white matter changes argues against CPMS.
- The age and lack of skin lesions argue against AT.
- *SPG7* mutation makes 1.5%–6% of the SPG family.
- This is an AR disease. Carriers are asymptomatic. Each sibling of an affected person has a 25% chance of being affected and a 50% chance of being a carrier.

SUGGESTED READING

Casari G, Marconi R. Spastic paraplegia 7. *Gene Rev*. 2010; December 23.

CASE 8.7: DYSARTHRIA AND SPASTICITY

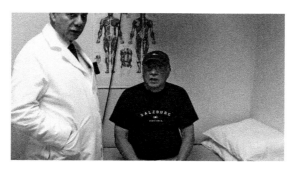

VIDEO 8.7

A 76-year-old man was referred to our center for slurring of speech suspicious of ALS. His examination is shown in the video.

The dysarthria is most likely caused by:

1. ALS
2. Cerebellar dysfunction
3. Progressive bulbar palsy
4. Psychogenic
5. Stroke

DIAGNOSIS

- A 1-year history of progressive slurring of speech. Examination revealed scanning speech, impaired rapid alternating movements of the fingers and hands, and cerebellar ataxia.
- He had normal bulk and strength of the tongue and no atrophy or fasciculations, but mild spasticity and jaw hyperreflexia.
- These features suggested a cerebellar syndrome with possible pyramidal dysfunction.
  - He had surgical removal of a benign tumor from the posterior fossa in his 50s and. A recent MRI of the brain revealed normal right cerebellar hemisphere and no vermis.
  - Patient had no risk factors to suggest ischemic insults to the cerebellum, and brain MRI did not show evidence of ischemic insults.
  - He had no history of smoking to suggest paraneoplastic cerebellar degeneration, and the history is too long for this condition.
  - There was no family history to suggest hereditary spinocerebellar ataxia (SCA).
  - Genetic testing for hereditary spinocerebellar degeneration was negative.
  - To look for an underlying genetic basis for this chronic cerebellar syndrome, whole exome sequencing was ordered and revealed pathogenic heterozygous mutations of the SPG and GBA genes.
    - The GBA gene encodes the lysosomal beta glugocerebrosidase, whose blood level was found to be abnormally low, but not low enough to be consistent with Gaucher disease.
- Autosomal-recessive cerebellar ataxia (ARCA) comprises a large and heterogeneous group of neurodegenerative disorders with more than 30 different forms currently recognized, many of which are also associated with increased tone and some of which have limb spasticity.
- Gaucher disease is a lysosomal storage disease resulting from a defect in the enzyme acid beta-glucosidase 1.
  - Beta-glucosidase 2 is an enzyme with similar glucosylceramidase activity.
  - Mutations of this enzyme are reportedly associated with ARCA and spastic ataxia, probably resulting in nonfunctional enzymes.
- The noted pathogenic mutation of SPG7 may have been responsible for the spasticity, at least partially. It is known to be associated with HSP.

SUGGESTED READING

Hammer MB, Eleuch-Fayache G, Schottlaender LV, et al. Mutations in GAB2 cause autosomal recessive cerebellar ataxia with spasticity. *Amer J Hum Genet* 2013;Feb 7 92:245–251.

CHAPTER 9

DYSPNEA

CASE 9.1: BREATHING DIFFICULTY AND INVOLUNTARY MOVEMENT

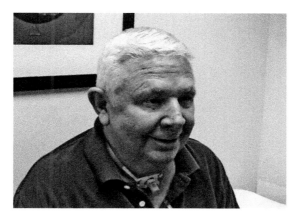

VIDEO 9.1

A 67-year-old man presented with a 10-year history of breathing difficulty. This disorder may be associated with:

1. Blepharospasm
2. Dysphagia
3. Airway obstruction
4. Spasmodic dysphonia
5. All of the above

DIAGNOSIS

- The examination showed involuntary facial contractions, blepharospasm, and bursts of breathing difficulty that seemed to be caused by laryngeal contractions. These findings are consistent with oromandibular dystonia. Other features include dysphagia, airway obstruction, and spasmodic dysphonia.
- Patients with dystonia may be referred to neuromuscular clinics due to respiratory problems.
- Movement disorders may be associated with different patterns of respiratory disorders.
  - Upper respiratory tract obstruction, diaphragmatic dysfunction, or both are the main ones.
- Spasmodic dysphonia may also cause upper airway obstruction. Sometimes the respiratory difficulty is severe enough to mandate a tracheostomy.
- The most common symptoms are stridor, gasping, dyspnea, and interrupted speech and paradoxical breathing.
- In this patient with craniocervical dystonia, the involuntary contraction of the posterior pharyngeal muscles and upper respiratory airways was associated with a paradoxical contraction of the vocalis muscles, mostly during inspiration, and the vocal cord adduction caused gasping.
- Desynchronized contraction of the diaphragm, chest, and upper respiratory airway muscles leads to dyspnea.

SUGGESTED READING

Mehanna R, Jankovic J. Respiratory problems in neurologic movement disorders. *Parkinsonism Related Disord* 2010;16:628–638.

CASE 9.2: RESPIRATORY FAILURE AND POSITIVE FACIOSCAPULOHUMERAL MUSCULAR DYSTROPHY (FSHD) DELETION

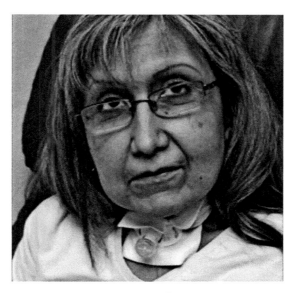

VIDEO 9.2

A 56-year-old woman presented with recurrent prolonged respiratory failure after viral upper respiratory tract infection (URTI) at least once a year. Creatine kinase (CK) level was 420 U/L. Electromyography (EMG) repeatedly showed myopathic units with fibrillations in the proximal arm and leg muscles and paraspinal muscles. Nerve conduction study (NCS) was normal. Arterial blood gas (ABG) analysis revealed hypercapnia, and pulmonary function testing (PFT) showed a restrictive pattern. Muscle biopsy showed only type II fiber atrophy, and diaphragmatic biopsy showed mild inflammation. She responded partially and temporarily to oral steroids and intravenous immunoglobulin (IVIG). There was no facial weakness or scapular winging, but there is mild pectoralis atrophy. Dry spot for acid alpha glucosidase (GAA) revealed normal activity. Facioscapulohumeral muscular dystrophy (FSHD) mutation analysis was positive for D4Z4 allel contraction.

The positive FSHD mutation in this case:

1. Is 100% specific
2. Should be confirmed by looking for a distal permissive gene
3. Is consistent with the shown typical clinical picture of FSHD
4. Should be confirmed by mutation analysis on muscle tissue

DIAGNOSIS

- FSHD is one of the most common genetic muscle diseases.
- Facial weakness, scapular winging, asymmetrical foot drop, and proximal weakness are common features.
- Respiratory compromise occurs very late in the course, and usually after the extremity weakness has become severe. Otherwise, respiratory compromise is so rare that its presence should call for reconsideration of the diagnosis.
- Genetic diagnosis of FSHD is based on identification of partial deletion of a large repetitive DNA element known as D4Z4 and is present in the subtelomeric region of chromosome 4q.
  - Each D4Z4 repeat is 3.3 Kb in size, and normal individuals typically have 10–100 D4Z4 repeats on each copy of chromosome 4q. In more than 95% of patients with FSHD, one copy of the 4q will have only 1–9 repeats.
  - Deletion of an integral number of D4Z4 repeats is necessary but not sufficient to cause FSHD.
  - Contraction must occur on the A variant (4qA) (Figure 9.2.1) in order for the D4Z4 mutation to be pathogenic.
- In atypical cases of FSHD, a positive deletion of D4Z4 should be supplemented by testing for the A variant.
- In this case, myopathies with respiratory failure as a common feature should be considered in the differential diagnosis, such as:
  - Adult onset nemaline myopathy
  - Myofibrillar myopathies
  - Acid maltase deficiency
  - Calpainopathy
  - Amyloid myopathy
  - Inflammatory myopathies

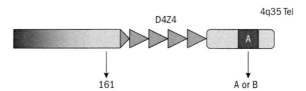

FIGURE 9.2.1 (A) variant (distal permissive gene) is essential for the diagnosis of FSHD.

Courtesy of Rabi Tawil, MD.

CASE 9.3: PERSISTENT RESPIRATORY FAILURE AFTER A CAR ACCIDENT

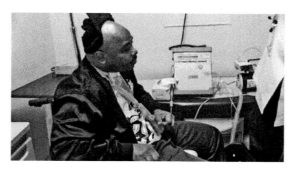

VIDEO 9.3

A 50-year-old man developed breathing difficulty after a car accident, which progressed to respiratory failure that required a tracheostomy. While he was in a long-term facility, his CK was found to be around 1,900 U/L repeatedly. His examination revealed mild proximal weakness. EMG showed proximal myopathic units with spontaneous paraspinal discharges. Muscle biopsy showed normal glycogen contents. Muscle and blood tissue acid alpha glucosidase activity was low. GAA sequence analysis confirmed mutation of the *GAA* gene. He improved slightly with GAA infusions.

The following are typical for this case except:

1. Predominant respiratory involvement
2. Irritative myopathy
3. Positive response to GAA
4. Low GAA activity in blood and muscle
5. Normal glycogen content in the muscle

DIAGNOSIS

- Among the myopathies that affect respiratory muscles early and out of proportion to the extremities and bulbar muscles, acid maltase deficiency is the most important.
- A total of 30% of cases present with respiratory failure that is usually triggered by infection.
- Headache, sleepiness, orthopnea, and dyspnea are common presenting features.
- All patients develop respiratory failure during evolution of the disease.
- The enzyme is a lysosomal housekeeper that is widely distributed in the tissue.
- In adult form, the enzyme activity is hugely reduced in muscle and white cells.
- Severity of disease correlates with enzyme activity.
- Autosomal recessive (AR), 17q23. Incidence: 2:100,000.
- Age: 10–60 years, with history of muscle cramps, fatigue, and mild muscle weakness for years.
- Expiration is more affected than inspiration, leading to weak coughing and atelectasis.
- Weakness is more proximal than distal. Scapular winging may lead to confusion with FSHD.
- Cardiomyopathy is common.
- EMG: irritative myopathy and paraspinal myotonic discharges.
- CK can be normal in adults.
- Muscle biopsy: glycogen deposition in cytoplasm and lysosomal vacuoles (positive acid phosphatase).
- Less glycogen deposition is seen in adults than in infants and juveniles, and atypically, cases of no glycogen accumulation may still show abnormal *GAA* activity.
- If clinically and electromyographically suspected, a dry blood spot is recommended.
- Intravenous (IV) recombinant alpha glucosidase is shown to improve strength, especially in young populations.
- Debrancher enzyme deficiency should be considered if GAA activity is normal. It can cause similar clinical and EMG pictures.

CASE 9.4: DYSPNEA AND SCAPULAR WINGING

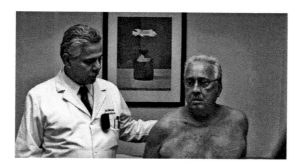

VIDEO 9.4

A 65-year-old man presented with acute right arm pain and dyspnea. Cervical magnetic resonance imaging (MRI) and brachial plexus MRI were normal. EMG showed denervation of the right rhomboid and diaphragm.

The most likely diagnosis is:

1. Parsonage-Turner syndrome
2. C3–C5 radiculopathy
3. Mononeuritis multiplex
4. Scapuloperoneal neuropathy
5. Hereditary neuropathy with liability to pressure palsy (HNPP)

DIAGNOSIS

- The acute and painful onset and the involvement of the dorsal scapular, axillary, and phrenic nerves suggest neuralgic amyotrophy.
- Neuralgic amyotrophy is a rare autoimmune inflammation of the brachial plexus.
- Sudden and severe burning pain in the shoulder and periscapular region for a few days, followed by weakness and atrophy of certain arm muscles, depending on the affected nerves.
- A similar syndrome affecting the lumbar plexus is reported. A total of 30% of cases are bilateral. A hereditary variant called *hereditary neuralgic amyotrophy* exists.
- Before weakness becomes obvious, the condition may be misdiagnosed as shoulder arthritis or herpes zoster.
- After weakness appears, other diagnoses are considered, such as cervical hereditary neuralgic amyotrophy (HNP), tumor of the spinal cord or brachial plexus, and thoracic outlet syndrome.
- Axillary, suprascapular, long thoracic, and musculocutaneous nerves are most commonly affected. Radial, anterior interosseus, median, ulnar, and phrenic nerves are next in frequency.
- Steroids provide no long-term benefit but may reduce pain and enhance tolerance to physical therapy.
- Pain management and rehabilitation are the mainstays of treatment. Most patients recover within 2 years with minimal residual deficit.

CHAPTER 10

WEAKNESS OF THE NECK MUSCLES

CASE 10.1: INABILITY TO HOLD HEAD UP

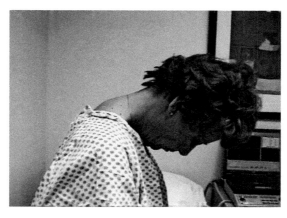

VIDEO 10.1

A 59-year-old woman presented with posterior neck pain and fatigability of neck extension evolved over 3 months. She soon developed slurring of speech and choking, especially in the evenings. Her examination showed weakness of the neck extensors and tongue atrophy with hyperreflexia.

Dropped head syndrome is a recognized manifestation of all of the following except:

1. MuSK myasthenia gravis (MG)
2. Amyotrophic lateral sclerosis (ALS)
3. Facioscapulohumeral muscular dystrophy (FSHD)
4. Polymyositis
5. Myotonia congenita (MC)

DIAGNOSIS

- The ability to hold the head up is made possible by at least five pairs of neck extensor muscles. It is a function that is taken for granted until it becomes defective.
- An average human head weighs 10 pounds. Animals have more developed neck extensors.
- Weakness of the neck extensors initially leads to the inability to lift the head off the pillow; therefore, the patient has to turn to the side before sitting up. With progression, it becomes hard to hold the head up for a long time, and then the head drops all the time so that the patient has to hold his chin up with his hands to be able to see forward.
- Excessive strain on the neck extensors leads to posterior cervical pain, which is a common early manifestation.
- The affected muscles appear atrophic, edematous, and are replaced by fat, as demonstrated by cervical spine magnetic resonance imaging (MRI).
- Common causes of dropped head syndrome include:
  - ALS: Weakness of the neck extensors is usually accompanied by bulbar dysfunction (dysphagia, dysarthria, dyspnea) and features of upper motor neuron (UMN) and lower motor neuron (LMN) lesions are seen. It is progressive, and diagnosis is hardly difficult. Mild creatine kinase (CK) elevation may deceivingly sway the diagnosis toward a myopathic process, but widespread denervation is usually evident by electromyography (EMG).
  - MG: Usually, fatigable diplopia and ptosis are present. In MuSK MG, dysphagia, fluctuating dysarthria, and tongue weakness and atrophy may lead to diagnostic confusion with ALS, which also shows a decremental response about 30% of the time. Even tongue fasciculation is reported in cases with MuSK MG. It is strongly recommended that MuSK antibodies are tested in patients with dropped head syndrome.
  - Inflammatory myopathies.
  - Metabolic myopathies such as acid maltase deficiency.
  - Adult onset nemaline myopathy with monoclonal gammopathy
  - FSHD.
  - Dystrophic myopathies like dysferlinopathy.
  - Chronic inflammatory demyelinating polyneuropathy (CIDP).
- After extensive evaluation, at least 25% of neck extensor weakness remains idiopathic [isolated neck extensor myopathy (INEM)].
- There are reports of response of INEM to immunomodulation. Some cases may represent restricted seronegative myasthenia, while others may represent restricted muscular dystrophy (MD) or axial myopathy.
- The finding of spontaneous activity in the cervical paraspinal muscles should not be overinterpreted. These changes can be secondary to the head drop, not primary.

SUGGESTED READING

Muppidi S, Saperstein DS, Shaibani A, Nations DP, Vernino S, Wolfe GI. Isolated neck extensor myopathy: is it responsive to immunotherapy? *J Clin Neuromuscl Dis.* 2010 Sep;12(1):26–29.

CASE 10.2: SPOTTING MONEY IN THE POST OFFICE

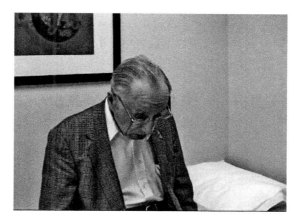

VIDEO 10.2

A 75-year-old man developed difficulty holding his head up that had been noticed a year earlier. There was no pain, diplopia, or ptosis. He had mild weakness of the hip flexors and fatigable weakness of the neck extensors. He told a story about a friend who spotted a lot of money since she developed a similar syndrome. Repetitive left spinal accessory nerve stimulation revealed a 15% decremental response of the left trapezius.

The most specific test for a treatable cause of dropped head syndrome is:

1. Muscle biopsy
2. FSHD mutation analysis
3. Acetylcholine receptor (AChR) antibodies
4. Repetitive nerve stimulation (RNS)
5. Striational antibodies

DIAGNOSIS

- This man was joking about a friend who spotted money many times in the post office during the Christmas season because she looked down all the time due to having a dropped head.
- Investigations of this patient revealed a very high AChR antibody titer. He responded well to prednisone.

The following investigations are appropriate in patients with dropped head syndrome:

1. CK activity: Marked elevation would suggest a myopathic process, while mild elevation would be nondiscriminatory.
2. Immunofixation protein electrophoresis (IFPE): Monoclonal gammopathy would suggest an adult-onset nemaline myopathy. However, monoclonal gammopathy can be normal in the elderly.
3. EMG to look for widespread denervation, which would suggest motor neuron disease (MND), and to look for signs of irritative myopathy.
4. MRI of the cervical and thoracic paraspinal (TPS) muscles to look for edematous and fatty changes.
5. Muscle biopsy: In the absence of peripheral muscle weakness and with normal CK and EMG, the utility of a muscle biopsy is questionable. Biopsy of paraspinal muscles has its limitations; in addition, these muscles are not standardized and their normal histology is not well characterized.
6. In the absence of neuromuscular etiology, a referral to a movement disorder clinic would be appropriate to rule out other causes such as Parkinson disease, anterocollis, and multi-system atrophy.

CASE 10.3: BENT NECK

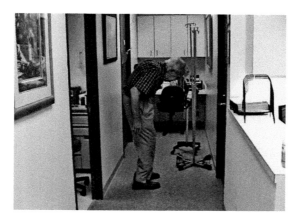

VIDEO 10.3

A 76-year-old man developed gait instability and abnormal head posture gradually over 10 years. He had no diplopia, dysphagia, or leg weakness. When he lay flat, his spine was fully extended. MG serology was negative. EMG revealed restricted thoracic and cervical spontaneous discharges (fibrillations and positive sharp waves).

The most likely diagnosis is:

1. Camptocormia
2. MG
3. ALS
4. Spine disorder
5. Parkinson disease

DIAGNOSIS

- The term *camptocormia* is derived from Greek *kamptos* (bend) and *kormos* (trunk). It refers to abnormal posture dure to hyperflexion of the thoracolumbar spine, which is relieved in the recumbent position, thus differing from those caused by spinal deformities. Early in the course, it becomes progressively difficult to maintain erect orthostatic posture. Later, the thoracolumbar flexion becomes fixed during walking.

- For decades, camptocormia was considered to be psychogenic because it was assumed by soldiers who could not cope with the stress of World Wars I and II; it may have been triggered by stooped posture while walking in the trenches.

- More recent studies revealed many causes for camptocormia:
  - Movement disorders such as Parkinson disease and dystonia. This patient had a normal arm swing and facial expression.
  - Neuromuscular disorders: Discussed in Case 10.2, these mostly include ALS, MG, and dystrophic and inflammatory myopathies
  - Spinal deformities
  - Psychogenic disorders

- Those associated with Parkinson disease may respond to botulinum toxin (BT) injection to the abdominal and neck muscles.

- Fatty infiltration of the paraspinal muscles would support a myopathic etiology.

- EMG is usually helpful to differentiate between a central and a peripheral etiology. However, paraspinal fibrillation and positive, sharp waves can be secondary to abnormal posture, and if restricted, do not have to imply a primary myopathic process.

- Like the case with INEM, many cases of camptocormia remain idiopathic. *Idiopathic thoracic extensor myopathy (ITEM)* is a term coined by Richard Barohn, MD, who speculated that it is a senile degenerative process of the TPS muscles. No treatment is available.

SUGGESTED READING

Shinjo SK, Ramos Torres SC, Radu AS. Camptocormia: a rare axial myopathy disease. *Clinics*. 2008 June;63(3):416–417.

CASE 10.4: PROGRESSIVE HEAD DROP

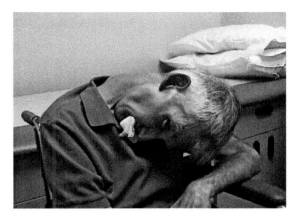

VIDEO 10.4

A 65-year-old man presented with progressive weakness of the neck extensors, dysarthria, dyspha-gia, and hypersialosis, developed over a year. He was hyperreflexic, and his tongue showed atrophy and fasciculation. He expired 3 months after Video 10.4 was filmed.

The most likely cause of dropped head syndrome in this case is:

1. Spinal muscular atrophy (SMA)
2. Primary lateral sclerosis (PLS)
3. ALS
4. MG
5. Parkinson disease

DIAGNOSIS

- In less than 2% of ALS patients, weakness of the neck extensors is the presenting feature of the disease.
- It is attributed to preferential degeneration of the motor neurons controlling the paraspinal muscles.
- These patients usually develop bulbar dysfunction early, and they may have a worse prognosis.
- The diagnosis of ALS is hardly a problem in these patients, who usually have clear UMN and LMN signs at the time of presentation.
- Dropped head causes social embarrassment and increased morbidity, and it interferes with coughing, clearing of secretions, and eating.
- A hard cervical collar may help, but only temporarily, and most patients find it inconvenient.
- An old method using a back stick, an abdominal belt, and a forehead band is employed by some patients.
- As the disease progresses, the dropped head, along with the wasting and weakness of the extremity muscles, renders the patient totally invalid.
- This patient continued to fight despite the terminal nature of his illness. He died from chest infection.
- Providing terminal care to ALS patients is a challenge to patients and their healthcare providers, and it lacks universally acceptable guidelines.

SUGGESTED READING

Gourie-Devi M, Nalini A, Sandhya S. Early or late appearance of "dropped head syndrome" in amyotrophic lateral sclerosis. *J Neurol Neurosurg Psych*. 2003;74:683–686. doi:10.1136/jnnp.74.5.683.

CASE 10.5A, B: DROPPED HEAD
AND CHEWING DIFFICULTY

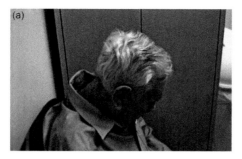

VIDEO 10.5A

An 83-year-old man developed the shown in Video 10.5A clinical picture over a month. The most likely cause of this dropped head syndrome is:

1. ALS
2. MG
3. Lambert-Eaton myasthenic syndrome (LEMS)
4. Polymyositis
5. Guillain-Barré syndrome (GBS)

DIAGNOSIS

- Weak neck extensor muscles can be the initial manifestation of MG, but it usually develops with other ocular and bulbar symptoms, such as diplopia, ptosis, dysarthria, dysphagia, dyspnea, and fatigability of the chewing muscles.
- It is imperative to test the fatigability of neck extensors in all myasthenics, even if they do not complain of weakness in these muscles. Increased fatigability of the neck extensors and triceps muscles is often used to differentiate MG from myopathies where weakness usually affects the neck flexors and deltoids.
- One has to be careful when performing repetitive neck flexion/extension testing in the elderly with severe cervical spondylosis and patients with a history of neck trauma.
- Dropped head due to MG is usually not as pronounced in the morning.
- MuSK antibodies–associated MG may present with dropped head as the main feature.
- The lack of ocular involvement and the atrophy of the tongue and pharynx may lead to diagnostic confusion with ALS.
- Dysarthria is not a differentiating feature, as it occurs in both diseases.
- Measurement of MuSK Ab is important in all cases of dropped head syndrome.
- A therapeutic steroid trial may be warranted in uncertain cases.
- Weakness and fatigability of neck extensors usually start improving within 3 weeks of initiation of steroids.
- Dropped head due to MG usually responds well to treatment of MG. This patient was placed on plasmapheresis and oral prednisone, and his symptoms resolved within 2 months (Video 10.5B).

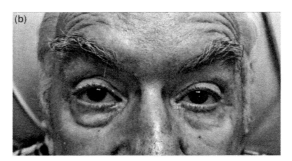

VIDEO 10.5B

CASE 10.6: NO MORE THAN DROPPED HEAD

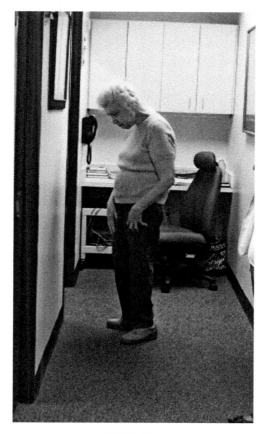

VIDEO 10.6

A 79-year-old woman presented with a 12-month history of neck discomfort and an abnormal stance. She had no proximal extremity weakness, dysphagia, dysarthria, diplopia, or ptosis. CK level was normal. AChR antibody testing was negative. EMG of the extremities revealed no myopathic units. EMG of cervical and thoracic paraspinal muscles showed fibrillations and positive, sharp waves. RNS testing was normal. MRI of the cervical and thoracic spine revealed atrophy and fatty replacement of the paraspinal muscles.

This is most likely a case of:

1. INEM
2. MG
3. Polymyositis
4. ALS
5. Camptocormia

DIAGNOSIS

- Dropped head syndrome can be caused by many neuromuscular disorders, and sometimes it is the presenting feature of these disorders, which could be myopathic, myasthenic, neuropathic, and motor neuronopathic.
- Sometimes weakness continues to be restricted to the cervical and sometimes TPS muscles, and evaluation fails to reveal a cause. This entity is called *isolated neck extensor myopathy (INEM)*.
- It usually affects the elderly population and presents with dropped head and kyphosis due to weakness and atrophy of the TPS muscles. Gait abnormality to adjust for the axial weakness is common.
- Posture is normal in the supine position, unlike patients with fixed contracture of the spine.
- Some of these cases are familial, while others are due to restricted MD or myopathy (axial myopathy).
- CK level is usually normal, and EMG may show myopathic units in the paraspinal muscles with spontaneous activity. Paraspinal muscle biopsy usually shows nonspecific myopathic findings.
- These EMG and pathologic findings should be interpreted with caution since most of these changes may be secondary to the altered head position.
- Rarely, paraspinal muscle biopsy shows specific findings like nemaline rods or many ragged red fibers, suggesting adult onset nemaline myopathy and mitochondrial disorders, respectively.
- Immunosuppression (e.g., steroids with or without azathioprine) is shown to be effective in some of these cases and is worth a trial.
- This case did improve with azathioprine.

SUGGESTED READING

Muppidi S, Saperstein DS, Shaibani A, Nations SP, Vernino S, Wolfe GI. Isolated neck extensor myopathy: is it responsive to immunotherapy? *J Clin Neuromuscl Dis.* 2010 Sep;12(1):26–29.

CASE 10.7: A TWISTED NECK AFTER BIRTH

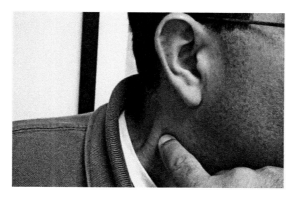

VIDEO 10.7

A 32-year-old man was born with forceps assistance and had multiple head and neck hematomas. As he grew up, he developed a head tilt to the left. Examination is shown in the video.

This is most likely a case of head tilt due to:

1. Cervical dystonia
2. Congenital torticollis
3. Axial myopathy
4. Cervical tic
5. Bad habit

DIAGNOSIS

- Abnormal head tilt can be a cause of referral to neuromuscular clinics due to suspicion of weakness.
- Weakness rarely leads to lateral tilt of the head, but it may lead to dropped head.
- Torticollis may be divided into:
  - Congenital muscular torticollis: This is due to birth injury of the sternocleidomastoid (SCM) muscles, resulting in fibrosis and turning of the head to the side of the contracted muscles. Sometimes this leads to deformity of the face, base of the skull, and cranium. Most of the time, it resolves spontaneously in few years. Otherwise, surgical myotomy may be needed.
  - Spasmodic torticollis: This is also called *cervical dystonia*. It is due to hyperactive cervical muscles. The head is turned away from the hyperactive muscle. It responds to BT.
  - Ocular torticollis: Weakness of the extraocular muscles leads to a corrective head tilt. A weak superior oblique leads to a head tilt away from the affected side. There is no restriction of the cervical motion otherwise.

CASE 10.8: DROPPED HEAD AND RIGIDITY

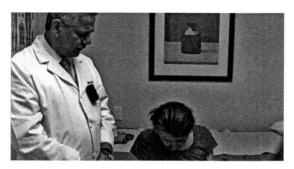

VIDEO 10.8

A 71-year-old woman presented with a 2-month history of difficulty walking and lifting her head. Her examination revealed normal neck extensor strength, cogwheeling, hypophonia, and hypomimia.

The most likely cause of dropped head in this case is:

1. ALS
2. Parkinson disease
3. MG
4. INEM
5. Camptocormia

DIAGNOSIS

- The most common cause of dropped head in the neuromuscular clinic is weakness of the neck extensors due to neuromuscular disorders such as myopathies, MG, and ALS.
- Some patients who are referred to the neuromuscular clinic do not have weakness of the neck extensors, and the cause of the head drop is dystonia of the neck flexors and abdominal muscles.
- Dropped head syndrome is common in multisystem atrophy and rare in Parkinson disease.
- Although it is mostly a chronic condition, acute deterioration has been reported.
- Response to anti-Parkinsonian medications is not consistent. BT is reported to be effective if injected into the neck flexors and abdominal muscles.

SUGGESTED READING

Kashihara K, Ohno M, Tomita S. Dropped head in Parkinson disease. *Mov Disord*. 2006 Aug;21(8):1213–1216.

CASE 10.9: DROPPED HEAD

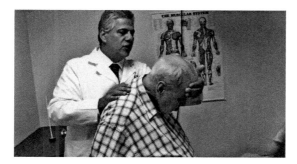

VIDEO 10.9

A 69-year-old man presented with a 6-month history of posterior neck pain during walking. He then could not hold his head up and had mild left ptosis and horizontal diplopia that resolved when he closed one eye. Examination is shown in the video.

The most specific and appropriate diagnostic test in this case is:

1. RNS
2. AChR antibody titer
3. EMG
4. Muscle biopsy
5. MRI of the cervical spine

DIAGNOSIS

- Dropped head syndrome is due to weakness of the neck extensors or dystonia of the neck flexors.
- Examination demonstrated weakness of the neck extensors.
- The most common neuromuscular causes are:
  - ALS
  - Myopathies
  - INEM
  - MG, suggested by diplopia and ptosis
- The most specific test is an AChR antibody titer.
- Prognosis of MG is good, and most patients regain full strength within 3 months of treatment.

CASE 10.10: FATAL FAMILIAL HEAD DROP

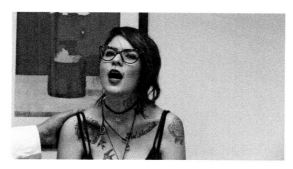

VIDEO 10.10

While on a flight picking her luggage 1.5 years earlier, she extended her neck. She had neck pain for a couple of weeks, and then difficulty holding her head up. She had difficulty holding her arms up and had mild Shortness of breath (SOB) on exertion 6 months later. Her mother died of the same symptoms at age 35, and her maternal aunt and grandfather had similar symptoms. There was atrophy of the arm muscles and areflexia in the arms, with normal reflexes in the legs. Tongue was normal. Forced vital capacity (FVC) was 900 cc. EMG showed diffuse denervation in the arms and TPS muscles. CK level was 90. Cervical spine MRI was normal.

Which familial ALS (FALS) is associated with neck extensor weakness the most?

1. ALS 1: *SOD1* mutations
2. ASL 4: senataxin mutations
3. ALS 6: *FUS* mutations
4. ALS 11: *FIG4* mutations
5. ALS 14: *VCP* mutations

DIAGNOSIS

- Genetic testing revealed *FUS* heterozygous pathogenic mutation, c.1572 G>C variant P.R524S.
- ALS 6 (*FUS* gene mutations) are characterized by the following:
  - They make up 5% of FALS and 0.5% of sporadic ALS cases (*SOD1* is responsible for 20% of FALS cases).
  - Early onset (25–70 years depending on subtype).
  - Cognitive impairment is not common.
  - More progressive and shorter survival than other FALS variants.
  - Bulbar, upper extremity, and neck extensor weakness are more pronounced than other FALS variants.
  - Autosomal-dominant (AD), autosomal-recessive (AR), or de novo mutations.

SUGGESTED READING

Yan J, Deng HX, Siddique N, et al. Frameshift and novel mutations in FUS in familial ALS and ALS/dementia. *Neurol.* 2010;75(9):807–814.

CASE 10.11: DEBILITATING PAINFUL NECK FLEXION

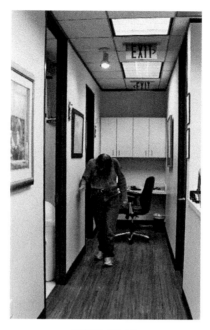

VIDEO 10.11

A 52-year-old healthy woman with a learning disability and anxiety presented with an acute inability to extend her neck that occurred a month ago intermittently, and then became constant. She lost 20 pounds due to inability to eat. There was no weakness in the extremities. She had no ocular or bulbar symptoms. MRI of the cervical spine was normal, but EMG could not be tolerated. CPK level was 1,200 IU/L. The patient refused to undergo muscle biopsy.

The likely diagnosis is:

1. Axial myopathy
2. Parkinson disease
3. Cervical dystonia
4. Camptocormia
5. MG

DIAGNOSIS

- Examination revealed restriction of neck extension because of pain. When she lay flat, the neck flexion was not corrected, which was very atypical of neuromuscular causes and was suggestive of skeletal deformity, dystonia, or rigidity.
- High CK level is likely secondary to strain caused by forced prolonged flexion of the neck. Initially, it suggested myopathy.
- Dropped head syndrome is a manifestation of
  - Neuromuscular disorders such as myopathies, MG, and ALS.
  - It can also be due to INEM. However, neuromuscular paraspinal weakness is usually correctable in the supine position.
- Movement disorders such as Parkinson disease also can cause dropped head syndrome. Patient has normal muscle tone and no tremor.
- Cervical dystonia, especially antecollis, may mimic dropped head syndrome, but such an acute onset is atypical.
- Movement disorder consultation confirmed cervical myotonia. She responded partially to BT injections.

CHAPTER 11

SCAPULAR WINGING

CASE 11.1: SCAPULAR WINGING
AND LOBULATED FIBERS

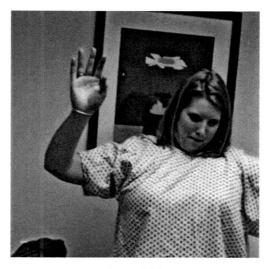

VIDEO 11.1

A 30-year-old woman presented with a slowly progressive arm weakness that started 7 years earlier. In addition to what is shown in the video, she had mild facial weakness. There was no family history of muscle disease. The creatine kinase (CK) level was 350 U/L, and electromyography (EMG) revealed 30% short-duration polyphasic units in the periscapular muscles. The muscle biopsy is shown in Figure 11.1.1. Facioscapulohumeral muscular dystrophy (FSHD) mutation analysis was negative.

Scapular winging in this case is most likely due to:

1. Limb girdle muscular dystrophy (LGMD) 2A (calpainopathy)
2. LGMD 2B (dysferlinopathy)
3. FSHD type 2
4. Scapuloperoneal syndrome (SPS)
5. Polymyositis

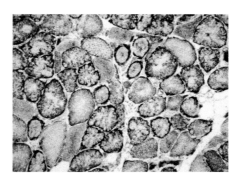

FIGURE 11.1.1 NADH-TR reaction, 100x.

DIAGNOSIS

- Muscle biopsy revealed active myopathy, with many lobulated fibers.
- Calpain-3 is a mostly calcium-dependent and muscle-specific enzyme that is important for cytoskeletal modeling. Its exact function is not clear.
- More than 60 pathogenic mutations of calpain-3 have been identified.
- It is the most common LGMD and affects children and adults (25% of dystrophies with normal dystrophin and sarcoglycans).
- The clinical picture may mimic FSHD due to scapular winging.
- It usually affects hamstrings and thigh adductors early. Magnetic resonance imaging (MRI) confirmation of preferential involvement of these muscles is diagnostically helpful.
- Periscapular and humeral muscles are usually affected a few years after onset.
- Distal and facial muscles are usually spared, unlike FSHD.
- Early elbow and calf contractures may lead to misdiagnosis of Emery-Dreifuss muscular dystrophy (EDMD).
- A total of 50% of patients are nonambulatory by age 20.
- No cardiac, intellectual, or respiratory involvement is expected.
- Longevity is normal.
- A total of 6% of patients have asymptomatic hyperCKemia.
- CK is normal or up to 20 times normal. EMG: myopathy with no muscle membrane irritability. Muscle biopsy: nonspecific myopathic features. Lobulated fibers are common, though nonspecific.
- Decreased enzyme activity in the muscle tissue is seen in 80% of cases; Western blot (WB) confirmation is necessary.
- Genetic confirmation is necessary because secondary calpain deficiency can be seen in dysferlinopathy and titinopathy.

SUGGESTED READING

Figarella-Branger D, El-Dassouki M, Saenz A, et al. Myopathy with lobulated muscle fibers: evidence for heterogeneous etiology and clinical presentation. *Neuromuscul Disord*. 2002 Jan;12(1):4–12.

CASE 11.2: SCAPULAR WINGING AFTER CERVICAL LYMPH NODE BIOPSY

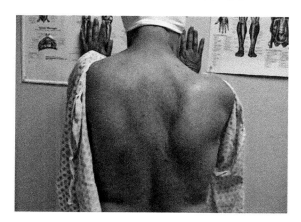

VIDEO 11.2

A 37-year-old woman who had had a cervical lymph node biopsy 3 months earlier presented with pain and stiffness of the right upper back muscles that did not respond to gabapentin. She developed tingling of the right little finger a couple of weeks earlier. A chiropractic manipulation gave her temporary relief. Examination is shown in the video.

EMG is expected to show denervation of:

1. Rhomboid
2. Trapezius
3. Serratus anterior
4. Levator scapulae
5. Supraspinatus

Tingling of the right little finger that developed later was most likely:

1. Not related to the scapular winging
2. Due to a related thoracic outlet syndrome
3. Due to a related focal ulnar neuropathy at the elbow
4. Due to an incidental C8 radiculopathy
5. Was associated with reduced ulnar compound muscle action potential (CMAP) amplitude

DIAGNOSIS

- The trapezius stabilizes the base of the scapula.
- It originates from the spinous processes of the cervical and thoracic vertebrae and inserts into the spine of the scapula.
- The spinal accessory nerve (SAN) branches from the third and fourth cervical roots.
- Surgical procedures in the posterior triangle of the neck can cause injury to the SAN due to its superficial location in that region.
- Patients rarely notice the winged scapula, and they usually present with periscapular pain and stiffness.
- Scapular winging is lateral. The scapula deviates laterally, unlike the medial winging seen in long thoracic neuropathy.
- Proximal lesions lead to sternocleidomastoid weakness as well.
- Depression of the shoulder is an important diagnostic clue.
- Shoulder droop may lead to thoracic outlet syndrome (TOS). This explains why the patient later developed little finger numbness. Typically, in neurogenic TOS, there is a reduction of the ipsilateral ulnar sensory nerve action potential (SNAP) and median CMAP.
- On nerve conduction study (NCS), stimulation of the right SAN did not produce a motor response (by comparison, the amplitude of the left CMAP was 6 millivolts).
- Needle examination showed active denervation changes in the right trapezius. Needle EMG of the right rhomboid and serratus anterior was normal.
- Surgical options include transfer of the levator scapula to the spine of the scapula, which has been reported to result in return of function and relief of pain.
- Levator scapulae is supplied by branches from the fourth and fifth cervical nerves, and frequently by a branch from the dorsal scapular nerve as well.

SUGGESTED READING

Bigliani LU, Compito CA, Duralde XA, Wolfe IN. Transfer of the levator scapulae, rhomboid major, and rhomboid minor for paralysis of the trapezius. *J Bone Joint Surg Am*. 1996 Oct;78(10):1534–1540.

CASE 11.3: PROGRESSIVE SCAPULAR WINGING AND SHORTNESS OF BREATH

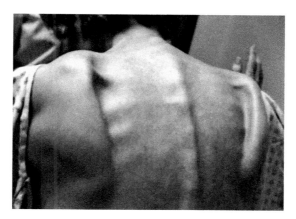

VIDEO 11.3

A 69-year-old female presented with a 6-month history of shortness of breath, weakness of the arms, and weight loss. Examination demonstrated atrophy of the periscapular muscles and winging of the scapulae, fasciculations of the arm muscles, hyperreflexia, and normal sensation. The CK level was 320 U/L. EMG showed active denervation of the proximal arm muscles and the cervical and thoracic paraspinal muscles.

Periscapular wasting and dyspnea in this case are features of:

1. Becker muscular dystrophy (BMD)
2. Motor neuron disease (MND)
3. Acid maltase deficiency
4. FSHD
5. Amyloid myopathy

DIAGNOSIS

- The scapulae play an important role in arm abduction and rotation. They are held in place by several muscles to ensure their stability during such movements.
- Scapular winging is a sign of weakness of one or more of the periscapular muscles.
- Laterally, the serratus anterior prevents the scapula from being displaced medially during arm movements. Medially, the rhomboids and trapezius muscles stabilize the scapulae.
- Lesions to these muscles or their nerve supplies may lead to scapular winging.
- Causes of winging of the scapulae include:
  - Diffuse muscle diseases that lead to symmetrical or asymmetrical weakness of the periscapular muscles, including:
    - FSHD
    - LGMD 2A
    - EDMD
    - Desmin myopathy
    - Centronuclear myopathy
  - Diffuse denervation:
    - Amyotrophic lateral sclerosis (ALS)
    - Spinal muscular atrophy (SMA), type 4
    - SPS
  - Focal nerve lesion:
    - Long thoracic neuropathy
    - Spinal accessory neuropathy
    - Dorsal scapular neuropathy
- While scapular winging is not usually a presenting sign in ALS, it is important to know that wasting of the periscapular muscles occurs commonly in ALS when upper limbs are involved. Scapular winging can easily be appreciated when the patient is disrobed for EMG.
- Diagnosis of ALS was suggested clinically by the presence of both upper motor neuron (UMN) and lower motor neuron (LMN) signs. EMG findings supported the diagnosis of ALS.
- Weakness of ventilatory muscles is common in these patients. Bulbar involvement will occur soon, if it is not already present by the time that periscapular wasting has occurred.
- Periscapular atrophy contributed to poor arm abduction in this case and thus compounded the patient's functional limitations.

CASE 11.4: SCAPULAR WINGING AND DEAFNESS

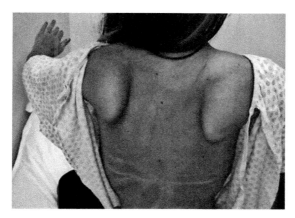

VIDEO 11.4

A 28-year-old woman presented with a 3-year history of arm weakness. She gradually developed right foot drop. Her mother noted hearing loss and inability to close her eyes completely during sleep. The CK level was 150 IU/L; EMG demonstrated myopathic motor units in the proximal arm muscles and in both tibialis anterior muscles. Ear, nose, and throat (ENT) evaluation demonstrated sensorimotor deafness, and an eye exam showed retinal telangiectasias.

The likely diagnosis is:

1. Davidenkow syndrome
2. Coats syndrome
3. Hopkins syndrome
4. Parsonage-Turner syndrome (PTS)
5. None of the above

DIAGNOSIS

- Coats syndrome is a rare extramuscular complication of FSHD associated with large D4Z4 contraction.
- High-frequency hearing loss and retinal telangiectasias are required for the diagnosis.
- Unilateral or bilateral sensorineural hearing loss is reported in 60% of FSHD patients, and more than 50% of patients have abnormal fluorescein angiography. Retinal vasculopathy may result in retinal detachment. If retinal vasculopathy is detected early, photocoagulation may prevent serious consequences. Annual hearing and ophthalmological examination is recommended.
- Coats syndrome occurs more frequently in female patients with FSHD with large D4Z4 contraction and has a widely variable age of onset (1–53 years).
- Males tend to develop symptoms earlier and more severely than females. By age 30 years, almost all males and only two-thirds of females exhibit symptoms of FSHD.

CASE 11.5: SCAPULAR WINGING AND BILATERAL FOOT DROP

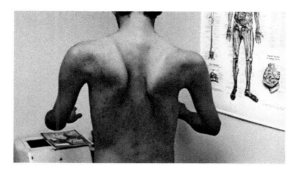

VIDEO 11.5

A 20-year-old Hispanic man presented with a 5-year history of arm weakness and tripping. His examination is demonstrated in the video.

SPS may be caused by all of the following except:

1. FSHD
2. Acid maltase deficiency
3. Myofibrillar myopathy (desminopathy)
4. Duchenne muscular dystrophy (DMD)
5. Scapuloperoneal neuronopathy

DIAGNOSIS

- SPS is defined by weakness of the shoulder girdle muscles, leading to bilateral scapular winging, and peroneal muscles, leading to bilateral foot drop.
- Many neuromuscular disorders may present with such a distribution, including:
  - Myotonic dystrophy
  - LGMD 2 A
  - Desminopathy
  - Acid maltase deficiency
  - Inclusion body myositis (IBM)
  - Myophosphorylase deficiency
  - Polymyositis
  - Congenital myopathies
  - Nonaka distal myopathy
  - FSHD
  - Hereditary neuropathy with liability to pressure palsy (HNPP)
  - Some cases of SMA
- Usually, the weakness spreads to other muscles that are characteristically involved in these diseases.
- After exclusion of these diseases, some patients continue to have unclassified scapuloperoneal weakness, and these are classified into two categories:
  1. Scapuloperoneal muscular dystrophy:
     - X-linked dominant SPS (hyalin body myopathy) localized to chromosome Xq. It is caused by mutation of the *FAHL1* gene.
     - Autosomal recessive form localized to 3p22
     - CK is slightly elevated, and EMG is myopathic. Muscle biopsy is nonspecific but can show hyaline bodies.
  2. Scapuloperoneal neuropathy (Dawidenkow syndrome):
     - Autosomal-dominant (AD) disease with scapuloperoneal weakness, distal sensory impairment, pes cavus, areflexia, and motor slowing.
     - In some cases, chromosome 17p11.2 deletions are found (a variant of HNPP).
- With genetic advances, this syndrome will yield to more specific genetic categories.
- The workup of SPS includes measurement of CK levels and an EMG to differentiate the myopathic from the neuropathic types. Genetic studies, and possibly a muscle biopsy, are also performed to define the diagnosis and rule out the other mentioned possibilities.

CASE 11.6: SCAPULAR WINGING AND SEVERE SHOULDER PAIN

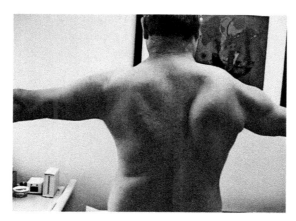

VIDEO 11.6

A 53-year-old man presented with sudden-onset, severe burning pain of the right shoulder that was preceded by cough and fever 2 weeks earlier. The patient lost the ability to raise his right arm 2 weeks later. EMG demonstrated denervation of the right serratus anterior and deltoid muscles.

The likely diagnosis is:

1. PTS
2. Long thoracic nerve injury
3. C5 cervical radiculopathy
4. Mononeuritis multiplex
5. Guillain-Barré syndrome (GBSs)

DIAGNOSIS

- Examination demonstrated mild atrophy of the right deltoid (suprascapular nerve) and prominent medial winging of the right scapula (serratus anterior, long thoracic nerve).
- PTS, or neuralgic amyotrophy, is due to an acute, patchy inflammation of the brachial plexus that may be triggered by a viral upper respiratory infection (URI), immunization, stress, surgery, or childbirth.
- Typically, it starts with severe nocturnal burning pain in the periscapular and shoulder regions that lasts for about 2 weeks, followed by weakness and atrophy of muscles supplied by one or more of the following nerves:
  1. Long thoracic nerve
  2. Axillary nerve
  3. Musculocutaneous nerve
  4. Suprascapular nerve
  5. Phrenic nerve
  6. Anterior interosseous nerve
  7. SAN
  8. Lingual nerve
- In 30% of cases, the other side is affected simultaneously or within a few weeks.
- EMG shows denervation of the affected muscles.
- NCS reveals loss of sensory responses of the affected nerves.
- Prognosis is good. Improvement starts a month after the onset, and maximum recovery may take up to 2 years.
- When the long thoracic nerve is affected, scapular winging is the main feature.
  - The winging is medial, meaning that the scapula moves medially when the arms are outstretched against a wall.
  - This is different from the lateral winging due to involvement of dorsal scapular or SANs.
    - Rhomboid weakness is more prominent when the arms are pushed posteriorly against resistance.
    - Trapezius weakness is associated with depressed shoulder and more winging when the arms are abducted.
- It is a self-limiting disease and steroids are not warranted. Judicious pain management is usually needed for severe pain, along with rehabilitation.

CASE 11.7: SUBACUTE SCAPULAR WINGING AND WEAKNESS OF FINGER FLEXORS

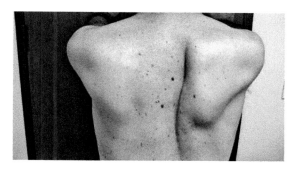

VIDEO 11.7

A 47-year-old man presented with acute unilateral shoulder pain, followed by right arm and finger weakness.

Weakness of the finger flexion in this case is most likely due to involvement of the following nerve:

1. Long thoracic nerve
2. Anterior interosseous nerve
3. Suprascapular nerve
4. Ulnar nerve
5. Median nerve, main trunk

DIAGNOSIS

- Anterior interosseus neuropathy (AIN) involves a motor branch of the median nerve above the elbow.
- It supplies flexor pollicis longus (FPL), flexor digitorum profundus (FDP) of the third and fourth fingers, and pronator quadratus (PQ).
- Dysfunction of these muscles leads to inability to produce the "OK" sign due to lack of flexion of the terminal phalanges of the first two fingers.
- The affected muscles can be tested via EMG. Median sensory response is normal because it branches off the median nerve proximal to the lesion.
- AIN is one of the common targets of PTS.
  - Other causes of AIN involvement include compression by pronator teres, bicipital tendon bursa, and trauma.
- Recovery occurs spontaneously in 50% of cases.
- In patients with Martin-Gruber anastomosis, atrophy of the intrinsic hand muscles (normally supplied by the ulnar nerve) can be diagnostically confusing.

CASE 11.8: FAMILIAL SCAPULAR WINGING

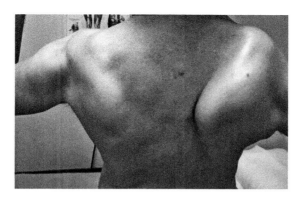

VIDEO 11.8

A 59-year-old man presented with a 10-year history of painless asymmetrical bilateral foot drop. A fraternal twin brother had similar symptoms. The CK level was 450 U/L, EMG was myopathic, and D4Z4 alleles were normal. Muscle biopsy revealed chronic myopathic changes with several inflammatory foci.

The most appropriate next test is:

1. *SMCHD1* gene mutation analysis
2. *DMPK* gene mutation analysis
3. Dystrophin staining in muscle
4. Calpain gene sequencing
5. Dysferlin WB analysis

DIAGNOSIS

- FSHD is an AD disease. Sporadic mutations occur in 20% of cases of FSHD 1 and 70% of cases of FSHD2.
- A total of 95% of FSHD patients have deletion of the *D4Z4* gene on chromosome 4. Severity of the disease correlates with the size of the mutation in FSDH 1, but not in FSHD 2.
- False positives may occur due to nonpathogenic contraction of the *D4Z4* gene. In atypical cases of FSHD, the pathogenicity of *D4Z4* mutations should be confirmed by looking for a permissive distal sequence (4qA).
- In 5% of FSHD cases, there is no contraction in the *D4Z4* gene, and yet they maintain an opening of the chromatin structure at the *D4Z4* locus. These cases are diagnosed as FSHD 2.
  - FSHD2 requires inheritance of two unlinked genetic factors: a permissive 4qA allele and a loss of function mutation of the *SMCHD1* gene, which is found on chromosome 18p11.
  - FSHD 2 presents similarly to FSHD 1. Onset age is usually older, though (more than 30 years).
  - Patients with severe weakness may have both FSDH 1 and FSHD 2 mutation.
  - Facial sparing, as in this case, occurs in 15% of cases and is usually associated with smaller deletions.
  - Muscle inflammation, as in this case, occurs in 75% of cases.

SUGGESTED READING

Lemmers RJ, Tawil R, Petek LM, et al. Digenic inheritance of an SMCHD1 mutation and an FSHD-permissive D4Z4 allele causes facioscapulohumeral muscular dystrophy type 2. *Nature Genet.* 2012;44:1370–1374.

CASE 11.9: SCAPULAR WINGING AND A CREATINE KINASE (CK) LEVEL OF 2,000 IU/L

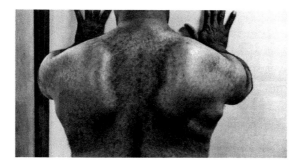

VIDEO 11.9

A 57-year-old man presented with a 5-year history of difficulty walking. Two years later, he could not lift his arms. Examination also showed elbow contractures and hearing loss. He had normal sural responses and myopathic EMG. The CK level was 2,000 U/L. Chest X-ray revealed cardiomegaly. Muscle biopsy showed chronic myopathic changes. There was no neurogenic atrophy or evidence of metabolic or mitochondrial myopathy. He did not know much about his parents' history.

Testing is most appropriate for which of the following?

1. Acid maltase activity in a dry blood spot
2. *FHL1* mutation
3. *FSHD* 2 gene mutation
4. *HNPP* mutation
5. Calpain muscle tissue staining

DIAGNOSIS

- Among the mentioned findings, the presence of contractures, cardiomegaly, and hearing loss suggested scapuloperoneal myopathy (SPM) due to *FHL1* gene mutation.
- Four-and-a-half LIM protein 1 (*FHL1*) mutation is the cause of four different phenotypes:
  - Reducing body myopathy
  - EDMD
  - X-linked myopathy characterized by postural muscle atrophy
  - SPM
    - It is an X-linked dominant disease.
    - Usual age of onset is late 20s.
    - Includes slowly progressive distal leg (foot drop) and proximal arm weakness.
    - Males are more severely affected than females and at an earlier age, and most of them become wheelchair bound.
    - Scapular winging.
    - Late-onset joint contractures.
    - Cardiomyopathy is a common cause of death.
    - Respiratory involvement is not common.
    - CK: 2–10 times normal.
    - Reducing bodies are seen in the muscle biopsy.
    - The pathogenic mechanism by which *FHL1* mutations cause human muscle disease is not clear. Despite heterogeneous phenotypes, a common pathogenic mechanism is suggested.

SUGGESTED READING

Wilding BR, McGrath MJ, Bonne G, Mitchell CA. FHL1 mutations that cause clinically distinct human myopathies form protein aggregates and impair myoblast differentiation. *J Cell Sci*. 2014;Mar 14; 127(10):2269–2281.

CHAPTER 12

PROXIMAL ARM WEAKNESS

CASE 12.1: CHRONIC PROXIMAL ARM ATROPHY

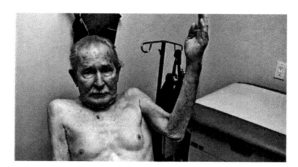

VIDEO 12.1

A 72-year-old man had developed progressive posterior neck pain and bilateral arm weakness that evolved over 3 years. He had atrophy of the deltoids and biceps and absent deep tendon reflexes (DTRs) in the arms and normal DTRs in the legs. Cervical magnetic resonance imaging (MRI) revealed a disc herniation at the C5–C6 level, for which he had cervical laminectomy. After surgery, weakness of the arms gradually increased and spread to the distal arm muscles. Rare fasciculation was noted in the deltoids. Electromyography (EMG) revealed chronic denervation of the proximal and distal bilateral arm muscles and normal bilateral leg muscles. Nerve conduction studies (NCSs) were normal. The creatine kinase (CK) level was 320 U/L, and cervical MRI continued to show moderate spondylosis.

The most likely explanation of these findings is:

1. Cervical spondylosis
2. Brachial amyotrophic diplegia (BAD)
3. Classic amyotrophic lateral sclerosis (ALS)
4. Multifocal motor neuropathy with conduction block (MMNCB)
5. Spinal muscular atrophy (SMA)

DIAGNOSIS

- BAD is an atypical and less progressive variant of motor neuron disease (MND) than classical ALS.
- It constitutes 10% of ALS cases.
- Age of onset is similar to classic ALS, but it has a longer median survival time (3–11 years).
- It is much more common in males (9:1) than classic ALS (1.5:1).
- It presents as progressive and painless weakness of the upper extremities and usually spares the lower extremities and the bulbar and respiratory muscles.
- One-third of patients develop weakness in the legs within several years of the diagnosis.
- It affects lower motor neurons (LMNs) only. Therefore, areflexia is observed.
- Mechanism of the disease is not clear.
- Differential diagnosis includes:
  1. Classic ALS: It is characterized by upper motor neuron (UMN) and LMN involvement and a more progressive course.
  2. MMNCB: Conduction block is usually found.
  3. Adult onset SMA: It is characterized by an earlier age of onset and a more chronic course. Fascicular atrophy with compensatory hypertrophy of muscle fibers is seen in muscle biopsy.
  4. Cervical spondylosis: It is characterized by radicular pain and numbness and abnormal cervical spine MRI and myotomal EMG abnormalities.
  5. Brachial plexopathy: It is characterized by sensory and motor symptoms along specific distribution and abnormal sensory responses of the affected branches.
  6. Inflammatory myopathies: Myopathic EMG is expected, as well as more severe CK elevation. Mild CK elevation is common in neurogenic conditions, including BAD.
  7. Postpolio syndrome: History of poliomyelitis is usually evident.

SUGGESTED READING

Pearlman S, Pourmand R. Evaluation of a patient presenting with progressive weakness and atrophy of the upper extremities. *JCNMD*. 2003;5(1):51–59.

CASE 12.2: ACUTE PROXIMAL ARM WEAKNESS

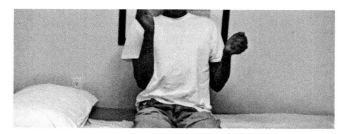

VIDEO 12.2

A 48-year-old man presented with a 2-week history of progressive painless weakness of the arms with no sensory symptoms. On examination, in addition to what is shown in the video, he had normal-to-brisk DTRs in all extremities and normal sensation. EMG revealed normal sensory responses (sural, ulnar, and median) and low amplitude of compound muscle action potentials (CMAPs) of the peroneal, tibial, median, and ulnar nerves, mild motor slowing of bilateral median and ulnar nerves, and active denervation of the proximal and distal muscles in all extremities and thoracic paraspinal muscles with a fast firing frequency. The CK level was 700 IU/L. Cerebrospinal fluid (CSF) analysis revealed a protein of 167 mg/dl, glucose of 54 mg/dl, and 152 white cells (mostly lymphocytes). HIV testing was positive. He recovered within 6 months of intravenous immunoglobulin (IVIG) and antiviral therapy.

This most likely diagnosis is:

1. Classical Guillain-Barré syndrome (GBS)
2. Vasculitis
3. Acute motor axonal neuropathy (AMAN)
4. Polymyositis
5. Chronic inflammatory demyelinating polyneuropathy (CIDP)

DIAGNOSIS

Neuromuscular manifestations of HIV infection are well recognized and can be the presenting features of HIV infection, as in this case. These syndromes include:

- Neuropathies
  - Sensory polyneuropathy:
    - Associated with chronic infection
    - Associated with antiviral therapy
  - Autonomic neuropathy
  - Demyelinating neuropathies: CIDP and GBS
  - AMAN
  - Peripheral nervous system vasculitis
- Myopathies:
  - Polymyositis
  - Inclusion body myositis (IBM)
  - Toxic myopathy
  - Nemaline myopathy
- Radiculopathy
- MND
- Myasthenia gravis (MG)
- The diffuse denervation and preserved sensory responses and hyperreflexia in this case suggested MND. However, the acute onset, the CSF findings, and the subsequent recovery suggested AMAN.
- Cases of diffuse fasciculations and bulbar involvement with recovery are reported with HIV infection, and they are termed *ALS-like disease.*
- Some typical ALS cases are reported in association with HIV infection, including relentless progression. No causal relationship was established.
- HIV is not known to invade UMNs or LMNs.
- Immune-mediated injury rather than direct viral invasion of the peripheral nerves is speculated in these cases.

SUGGESTED READINGS

Harrison T, Smith B. Neuromuscular manifestations of HIV/AIDS. *JCNMD*. 2011;13(2):68–84.

MacGowan DJ, Scelesa SN, Waldron M. An ALS-like syndrome with new HIV infection and complete response to antiretroviral therapy. *Neurol*. 2001 Sep 25;57(6):1094–1097.

CASE 12.3: PROXIMAL ARM WEAKNESS AND FASCICULATION

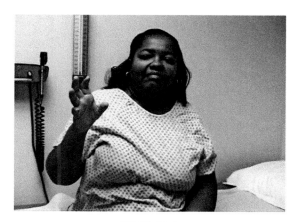

VIDEO 12.3

A 35-year-old woman presented with an 18-month history of arm weakness. Examination revealed (in addition to what is shown in the video) areflexia in the arms and legs and normal sensation. The CK level was 430 U/L. EMG revealed active denervation of the proximal and distal bilateral arm muscles and thoracic paraspinal muscles, with rare polyphasic fasciculation in the biceps muscles. Cervical MRI revealed moderate cervical spondylosis. Examination 8 years later revealed atrophy and fasciculation of the tongue, severe proximal and distal weakness of the arms, and only mild weakness of the legs. She was hyperreflexic in the legs.

The initial findings are mostly consistent with the diagnosis of:

1. BAD
2. Cervical polyradiculopathy
3. Myositis
4. Kennedy disease
5. SMA

DIAGNOSIS

- BAD is a variant of ALS where weakness starts in the proximal arm muscles, usually bilaterally.
- It is a segmental variant of progressive muscular atrophy (PMA), with only LMN lesions, so the arms are usually areflexic.
- It constitutes 10% of ALS cases, and it is important to recognize because of its relatively increased longevity compared to classic ALS.
- Age range: 35–68 years.
- Disease duration ranges from 3–11 years.
- Eventually, 33% of patients develop weakness in the legs. Bulbar dysfunction is rare.
- *Man in the barrel syndrome* refers to bilateral proximal arm weakness and atrophy without leg weakness.
- Neuromuscular causes of man in the barrel syndrome include:
  - MND
    - BAD
    - HIV-associated MND
    - Monomelic amyotrophy (MMA)
    - SMA
  - Multifocal motor neuropathy
  - Bilateral brachial plexopathy
  - Cervical polyradiculopathy (C5 and C6)
  - Myopathic:
    - Limb girdle muscular dystrophy (LGMD)
    - Facioscapulohumeral muscular dystrophy (FSHD)
    - Polymyositis (brachiocervical inflammatory myopathy)
- This case progressed to full-blown ALS few years latter, an outcome that is recognized in some cases of BAD.

CASE 12.4: PROXIMAL WEAKNESS AND AREFLEXIA

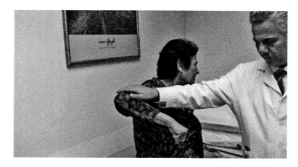

VIDEO 12.4

A 72-year-old woman presented with a 6-month history of fatigue, difficulty walking and getting in and out of the car, and inability to reach up to the kitchen shelves. She lost 25 pounds. Examination is shown in the video.

The following findings are highly consistent with the diagnosis except:

1. Proximal weakness
2. Xerostomia
3. Diminished or absent DTRs at rest
4. Facilitation of CMAP and DTRs with exercise
5. Decremental response with high-frequency stimulation

DIAGNOSIS

- Examination showed proximal weakness and areflexia that were facilitated with exercises.
- Patients with LEMS are usually referred to neuromuscular clinics due to suspected myopathy because they present with proximal weakness.
- Characteristically, strength improves with repeated testing.
- LEMS rarely starts with ocular or bulbar symptoms. If diplopia is present at the onset, one will have to rule out a concomitant MG.
- Sensory symptoms are common, and they are distal and symmetrical.
- Dry mouth, constipation, and anhidrosis are common due to dysautonomia.
- Absent DTRs are common, and their enhancement with exercise is typical.
- Weight loss is common in paraneoplastic LEMS.
- Only 50% of cases are associated with neoplasm (mainly small cell lung cancer), and they are characterized by:
  - Male predominance (70% of cases)
  - History of smoking
  - Weight loss and dysautonomia being more common
  - Life expectancy means life span
- A total of 85% of cases are associated with voltage-gated calcium channel (VGCC) antibodies.
  - VGCC antibodies occur in 40% of paraneoplastic cerebellar syndrome cases.
  - They are falsely positive in 3% of the population.
- Other paraneoplastic antibodies are commonly positive, like anti– glutamate acid decarboxylase (GAD), anti-Hu, antinicotinic acetylcholine receptor (AChR), and anti–voltage-gated potassium channel (VGKC) antibodies.
- A small CMAP amplitude that facilitates at least 100% with exercise is characteristic.
- It is advised to test for postexercise facilitation whenever a generalized decrease in CMAP is noted.
- CMAP decrement with slow (3–5-Hz) repetitive nerve stimulation (RNS), and CMAP increment with rapid (50-Hz) RNS is characteristic.
- Associated cancers include:
  - Small-cell lung cancer (SCLC)
  - Lymphoproliferative neoplasia, such as lymphoma
  - Other tumors, such as thymoma
- LEMS onset is 0.5–5 years before neoplasm is detected.
- If no neoplasm is noted initially, annual screening for cancer is advised.
- 3,4-diaminopyridine, up to 20 mg tid, is relatively effective for symptomatic treatment.
- IVIG, plasma exchange (PLEX), and rituximab are commonly used.

SUGGESTED READING

Sanders DB, Massey JM, Sanders LL, Edwards LJ. A randomized trial of 3,4 DAP in LEMS. *Neurol*. February 8;54(3):603–607.

CASE 12.5: THE PATIENT IN CASE 12.4 AFTER TREATMENT

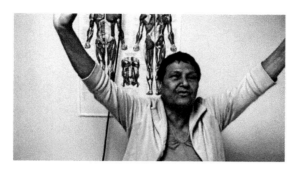

VIDEO 12.5

Video 12.5 shows the patient in Case 12.4 after treatment with plasmapheresis and rituximab. LEMS usually responds very well to:

1. 3,4-diaminopyridine
2. Intravenous immunoglobulin (IVIG)
3. Intravenous (IV) steroids
4. Plasmaphoresis
5. None of the above

DIAGNOSIS

- LEMS does not usually respond very well to any of the mentioned modalities. Most patients require substantial and prolonged use of immunosuppressive therapy to achieve modest improvement of symptoms.
- Clinical severity does not correlate with the level of VGCC antibodies.
- To increase the acetylcholine (ACh) available at the postsynaptic membrane, one will have to:
  - Reverse pathological attacks against the calcium channels in the presynaptic membrane (immunomodulatory therapy).
  - Interfere with the ACh release mechanism (symptomatic therapy)
  - Decrease ACh degradation by choline esterase
- 3,4-diaminopyridine prolongs depolarization of the presynaptic membrane and thereby increases calcium entry to the presynaptic terminal and results in release of ACh.
  - It improves both motor and autonomic dysfunction.
  - The maximum dose is 20 mg QID.
  - It is not approved by the U.S. Food and Drug Administration (FDA) yet, but it can be obtained from compounding pharmacies.
- Acetylcholinesterase (AChE) inhibitors reduce the metabolism of ACh and thereby increase the amount available at the binding sites. Alone, they have a marginal effect. They are commonly used along with 3,4- diaminopyridine.
- Immunologic therapies:
  - Are reserved for severe symptoms that do not respond to 3,4- diaminopyridine.
  - Prednisone, azathioprine, IVIG, PLEX, and rituximab are all reported to be effective to some extent.
- Cases of LEMS that are not associated with malignancies have a better survival rate.
- Treatment of the underlying malignancy may lead to remission of LEMS. Unfortunately, most of the associated cancers are not curable.

SUGGESTED READING

Maddison P, Lang B, Mills K, Newsom-Davis J. Long term outcome in Lambert-Eaton myasthenic syndrome without cancer. *J Neurol Neurosurg Psych.* 2001;70:212–217.

CASE 12.6: CHRONIC PROXIMAL ARM WEAKNESS

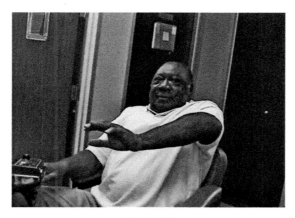

VIDEO 12.6

A 60-year-old man presented with a 15-year history of difficulty climbing stairs and lifting his arms. The symptoms gradually progressed. He had no distal weakness, reflex abnormalities, dysphagia, or abnormal sensory findings. He had three healthy daughters. The CK level was 2,200–3,300 U/ L. EMG revealed many short-duration and polyphasic units in the proximal arm and leg muscles. There were no spontaneous discharges. Muscle biopsy showed remarkable variation of fiber size and shape, many internal nuclei, split fibers, and rare necrotic fibers. There was no inflammation. Dystrophic protein immunohistochemistry and Western blot (WB) analyses were negative, including for dystrophin, sarcoglycans, dysferlin, calpain, and caveoline.

This case is classified as:

1. Polymyositis
2. Becker muscular dystrophy (BMD)
3. Myotonic dystrophy
4. LGMD, undetermined type
5. FSHD

DIAGNOSIS

- LGMD is a descriptive term that was popular when muscle diseases were classified according to the distribution of weakness. Current classification mostly relies on the genetic profile (see Box 12.6.1).

BOX 12.6.1 Classification of LGMDs

- Autosomal dominant:
  - LGMD 1A 5q22.3–31.3 Myotilin
  - LGMD 1B 1q11–21 Lamin A/C
  - LGMD 1C 3p25 Caveolin-3
  - LGMD 1D 7q36.3 DNAJB6
  - LGMD 1E 2q35 Desmin
  - LGMD 1F 7q32 TNPO3
- LGMD IG 4q21 HNRPDL
- LGMD IH 3p23
- Autosomal recessive:
  - LGMD 2A 15q15.1–21.1 Calpain-3
  - LGMD 2B* 2p13 Dysferlin
  - LGMD 2C 13q12 -Sarcoglycan
  - LGMD 2D 17q12–21.3 -Sarcoglycan
  - LGMD 2E 4q12 -Sarcoglycan
  - LGMD 2F 5q33–34 -Sarcoglycan
  - LGMD 2G 17q11–12 Telethonin
  - LGMD 2H** 9q31–33 E3-ubiquitin-ligase (TRIM 32)
  - LGMD 2I 19q13 Fukutin-related protein (FKRP)
  - LGMD 2J 2q31 Titin
  - LGMD 2K 9q31 POMT1
  - LGMD 11p 14 ANO5
  - LGMD 2M 9q31 Fukitin
- 2N 14q24 POMT2;
- 2O 1p32 POMGnT1
- 2P: 3p2 DAG1
- 2Q: 8q24 Plectin
- 2R: 2q35 Desmin
- 2S: 4q35 TRAPPC11
- 2T: 3p21 GMPPB
- 2U 7p21 ISPD
- 2V: 17q25 GAA
- 2W: 2q14 LIMS2
- 2X: 6q21 POPDC1
- 2Y: 1q25 TOR1AIPI
- 2Z: 3q13 POGLUT1

- LGMD was a kind of "wastebasket" for all nonclassified myopathies.
  - In the last decade, most of the contents of the so-called basket have become genetically oriented.
  - Molecular advances identified the muscle cell membrane's components and their functions.
  - Deficiency of various proteins lead to different types of LGMD, and the genes that code for most of these proteins have been identified. At least 35 types of LGMD are recognized.
  - While treatment of LGMD has not significantly changed in the last 50 years, the molecular and genetic basis of many of these disorders has become clear, and hopefully this is a step toward a curative approach through genetic engineering and stem cell transplantation.
- Genetic advances have limited the utility of muscle biopsy in the diagnosis of most of these disorders. If the phenotype suggests a specific type of LGMD, then a blood sample may be adequate for the diagnosis.
- Even the most exhaustive investigations leave 30% of LGMD unclassified.
- Even when a specific form of LGMD is suspected, many insurance companies deny payment because such a diagnosis does not change management. The impact of a specific diagnosis on the prognosis of the disease and genetic counseling should be emphasized to facilitate insurance payment.
- The exact defect in the presented case was not identified. The frozen muscle tissue, along with other tissue, is awaiting a new round of studies based on the newly identified defects or a research protocol. Whole exome sequencing is a useful tool for identifying types of LGMD.

SUGGESTED READINGS

Amato A, Russell J. *Neuromuscular Disorders*. New York: McGraw-Hill; 2008.

Neuromuscular.wustl.edu

CASE 12.7: PROXIMAL ARM WEAKNESS AND CARDIOMYOPATHY

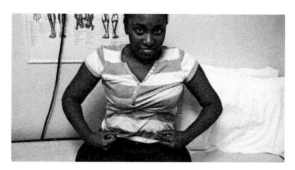

VIDEO 12.7

A 25-year-old woman presented with symptoms starting at age 10 years, which consisted of difficulty arising from chairs and lifting her arms to style her hair. Progressively, she became weaker and she developed bilateral foot drop and mild quadriceps weakness. She developed orthopnea. Echocardiogram revealed an ejection fraction of 30%. EMG revealed many short-duration polyphasic units in the proximal and distal muscles of the arms and legs and no spontaneous discharges in the thoracic paraspinal muscles. CK level was 1,840–2,300 U/L repeatedly. Muscle biopsy showed end stage muscle disease with few fibers with rimmed vacuoles.

In this case of LGMD, the following features suggest Telethonin mutation:

1. Cardiomyopathy
2. Quadriceps weakness
3. CK level
4. Vacuoles in the muscle biopsy
5. All of the above

DIAGNOSIS

- Telethonin is localized to skeletal and cardiac muscles, and it is a substrate of the serine kinase domain of titin.
- Age of onset is 9–15 years.
- Weakness affects proximal and distal leg muscles (quadriceps and tibialis anterior) and proximal arm muscles. Facial and neck muscles are usually saved.
- Patients progress to a nonambulatory state in the third or fourth decade of life in 40% of cases.
- Cardiomyopathy occurs in 50% of cases.
- The CK level increases 3-fold to 30-fold.
- Muscle pathology usually shows dystrophic myopathy, lobulated fibers, rimmed vacuoles, and absent Telethonin staining.
- Genetic advances have made muscle biopsy not the first diagnostic option. Most LGMD genetic panels test for Telethonin mutations.

CASE 12.8: PROXIMAL WEAKNESS AND HARD BREASTS

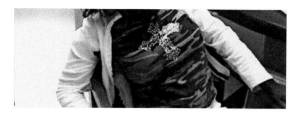

VIDEO 12.8

A 50-year-old woman with chronic renal failure has been on hemodialysis for 5 years. She had multiple gadolinium-enhanced MRIs for chronic lower back pain. She became unable to raise her arms and legs, which evolved over 6 months. She had no dysphagia. She was found to have hard skin and breasts, and her CK level and EMG were normal.

The most likely diagnosis is:

1. Scleroderma
2. Polymyositis
3. Nephrogenic systemic sclerosis (NSS)
4. Polymyalgia rheumatica
5. Systemic calcinosis

DIAGNOSIS

- NSS is a dramatic hardening of the skin and subcutaneous tissue that is reported in uremic patients who get gadolinium contrast. The deposited mucin, collagen, and elastic fibers are produced by activated fibroblasts.
- There is evidence that sclerosis goes beyond the skin and subcutaneous tissue. Muscle involvement is documented. Reported axonal neuropathy also may be related to uremia.
- The CK level is usually low due to decreased muscle mass, and EMG is either normal or shows mixed short- and long-duration units consistent with chronic myopathy.
- Other disorders with a similar picture include amyloidosis, scleromyxedema, systemic sclerosis, and eosinophilic fasciitis, and graft vs. host disease (GVHD) should be considered.
- The exact pathogenesis is not clear, and some patients with uremia develop NSS without being exposed to gadolinium.
- Renal transplantation may improve outcomes; otherwise, there is no cure for this condition. Steroids, PLEX, and IVIG are reported to cause transient improvement.

SUGGESTED READING

Keyrouz S, Rudnicki SA. Neuromuscular involvement in nephrogenic systemic fibrosis. *J Clin Neuomuscul Dis*. 2007 Dec;9(2):297–302.

CASE 12.9: RECURRENT PROXIMAL WEAKNESS AND AREFLEXIA

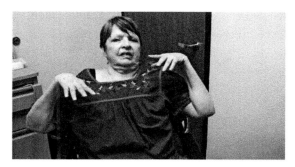

VIDEO 12.9

A 70-year-old woman presented with a 1-week history of progressive weakness of the arms and legs. Examination also showed mild distal sensory impairment and diffuse areflexia. EMG revealed moderate motor slowing with conduction block in various nerves. F responses were around 90 ms in the legs. CSF protein was 180 mg/dl. She progressed for a month and then recovered almost completely with aggressive PLEX therapy. The symptoms returned after a few months, and she continued to need monthly PLEX for maintenance of improvement.

Which of the following is correct?

1. The second episode was not related to the first one.
2. The first episode was GBS.
3. The first episode was part of CIDP.
4. The patient had GBS at both times.
5. None of the above.

DIAGNOSIS

- The diffuse loss of reflexes and severe proximal weakness and motor slowing with conduction block and elevated CSF protein level suggested an inflammatory demyelinating neuropathy. The temporal profile of the first episode suggested GBS, as there was no more progression after 4 weeks from the onset.
- Recurrence of the disease a few months later indicated that the first episode was most likely part of relapsing remitting CIDP. About 2%–4% of patients who are diagnosed initially with GBS turn out to have CIDP as the future course unfolds.
- Distinguishing acute onset CIDP from fluctuating GBS is difficult but important because steroids are contraindicated in GBS and maintenance treatment is often needed in CIDP. The prognosis and associated diseases are not the same.
- If worsening occurs within 8 weeks of the onset of symptoms, differentiation is not very easy. CIDP is usually the diagnosis if the disease relapses after 8 weeks of the first episode.
- Features that favor the diagnosis of GBS are facial involvement and dysautonomia. The presence of significant distal sensory impairment and loss of sural responses are more indicative of CIDP.

SUGGESTED READING

Ruts L, Drenthen J, Jacobs BC, van Doorn PA; Dutch GBS Study Group. Distinguishing acute-onset CIDP from fluctuating Guillain-Barre syndrome: a prospective study. *Neurol.* 2010 May 25;74(21):1680–1686.

CASE 12.10: PROGRESSIVE PROXIMAL WEAKNESS AND CARDIOMYOPATHY

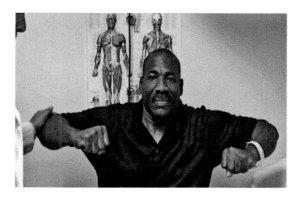

VIDEO 12.10

A 54-year-old-man presented with progressive shortness of breath of a few months' duration. His ejection fraction was 20% and coronary arteriogram was normal. The CK level was 3,400 U/L. Myocardiac biopsy revealed endomysial inflammation. A left ventricular assist device was inserted. No cause was found for the increased CK level. After several admissions to the hospital, he was found to have proximal weakness. Glucosidase acid alpha dry blood spot was negative. Muscle biopsy (Figs. 12.10.1 and 12.10.2) showed inflammatory myopathy. Extremity strength normalized with steroids, but not the congestive cardiac failure (CCF). He was placed on the cardiac transplantation list.

Which of the following are true about cardiac/pulmonary involvement in myopathy?

1. Cardiomyopathy can be the presenting feature of polymyositis.
2. Cardiomyopathy and inflammatory myopathy can be explained by dystrophinopathy.
3. Dyspnea out of proportion to muscle weakness is seen in acid maltase deficiency.
4. His muscle weakness was all due to CCF.
5. Cardiac involvement associated with polymyositis is usually responsive to treatment of the disease.

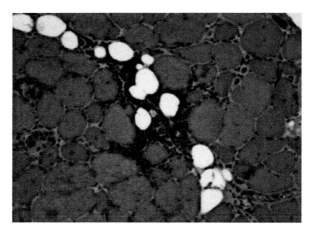

FIGURE 12.10.1 Muscle biopsy: H&E stain: endomysial inflammation.

DIAGNOSIS

- Cardiac involvement is the most common cause of death in polymyositis, and it can be the presenting feature.
- Cardiac involvement usually is not reversible, but early detection may improve the prognosis.
- In addition to inflammatory myopathies, there are other myopathies with cardiac involvement that should be considered, such as:
  - ◆ Dystrophinopathies: Inflammatory features in muscle biopsy are not uncommon. CK elevation is remarkable.
  - ◆ Pompe disease: Respiratory muscle weakness is out of proportion to proximal muscle weakness. CK level may be normal or only slightly elevated.
  - ◆ Nemaline myopathy.
  - ◆ Amyloidosis.
  - ◆ Carnitine disorders.

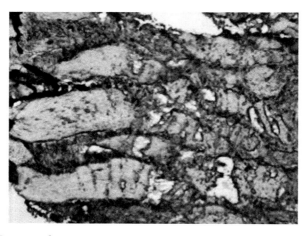

FIGURE 12.10.2 MHC 1 upregulation.

CASE 12.11: UNILATERAL-ONSET SEVERE BICEPS WEAKNESS

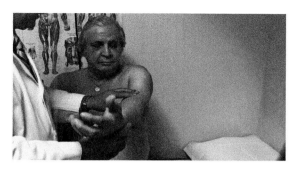

VIDEO 12.11

A 70-year-old man presented with an 8-month history of left arm weakness. He developed bilateral hip flexor weakness 6 months later. Examination is shown in the video. He had had cervical C5 laminectomy 10 years earlier. Recent cervical MRI showed moderate spondylotic changes. He had no sensory or bulbar findings.

The following possibilities should be entertained in the initial presentation:

1. Cervical polyradiculopathy
2. MMNCB
3. ALS
4. MG
5. Myopathy

DIAGNOSIS

- Asymmetric, purely motor arm weakness is a clinical challenge, especially at the onset.
- There is no myopathy with this pattern (unilateral biceps and bilateral deltoids weakness at onset), and MG causes more triceps than biceps weakness.
- C7 radiculopathy and bilateral C5 radiculopathy are a consideration, but the spread of the weakness to the legs defeated this possibility unless one considers two pathological processes.
- MMNCB is suggested by the weakness of the left biceps, but the weakness is proportional to atrophy and the reflexes are brisk. No conduction block was identified. Instead, there was diffuse denervation in the arms and thoracic paraspinal (TPS) muscles with normal sensory responses.
- Within a year, the patient developed weakness in the legs and more diffuse weakness and hyperreflexia in the arms, confirming the diagnosis of ALS, which may present very asymmetrically mimicking focal pathology.

CASE 12.12: CHRONIC UNILATERAL ARM ATROPHY

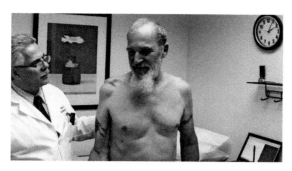

VIDEO 12.12

A 61-year-old man presented with a 2-year history of progressive, painless weakness and atrophy of the right C5 and C6 muscles with normal sensory exam and sensory responses, including the lateral antebrachial cutaneous nerve of the arm. The right biceps and Brachioradialis reflex are absent compared to the triceps reflex, which is normal. He is a smoker and recently was diagnosed with carcinoma of the prostate. MRI of the brachial plexus was negative. Cervical spine MRI revealed no significant pathology. NCS revealed normal sensory responses, including lateral antebrachial cutaneous, and median nerves. The CMAP of the left median nerves was reduced. Needle EMG revealed chronic denervation of the right supraspinatus, deltoid, biceps, and brachioradialis only. MRI of the cervical spine and brachial plexus revealed mild, age-appropriate spondylitic changes. CSF examination was normal, and the GM1 antibody titer was negative.

This is most likely a case of:

1. MMNCB
2. MMA
3. ALS
4. Cervical polyradiculopathy
5. BAD.

DIAGNOSIS

MMA

- The clinical picture is that of chronic, progressive pathology restricted to the C5 and C6 nerve roots or motor neurons clinically and by EMG.
- This is a case of MMA (monomelic amyotrophy)
- Multifocal motor neuropathy is not proximal or primarily axonal.
- Brachial plexitis is painful and does not progress for long. Sensory responses are usually affected.
- ALS does not remain that restricted 2 years from the onset. The stable nature of the symptoms is reassuring.
- BAD may present with unilateral involvement first, but such a restricted pattern is not usual (neurology March 1999). However, this entity overlaps with MMA.
- MMA (Hirayama disease) typically starts at 15–25 years of age and progresses for 1–4 years. It is often predominant in one arm, and in 97% of cases, it is distal along C8–T1 myotomes. The predominant proximal form occurs in 3% of cases. These cases may represent a different entity than Hirayama in terms of pathogenesis and prognosis. The age of onset is typically the fifth decade.
- Classification of chronic LMN disorders is still arbitrary and descriptive, and there is significant overlap among its entities. Many of these entities defy the original description and may evolve into different entities with time, so it is imperative that these cases are monitored clinically and named differently as they progress. What appears to be MMA or BAD may evolve into ALS and what appears to be progressive MND may arrest within 2–4 years.

SUGGESTED READINGS

Goudie-Devi M, Nalini A. Long term follow up of 44 patients with brachial monomelic amyotrophy. *Acta Neurol Scand*. 2003 Mar;107(3): 215–220.

Katz JS, Wolfe GI, Andersson PB, et al. Brachial amyotrophic diplegia: a slowly progressive motor neuron disorder. *Neurol*. 1999 Sep 22;53(5):1071–1076.

CASE 12.13: ARM WEAKNESS AFTER TRAUMA

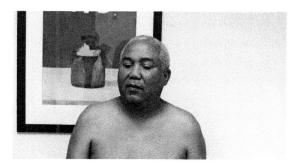

VIDEO 12.13

Sensation was normal. EMG revealed chronic distal and proximal denervation of the arm muscles. CSF examination was normal. Genetic study for SMA 5q variants was negative. Cervical spine flexion MRI was normal.

The mentioned clinical scenario is mostly consistent with:

1. BAD
2. ALS
3. Hirayama disease
4. SMA
5. West Nile viral infection

DIAGNOSIS

- A 56-year-old man with a 10-year history of slowly progressive, painless proximal and distal, symmetrical, bilateral upper-extremity weakness, atrophy, and areflexia with no sensory findings.
- Sensory responses were normal, and EMG revealed diffuse denervation in the upper extremities.
- There is no bulbar involvement or spread of weakness to the lower extremities.
- CSF exam was normal, and genetic testing for SMA was negative. Flexion cervical spine MRI was negative.
- This is a case of BAD, which is a form of slowly progressive LMN disease, most likely degenerative in nature. Preceding trauma is common in all acquired MNDs:
  - Onset: 45–76 years.
  - A total of 80% of cases are in males.
  - Sporadic.
  - The face and legs are spared.
  - The 50% survival rate is more than 5 years.
- Differential diagnosis includes:
  - Hirayama disease. This condition typically affects the C8–T1 muscles. The age of the patient and normal cervical flexion MRI are counter to this possibility.
  - SMA. There is no family history. The duration is too short. Genetic testing was negative. Rare non–5q SMA may be missed unless whole exome sequencing is obtained.
  - Kennedy disease. Genetic testing for mutations in androgen receptors was negative.
  - MMNCB. There was no conduction block. Instead, there was evidence of diffuse denervation in the upper extremities.
  - West Nile viral infection. The onset was not acute, and progression continued for a long time. CSF examination was normal.

SUGGESTED READING

Pestrok A, Chaudhry V, Feldman EL, et al. Lower motor neuron syndromes defined by patterns of weakness, nerve conduction abnormalities, and high tier of antiglycolipid antibodies. *Ann Neurol*. 1990 Mar;27(3): 316–326.

CASE 12.14: CAN'T RAISE ARMS

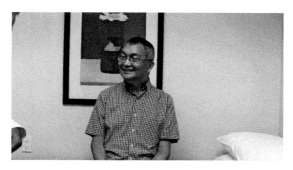

VIDEO 12.14

A 70-year-old man presented with 8 months' history of progressive, painless inability to lift his arms. Examination is shown in the video. The CK level was 420 IU/L, and EMG revealed diffuse denervation of the arms and TPS muscles. Sensory responses in the arms are normal. Cervical spine MRI showed age-appropriate spondylosis. There is no significant family history.

The most likely explanation for the areflexic arm weakness is:

1. Cervical polyradiculopathy
2. SMA
3. PMA
4. LGMD
5. Severe shoulder arthritis

DIAGNOSIS

- Progressive weakness and atrophy of the arm muscles (which may start unilaterally), with no pain or sensory symptoms and with normal sensory responses and absent DTRs, suggest MND.
- The short duration and progression suggest PMA, which is a degenerative LMN disorder.
  - It constitutes 4% of MNDs.
  - It has a better prognosis than ALS (the 5-year survival rate is 33%, as opposed to 20% for ALS). Some cases last for decades.
  - A total of 22% of cases evolve into ALS within 61 months of the diagnosis. The appearance of UMN signs such as spasticity, hyperreflexia, and upgoing toes would indicate such progression.
  - It may start in the legs or the arms, proximally or distally. In this case, it started in the proximal arm muscles, leading to what is described as *flail arms syndrome, man in the barrel syndrome*, or *BAD*.
  - PMA patients do not develop the cognitive impairment that is sometimes seen in ALS.
  - lSince SMA patients do not have UMN signs, they do not meet the El Escorial criteria (EEC) for definite or probable ALS and thus are not eligible for most ALS clinical trials.
  - The term *PMA* is not recognized by most insurance companies, and therefore these patients are deprived from the services associated with the diagnosis of ALS. So it may be more conducive to call it *LMN-dominant ALS.*
  - Management of PMA follows the same guidelines of ALS management.

SUGGESTED READINGS

Kim WK, Liu X, Sandner J, Pasmantier M, Andrews J, Rowland LP, Mitsumoto H. Study of 962 patients indicates progressive muscular atrophy is a form of ALS. *Neurol.* November 17, 2009 73(20) 1686–1692.

Wijesekera LC, Mathers S, Talman P, Galfrey C, Parkinson MH, Ganesalingham J. Natural history and clinical features of the flail arm and flail leg ALS variants. *Neurol.* 72(12): 1087–1094.

CASE 12.15: DROPPED HEAD AND WEAK ARMS

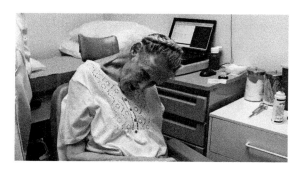

VIDEO 12.15

A 70-year-old woman with progressive arm weakness and inability to lift her head of 1 year's duration.

The most important test to establish the diagnosis of this disease is:

1. MRI of the cervical spine
2. CK level
3. EMG
4. Muscle biopsy
5. Genetic testing

DIAGNOSIS

- Progressive severe weakness of the neck extensors and upper extremities, hyperreflexia of even the weak muscles, fasciculation of the left arm muscles, mild weakness of the lower extremities, and normal sensation suggest ALS.
- The tongue was weak but did not show fasciculation or atrophy. There was no extraocular muscle weakness.
- EMG confirmed widespread denervation with normal sensory responses.
- Forced vital capacity was 0.75 liters, which was a bad prognostic sign.
- The patient met the EEC for definitive ALS.
- Prognosis was poor because of the age, bulbar involvement, and decreased vital capacity.
- Dropped head syndrome can be the presenting feature of ALS or may develop any time in the course of the disease.
- Neck muscle weakness is a bad prognostic sign because it correlates with bulbar involvement.

CASE 12.16: PROGRESSIVE ARM WEAKNESS AND ATROPHY

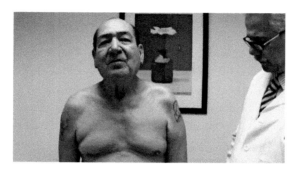

VIDEO 12.16

A 72-year-old man presented with progressive, painless left arm weakness of 6 months' duration. The CK level was normal. Left median and ulnar motor nerves were nonconductible. Sensory counterparts were normal. Needle EMG showed chronic diffuse denervation in the arms. Cervical spine MRI revealed moderate spondylosis. There was no cord compression.

The most likely diagnosis is:

1. MMNCB
2. Hirayama disease
3. BAD
4. SMA
5. Cervical polyradiculopathy.

DIAGNOSIS

- Progressive proximal and distal weakness of the left arm muscles and, to a lesser extent, the right arm muscles, fasciculation and atrophy, and increased reflexes in the weak muscles are all suggestive of ALS.
- Normal sensory responses and diffuse denervation in both arms support this diagnosis.
- Cervical spondylitic changes may have contributed to, but are unlikely the major cause of, the symptoms because of the lack of pain and radicular symptoms.
- Hirayama disease is a form of MND that starts insidiously and plateaus within 2–5 years and is more common in India and Japan. Typical cases appear much earlier in age (15–25 years) and affects the C8–T1 myotomes.
- BAD is a descriptive term for progressive, usually bilateral proximal arm weakness and atrophy (man in the barrel syndrome). It may start in one arm. It usually represents an ALS variant such as PMA and may follow a long course. In other times, it soon evolves into a full-blown ALS picture, as in this case.
- MMNCB is a consideration. Severe atrophy precluded testing for conduction block. No conduction block was found on the right side with Erb's point stimulation. Such a proximal onset and diffuse denervation and hyperreflexia are not features of this condition.

SUGGESTED READING

Jawdat O, Statland JM, Barohn RJ, Katz J, Dimachkie, MM. ALS regional variants (brachial amyotrophic diplpegia, leg amyotrophic diplegia, and isolated bulbar ALS). *Neurol Clin.* 2015 Nov;33(4):775–785.

CHAPTER 13

PROXIMAL LEG WEAKNESS

CASE 13.1: PROXIMAL WEAKNESS
WITH NONINFLAMMATORY MUSCLE NECROSIS

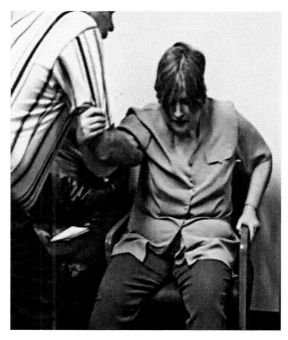

VIDEO 13.1

A 50-year-old woman had progressive, proximal weakness in the arms and legs and myalgia that evolved over a year. There was no dysphagia or weight loss. She has never been on statins. Creatine kinase (CK) levels were 5,000–7,000 U/L. Electromyography (EMG) showed small, polyphasic motor unit action potentials (MUAPs) with paraspinal fibrillations. Erythrocyte sedimentation rate (ESR) was 50 mm/hour. The antinuclear antibody (ANA) titer was negative. Multiple muscle biopsies within 1 year revealed many necrotic fibers with no inflammation. Immunohistochemical studies for muscular dystrophy (MD)–related proteins were normal. She did not respond to a 6-week course of 80 mg of prednisone. She responded to intravenous immunoglobulin (IVIG) by 50%, but only for 3 months. Repeat IVIG did not help. Response to plasma exchange (PLEX) was modest and transient. Azathioprine for 6 months did not help.

Such an acute, refractory, irritative proximal myopathy and high CK level should raise the possibility of:

1. Polymyositis
2. Signal recognition particle (SRP) antibody–associated myopathy
3. Inclusion body myositis (IBM)
4. 3-hydroxy-3-methylglutaryl-CoA reductase (HMGCR) antibody–associated myopathy
5. Metabolic myopathy

DIAGNOSIS

- The SRP antibody titer was remarkably elevated.
- SRP antibody–associated myopathy is a variant of necrotizing myopathy (NM) in which muscle fiber necrosis is the dominant feature, with little evidence of inflammation in the muscle biopsy.
- Myopathy associated with antibodies to SRP (anti-SRP myopathy) is regarded as an immune-mediated NM based on histological findings, and it has been clinically characterized by severe muscle weakness, marked elevation of serum CK levels, and poor response to corticosteroid therapy.
- It affects females more than males, and the age range is 36–51 years.
- Symmetric proximal weakness of the legs and arms evolves over months to a severe degree.
- Myalgia is common.
- No skin rash is expected.
- The CK level is usually more than 20 times normal.
- EMG shows small, polyphasic MUAPs with a variable degree of muscle membrane irritability appearing as fibrillations and positive, sharp waves, mostly in the thoracic paraspinal (TPS) muscles.
- Usually refractory to treatment.
- Muscle biopsy usually reveals evidence of myopathy with many necrotic fibers and a reduced number of endomysial capillaries. Inflammation, if present, is scarce.
- SRP antibodies are remarkably increased.
- Some experts consider this as a part of the spectrum of polymyositis, and the lack of inflammation is due to sampling error.
- In this case, the patient had three biopsies from different muscles at different times over a year, and none showed inflammation. Increased expression of MHC-1 in the nonnecrotic muscle fibers is a characteristic findings and a pathological marker of an immune mediated process.
- Prognosis is poor. Most patients end up wheelchair-bound within 2 years.
- HMGCR antibody–associated myopathy may present similarly especially in patients exposed to statins.

SUGGESTED READING

Suzuki S, Hayashi YK, Kuwana M, Tsubaraya R, Suzuki N, Nishino I. Myopathy associated with antibodies to signal recognition particle. *Arch Neurol.* 2012;69(6):728–732.

CASE 13.2: PROXIMAL WEAKNESS AND SENSORY ATAXIA

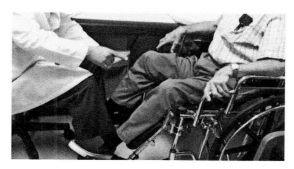

VIDEO 13.2

A 71-year-old man had progressive foot and hand numbness and severe weakness of the arms and legs. The symptoms evolved over 6–9 months. In addition to what is shown in Video 13.2, he had diffuse areflexia and sensory ataxia. Nerve conduction study (NCS) revealed severe asymmetrical slowing with prolonged distal latencies and multiple conduction blocks. The cerebrospinal fluid (CSF) protein level was 92 mg/dl. The immunoglobin G (IgG) synthesis rate was increased. Immunofixation protein electrophoresis (IFPE) revealed an immunoglobin M (IgM) spike.

Chronic inflammatory demyelinating polyneuropathy (CIDP) can be associated with all the following tumors except:

1. Lymphoma
2. HIV infection
3. Lung cancer
4. Paraproteinemias
5. Multiple myeloma

DIAGNOSIS

- CIDP is an autoimmune disease.
- The immune attack is directed against an antigen in the myelin of the peripheral nerve.
- As with other autoimmune disorders, CIDP patients are more likely to have other autoimmune diseases personally or in their family members.
- The precipitating events are not always clear, but it is believed that viral infections set the immune system off or make certain components of the myelin antigenic:
  - Viral disorders like HIV and hepatitis C
  - Monoclonal proteins
  - Graft versus host disease
  - Lymphoma
  - Interferon treatment
  - TNF-alpha antagonists: infliximab, etanercept
  - Diabetes mellitus (DM): It is not clear if DM is a risk factor for CIDP.
- Monoclonal gammopathies:
  - A total of 15%–20% of CIDP cases are associated with the M protein.
  - Before calling it *monoclonal gammopathy of unknown significance (MGUS)*, one has to rule out malignant features.
  - Malignant transformation occurs in 25% of cases at 10 years and should be watched for.
  - Features that favor MGUS are:
    - Kappa more than lambda
    - Less than 3 gm/dl protein concentration
    - No monoclonal band in the urine
    - BM plasma cells less than 5%
    - Normal skeletal survey
    - No organomegaly
- All the mentioned disorders are associated with CIDP except for lung cancer, which is associated with paraneoplastic neuropathy, which is usually sensory.

CASE 13.3: RESOLUTION OF WEAKNESS WITH PLASMA EXCHANGE (PLEX)

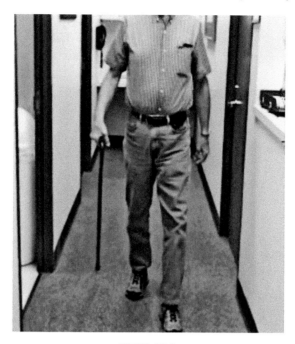

VIDEO 13.3

The patient in Case 13.2 did not respond to intravenous (IV) solumedrol and responded partially to IVIG. He responded to PLEX, and after 6 months of treatment, he walked unassisted.

What percentage of CIDP patients respond to PLEX as a first-line treatment?

1. 20%
2. 40%
3. 60%
4. 80%
5. 100%

DIAGNOSIS

- PLEX is shown in multiple studies to be as effective as IVIG for the treatment of CIDP.
- A total of 80% of virgin CIDP cases respond to PLEX, but 66% of them relapse within 2 weeks of discontinuation. All cases improve with subsequent interval PLEX therapy. Long-term immunosupression with azathioprine or similar agents may be needed to reduce reliability on PLEX.
- IVIG is used as the first line of treatment due to the perceived high risk of complications of PLEX and more availability of IVIG. A total of 50% of IVIG refractory cases respond to PLEX.
- However, with the availability of smaller and well-computerized PLEX machines that can be made available on an outpatient basis, PLEX can be given the same consideration as IVIG. The complication rate is comparable to IVIG and is mostly related to venous access.
- The best outcome measure in CIDP is proximal weakness. Sensory ataxia, distal weakness, and deep tendon reflexes (DTRs) are the last to improve.
- Patients that may benefit from PLEX more than IVIG include ones with:
  - Congestive cardiac failure: Fluid volume can be adjusted to negative during PLEX, but fluid overload can easily be precipitated by IVIG.
  - Renal impairment, especially in diabetics: IVIG may worsen renal function, but PLEX does not.
  - Recurrent deep vein thrombosis (DVT).
  - In CIDP cases, IgG monoclonal gammopathy is more responsive to PLEX than IgM monoclonal gammopathy.

SUGGESTED READING

Hahn CF, Bolton CF, Pillay N, et al. Plasma-exchange therapy in chronic inflammatory demyelinating polyneuropathy: a double blind, sham-controlled, crossover study. *Brain*. 1996;119:1055–1066.

CASE 13.4: ACUTE MYALGIA AND ELEVATED CREATINE KINASE (CK) LEVEL

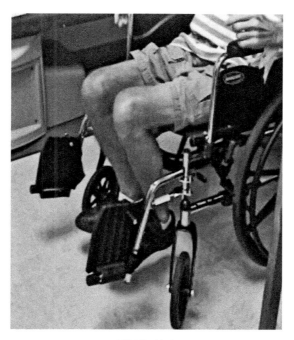

VIDEO 13.4

A 65-year-old man had subacute myalgia and progressive proximal weakness in the arms and legs. The CK level was 7,500 U/L. EMG is shown in Video 13.4. Muscle biopsy showed severe muscle necrosis with no inflammation, SRP antibodies were positive. Response to steroids was poor.

The most likely diagnosis is:

1. Polymyositis (PM)
2. Vasculitis
3. NM
4. IBM
5. Viral myositis

DIAGNOSIS

- EMG revealed many polyphasic, short-duration units with early recruitment and pseudo-myotonic discharges, suggesting an irritative myopathic process.
- NM is a separate myopathic entity that has some similarities with polymyositis.
- It is characterized by:
  - Subacute onset of myalgia
  - Progressive proximal weakness
  - Remarkably elevated CK
  - Irritative myopathic EMG pattern; TPS muscles are usually rich in PSWs, fibrillations, and pseudomyotonic discharges
- Muscle biopsy shows extensive muscle fiber necrosis with sparse or no inflammation.
  - The pathology is different from that of polymyositis by showing membrane attack complex deposition on blood vessels and depletion of capillaries. The latter finding is seen in dermatomyositis, but in this case, there is no perifascicular atrophy or endomysial inflammation.
  - Complement deposition on the blood vessels has suggested an autoimmune microangiopathy.
- SRP antibodies are elevated in at least a third of NM cases.
- NM may also be associated with mixed connective tissue disease (MCTS), statin exposure (HMGCR antibody–associated myopathy), and internal malignancy like lung cancer and renal cell carcinoma.
- Incidence of malignancy in NM is much less than in dermatomyositis.
- HMGCR antibody–associated myopathy:
  - Statin therapy: Statins may induce an autoimmune NM. A recent study showed that the number of blood vessels with C5b9 deposition and the number of patients with destroyed blood vessels is very small; therefore, another mechanism should be sought.
  - HMGCR antibodies are usually positive.
- NM is not as responsive to immunomodulation as polymyositis and dermatomyositis. A steroid-sparing agent is usually needed along with steroids. It also responds to IVIG and immunosupression. Rituximab is reported to be effective in some cases.

SUGGESTED READINGS

Mohassel P, Mammen AL. Statin-associated autoimmune myopathy and anti-HMGCR autoantibodies. *Muscle & Nerve*. 2013 Oct;48(4):477–483.

Shimizu J, Maeda M, Date H, Tsuji S. Pathological changes of necrotizing autoimmune myopathy associated with anti-signal recognition particle antibody (P07.044). *Neurology*. 2013 Feb 12;80(7).

CASE 13.5: NECROTIZING MYOPATHY (NM) RESPONDING TO TREATMENT

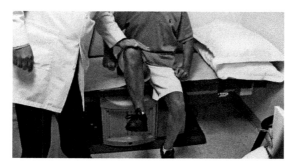

VIDEO 13.5

The patient in Case 13.4 improved after treatment with IVIG and azathioprine. He relapsed a few months later.

NM:

1. Is as responsive to treatment as polymyositis.
2. More aggressive treatment than polymyositis is frequently needed.
3. Steroids alone usually are enough to suppress the disease.
4. The treatment resistance rate is similar to that of IBM.
5. It has a strong association with internal malignancy.

DIAGNOSIS

- Some NM cases respond to treatment in a similar way as polymyositis. These probably are polymyositis cases that did not show inflammation in the muscle biopsy due to sampling errors or modification of pathology by partial treatment.
- Real cases of NM are usually more aggressive and less responsive to treatment, and often polypharmacy is needed.
- Discontinuation of myotoxic agents is crucial. Statins are the most common of these agents.
- Identification and treatment of any underlying autoimmune disease, such as systemic lupus erythematosus (SLE) or vasculitis, and malignancy is a key.
- The risk of malignancy is slightly increased.
- They respond to treatment better than IBM.
- Cases that are associated with adult-onset nemaline myopathy are usually resistant.

CASE 13.6: A DIABETIC WITH THIGH PAIN AND WEAKNESS

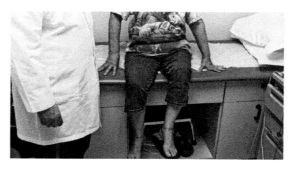

VIDEO 13.6

A 55-year-old diabetic woman presented with subacute severe right pelvic and anterior thigh pain that was followed by weakness of bilateral quadriceps, and then, 2 months later, by weakness of the hip flexors. She had no ankle or knee reflexes. Lumbosacral (LS) magnetic resonance imaging (MRI) showed mild degenerative disease of the spine. Her DM was well controlled.

The most likely diagnosis was:

1. LS polyradiculopathy
2. Vasculitis
3. Atypical polymyositis
4. Diabetic amyotrophy
5. Arachnoiditis

DIAGNOSIS

- Diabetic amyotrophy (diabetic LS radiculoplexus neuropathy) is a characteristic syndrome that mostly affects diabetic patients and constitutes about 1% of diabetic neuropathies.
- Diabetic neuropathies are grouped into two main categories according to their pathology:
  - Metabolic/ischemic mechanisms explain the most common distal sensory diabetic neuropathy.
  - Microvasculitic mechanism explains diabetic amyotrophy and diabetic third cranial nerve palsy.
- The microvasculitic type is called so because it is pathologically characterized by microvasculitis. Unlike metabolic/ischemic type, it occurs usually in well-controlled DM and in patients with minimal end organ damage (retinopathy, nephropathy).
- Other causes of thigh pain in diabetic patients should be considered, including:
  - L3 radiculopathy: The L3 nerve root is not a common target for degenerative spine disease, but it can lead to severe anterior thigh pain.
  - Diabetic muscle infarction: It usually affects the quadriceps muscles and presents with pain and indurated swelling in the anterior thigh. An MRI of the area shows infraction of the muscle.
  - Meralgia paresthetica: Severe lateral thigh pain due to entrapment of the lateral femoral cutaneous nerve is common in diabetic patients. Knee jerk and quadriceps strength are preserved.
- Diabetic amyotrophy may be as benign as a transient thigh pain that does not even reach the attention of the physician.
  - However, more than a third of the cases are bilateral, and 15% of cases lead to bilateral foot drop and 12% spread to the arms (diabetic cervical radiculoplexus neuropathy) and chest and abdomen (diabetic thoracoabdominal radiculopathy).
- The progression of pain and weakness, despite good diabetes control, causes significant frustration.
- Lumbar surgery is frequently performed due to the presence of incidental LS degenerative spine disease.
- Most cases regain significant strength, but it may take a year for recovery to start and 2 years to reach the maximum.

SUGGESTED READING

Shaibani, A., Jabari, D. Diabetic amyotrophy. *Medlink Neurol.* 2016.

CASE 13.7: QUADRICEPS WEAKNESS AND CALF HYPERTROPHY

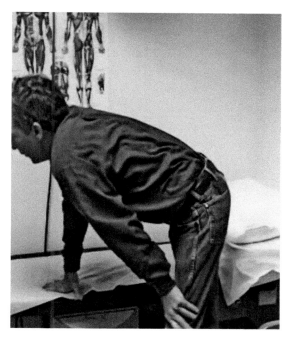

VIDEO 13.7

A 37-year-old man had stopped dancing due to his knees buckling 10 years earlier. He fell frequently. Gradually, he could not arise from a chair without using his hands. His hand grips have gotten weaker, and he was found to have large calves. The CK level was 4,100 U/L. His older brother had similar problems. His parents were healthy.

The most likely cause of quadriceps weakness in this patient is:

1. Dysferlinopathy
2. Dystrophinopathy
3. Calpainopathy
4. Myotilinopathy
5. Cavuolinopathy

DIAGNOSIS

- Becker muscular dystrophy (BMD) should be considered in the differential diagnoses of several presentations in male adults, including limb girdle weakness, isolated quadriceps weakness, asymptomatic hyperCKemia, muscle cramps, rhabdomyolysis, and cardiomyopathy. The diagnosis is not difficult when all these abnormalities exist in the same patients, but they may be present individually, and in these cases, the diagnosis is usually delayed.
- The lack of family history is not exclusive, as 10% of cases are due to spontaneous mutation.
- Calf pseudohypertophy is a useful sign.
- The most common presentation is walking difficulty after age 15 years. A total of 50% of patients lose the ability to walk by age 40.
- CK elevation is usually 20–200 times normal. EMG is myopathic in the affected muscles.
- MRI has become a popular tool in neuromuscular clinics in the last decade. It was used in this case to demonstrate the fatty replacement of calf muscles. Muscle ultrasound (US) is being increasingly used for this purpose as well.
- Muscle biopsy shows dystrophic myopathy. Dystrophin decreases uniformly or in a patchy pattern, unlike with Duchenne muscular dystrophy (DMD), where it is absent. Western blot (WB) analysis typically reveals a decreased amount or size of dystrophin.
- There is a 50% chance that the daughters of this man will be carriers. Carriers are usually asymptomatic, but they may display mild weakness or muscle pain. The more sensitive way to diagnose carriers is WB analysis, not CK or muscle biopsy. Genetic testing has become affordable enough to be the test of choice for the diagnosis of dystrophinopathies, including carrier states.
- While steroids are commonly used to treat DMD patients, they are not recommended in BMD except in very progressive cases.
- The exon-skipping strategy provides hope for treating dystrophinopathies and has demonstrated efficacy in producing traces of dystrophin in some DMD cases that formed the basis for the recent approval of eteplirsen by the U.S. Food and Drug Administration (FDA).
- An annual ECG is recommended to detect conduction abnormalities early.

SUGGESTED READING

Young CS. Exon skipping therapy. *Cell.* Nov. 17, 2016;167(5):1144.

CASE 13.8: DYSTROPHIC MYOPATHY WITH INFLAMMATION

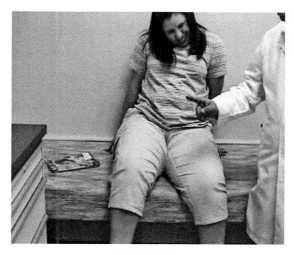

VIDEO 13.8

A 32-year-old woman had a 7-year history of difficulty climbing stairs, followed by weakness of the hand grips and frequent falls. The CK level was 3,000–9,000 U/L and EMG revealed myopathy with TPS fibrillations. Muscle biopsy revealed chronic myopathy with lymphocytic inflammatory changes. She did not respond to 6 months of IVIG treatment and 1 year of treatment with methotrexate. There is no family history. Our neuromuscular exam revealed the following medical research council (MRC) power grades: hip flexion: 0; knee extension: 3; knee flexion: 3; ankle extension: 2; ankle flexion: 3; wrist extension: 4; finger flexion: 3; neck flexion: 4; neck extension: 5. There was no facial weakness or scapular winging.

These findings are consistent with:

1. Dysferlinopathy
2. Dystrophinopathy
3. Calpainopathy
4. Caveolinopathy
5. Myotilinopathy

DIAGNOSIS

- Patients with dysferlin mutations may present to the neuromuscular clinic with different phenotypes.
- A total of 80% of cases present as progressive atrophy of the calf muscles and loss of ankle reflexes, or Miyoshi myopathy (unlike other MDs, which usually lead to hypertrophy of the calves and preserved ankle reflexes).
- A total of 8% of cases present with progressive limb girdle muscle weakness, as did this case.
- A total of 6% of cases present with asymptomatic hyperCKemia. Some cases present with weakness of the tibial muscles.
- CK is usually 35–200 times higher, and EMG shows myopathy in the weak muscles.
- Muscle biopsy shows dystrophic changes and endomysial inflammation, which may lead to erroneous diagnosis of polymyositis.
  - There is no invasion of nonnecrotic muscle fibers, and mycobacteria avium complex (MAC) deposition on the sarcolemma of the nonnecrotic fibers is noted.
  - Dysferlin immunostaining reveals sarcolemmal absence of dysferlin. Since this can be done on white blood cells (WBCs), there is no need for muscle biopsy if dysferlinopathy is clinically suspected.
- Dysferlinopathy is an autosomal-recessive (AR) disease. Symptomatic carriers with a single mutation in the dysferlin gene are reported, suggesting that some cases are autosomal dominant (AD).
- Dysferlinopathy makes up 1% of MDs. No cardiac involvement is reported.
- Calpainopathy is usually associated with eosinophilic myositic picture, but inflammation in the case was lymphocytic.
- Dysferlinopathy patients sometimes have interstitial amyloidosis in muscle biopsies, mimicking light chain amyloidosis.

SUGGESTED READING

Spuler S, Carl M, Zabojszcza J, et al. Dysferlin-deficient muscular dystrophy features amyloidosis. *Ann Neurol.* 2008 Mar;63(3):323–328.

CASE 13.9: THIGH AND INTERCOSTAL PAIN

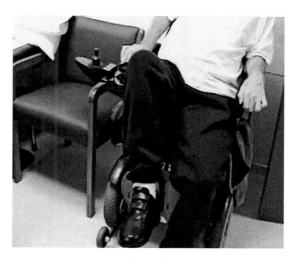

VIDEO 13.9

A 65-year-old man with well-controlled DM had developed subacute severe right pelvic and thigh pain that took him to the emergency room several times. The pain spread to the other side 2 weeks later, and he noticed weakness and atrophy of the quads. A month later, he developed bilateral foot drop, and 1 month after that, intercostal pain. EMG revealed axonal polyneuropathy and denervation of the quads. CSF protein was 85 mg/dl.

The picture is very consistent with:

1. Systemic vasculitis
2. Diabetic amyotrophy
3. Compressive LS radiculopathy
4. IBM
5. BMD

DIAGNOSIS

- Diabetic amyotrophy is a unique form of diabetic neuropathy that affects patients with type 2 DM.
- It mostly occurs in middle or later age. This can be a diagnostic challenge, especially when it is the presenting feature of diabetes.
- Usually, DM is controlled and there is no associated retinopathy or nephropathy.
- Commonly, it presents with sudden, sharp, and unilateral hip and pelvic pain, followed a couple of weeks later by weakness of the thigh extensors and gradual wasting of the quadriceps. Usually, pain subsides within weeks, but weakness and wasting continues.
- There is a wide range of severity that cannot be predicted by the age of the patient or the degree of diabetes control. Most of the time, the disease is mild and recovery occurs within months.
- In about one-third of cases, symptoms spread to the other thigh muscles.
- Surgical laminectomy is commonly done due to the presence of incidental spondylotic changes.
- Weakness may spread to the distal muscles, leading to unilateral or bilateral foot drop, raising the possibility of vasculitis.
- Patients need heavy doses of analgesia in the first few weeks, but disability from weakness becomes the main concern later.
- Progression may continue for as long as 18 months. Bulbar and respiratory involvement is rare.
- Dyck recently described a painless variant with identical pathology (Graces-Sanchez et al., 2011).
- Pathological studies confirmed that microvasculitis is the hallmark of this process, and that explains the severe pain and acute onset. A similar syndrome is noticed in nondiabetics. An offensive antigen is not identified yet.
- It is important to diagnose this condition to avoid unnecessary investigations and procedures and to be able to reassure patients about the favorable outcome. Most people significantly and spontaneously recover, but it may take 2 years for maximum recovery to happen.

SUGGESTED READING

Graces-Sanchez M, Laughlin RS, Dyck PJ, et al. Painless diabetic motor neuropathy: a variant of diabetic lumbosacral radiculoplexus neuropathy? *Ann Neurol.* 2011 Jun;69(6):1043–1054.

CASE 13.10: PROXIMAL WEAKNESS AND HYPERREFLEXIA

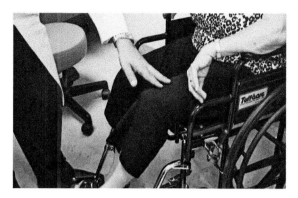

VIDEO 13.10

A 66-year-old woman had a 5-year history of difficulty climbing stairs. She was referred for a muscle biopsy because of proximal leg weakness. In addition to what is shown in the video, she had sensory ataxia and hyperreflexia in the legs. Arms had normal strength, reflexes, and sensation. She had a normal CK level and EMG of the proximal leg muscles. Cervical MRI revealed mild spondylosis with no evidence of cord compression.

The most appropriate next step is:

1. Muscle biopsy
2. Thoracic MRI
3. CSF examination
4. LS MRI
5. Brain MRI

DIAGNOSIS

- Imaging of the thoracic spinal cord is often missed in evaluation of patients with sensory ataxia and hyperreflexia due to the infrequent involvement of the thoracic cord with spondylotic myelopathy compared to the cervical cord. However, lesions such as herniated disc, meningeoma, metastatic tumors, and lymphoma are important causes of thoracic myelopathy.
- After exclusion of compression myelopathies, investigations should be directed to noncompressive causes such as B_{12} deficiency, copper deficiency, adrenal myeloneuropathy, hereditary spastic paraplegia (HSP), tropical spastic paraplegia, HIV vacuolar myelopathy, and so on.
- The confinement of the symptoms and signs to the legs raised the possibility of thoracic myelopathy despite the lack of a clear sensory level. Thoracic spine MRI did reveal T5 cord compression by a large herniated disc.
- Commonly, an MRI of the LS area is ordered to look for an explanation of sensory and motor symptoms restricted to the legs with hyperreflexia. However, the spinal cord ends at the L1 level, and pathology below that level would not explain the hyperreflexia and ataxia.

CASE 13.11: PROXIMAL WEAKNESS AFTER BONE MARROW TRANSPLANTATION

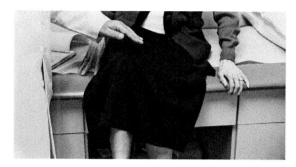

VIDEO 13.11

A 56-year-old woman had a history of allogenic bone marrow transplantation for myelofibrosis 2.5 years earlier, with previous use of tacrolimus. She presented with subacute myalgia, weakness, fever, and skin induration. Examination revealed induration of skin, moderate proximal weakness, and normal sensation. The CPK level was 1,200 U/L. EMG revealed irritative myopathy. Muscle biopsy is shown in Figures 13.11.1 and 13.11.2.

The following should be considered in the differential diagnosis:

1. Idiopathic polymyositis
2. Graft vs. host disease (GVHD)–associated polymyositis
3. Tacrolimus-induced polymyositis
4. Dermatomyositis
5. IBM

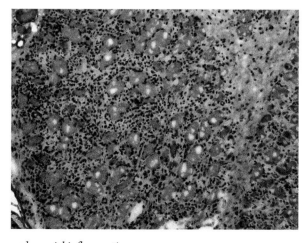

FIGURE 13.11.1 Severe endomysial inflammation.

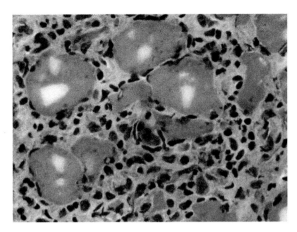

FIGURE 13.11.2 Severe endomysial inflammation.

DIAGNOSIS

- GVHD is a major complication of bone marrow transplantation, and it can mimic autoimmune diseases like scleroderma, dermatomyositis, polymyositis, medication-induced myositis, and sicca syndrome.
- GVHD develops in 33%–64% of allogenic stem cell transplantation (SCT) and is more common with advancing age and in patients with a history of acute GVHD.
- It is a multiorgan disease that can develop months to years after the graft.
- Involvement of skeletal muscles is rare (less than 1% of patients who undergo bone marrow transplantation) and even more rare when skeletal muscles are the main target. The incidence of myositis is not related to the underlying disease that was treated with bone marrow transplantation.
- A study has shown that GVHD-induced myositis developed anywhere between 7 and 55 months after transplantation.
- CK ranged between 454 and 8,400 U/L.
- EMG showed irritative myopathy.
- Muscle biopsy showed inflammatory myopathy in 80% of cases.
- All patients have involvement of other organs, mostly the skin and liver. The skin lesions are different from those of dermatomyositis. The skin is diffusely indurated and firm, with mild erythema.
- They respond well to steroids and azathioprine or cyclosporine.
- Tacrolimus is reported to cause polymyositis, but no skin lesions are reported. Yet, it may be better to replace it with another immunosuppressive agent in this case.
- Pathological identification of the type of cells in the muscle lesions can determine if the cells are donor related, thus confirming GVHD.

SUGGESTED READINGS

Allen JA, Greenberg SA, Amato AA. Dermatomyositis-like muscle pathology in patients with chronic graft-ver-sus-host disease. *Musc Nerve*. 2009;40:643–647.

Stevens AM, Sullivan KM, Nelson JL. Polymyositis as a manifestation of chronic graft-versus-host disease. *Rheumatol*. 2003;42:34–39.

CASE 13.12: PROXIMAL WEAKNESS AND UNEXPECTED MUSCLE BIOPSY FINDINGS

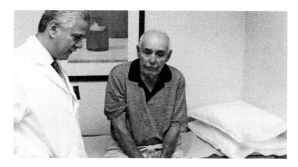

VIDEO 13.12

A 77-year-old man presented with a 1-year history of weakness in the arms and legs and numbness in the feet. He was on atorvastatin for years. He drank three glasses of wine every evening. He had multiple decompressive LS and cervical spine surgeries. Examination revealed weakness of the hip flexors and deltoids, sensory impairment in the feet, and absent ankle reflexes. The CK level was normal. IFPE revealed IgG lambda spikes. ANA was negative and SR was normal. EMG revealed 30% short-duration units in the hip flexors, NCS revealed axonal neuropathy, and CSF was normal.

The proximal weakness is likely related to:

1. CIDP
2. Radiculopathy
3. Myopathy
4. Statin-induced autoimmune myopathy
5. Alcohol-related myopathy.

Muscle and nerve involvement is a feature of all of the following except:

1. Vasculitis
2. Amyloidosis
3. Statin therapy
4. Alcoholism
5. Sarcoidosis

DIAGNOSIS

- Proximal weakness and myopathic EMG are consistent with proximal myopathy. Sensory impairment in the feet and absent ankle reflexes suggested neuropathy, which was confirmed by NCS to be axonal.
- The patient drank three glasses of wine a night. This may have contributed, but it is unlikely to be the sole cause.
- The appearance of neuropathic symptoms with myopathic symptoms suggested an inflammatory condition such as vasculitis or a systemic condition such as amyloidosis or sarcoidosis. He had no pain, renal impairment, or respiratory symptoms. ANA was negative and SR was normal.
- IgG lambda spikes can be normal in 3% of the elderly but can lead to amyloidosis.
- Remotely, the proximal weakness may be secondary to CIDP, but NCS did not support this possibility.
- While statins may worsen muscle diseases, I doubt that the whole symptomatology in this case is related to them. Increased risk of neuropathy by statin is controversial.
- The patient has had multiple back surgeries. Lumbar polyradiculopathy may cause patchy proximal weakness in the legs, but he has no radicular symptoms and EMG showed no denervation.
- Left vastus lateralis muscle biopsy revealed Congo red positive material in the vascular wall (amyloid deposits) (Fig 13.12.1). There were no myopathic changes. Mass spectrometry revealed peptide sequences consistent with transthyretin (TTR) amyloidosis. Genetic sequencing of the *TTR* gene revealed no mutations. This was considered a wild TTR amyloid deposition in the muscles. He was treated with diflunisal. It was not clear if deposition of amyloid in the muscles was the cause of weakness. No other causes of myopathy were found.

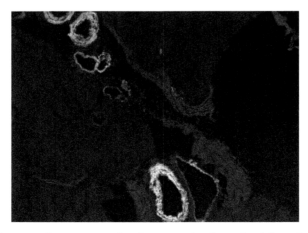

FIGURE 13.12.1 Left biceps uscle tissue stained with congo red and visualized through a rhodamine filter under fluorescent light (400X)

CASE 13.13: WEAKNESS YEARS AFTER THYMECTOMY

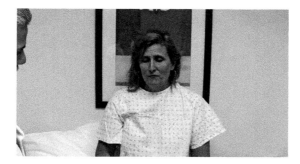

VIDEO 13.13

A 49-year-old woman with a history of thymoma that was resected in 2006 and treated with radiation presented 10 years later with leg and arm weakness. She had no diplopia, ptosis, or dysarthria. RNS test of the left SAN is shown in Figure 13.13. 1.

The Figure 13.13.1 is highly suggestive of:

1. MG
2. LEMS
3. Myopathy
4. Recurrence of thymoma
5. None of the above

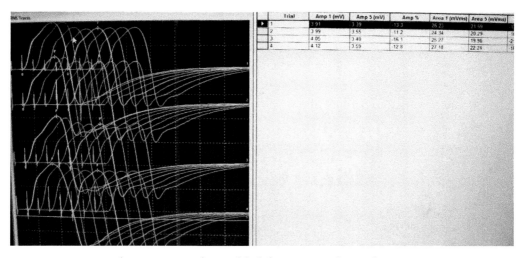

FIGURE 13.13.1 image showing tracing of RST of the left trapezius with 3 Hz frequency.

DIAGNOSIS

- This patient presented with a 4-month history of fluctuating, slowly progressive proximal weakness in the arms and legs.
- Physical examination revealed significant proximal weakness in the arms and legs with fatigability of the triceps muscles.
- RNS of the left SAN revealed a decremental response with postexercise exhaustion.
- Binding acetylcholine receptor (AChR) antibody titer was 32.9 no/L. The CK level was 74 U/L. EMG revealed no myopathic findings.
- These findings were very strongly suggestive of generalized myasthenia gravis (MG) despite the lack of ocular findings.
- It is well reported that MG may follow thymectomy for tumors. The thymus plays an inhibitory role on a subset of lymphocytes, and release of that inhibition predisposes thymectomyzed patients to autoimmune diseases like neuromyelitis optica (NMO), SLE, and MG.
- LEMS may present like myopathy, but the patient denies weight loss and her reflexes are normal. LEMS screening revealed no facilitation with exercise.
- Polymyositis is possible alone or with myasthenia. CK levels and EMG were normal.
- A total of 5 %–10% of patients with myasthenia present with purely proximal weakness similar to myopathy.
- Since myasthenia and related syndromes (LEMS, CMS, etc.) may present with a myopathy picture, it is recommended to perform RST with at least atypical or refractory myopathies.

CASE 13.14: FATIGUE AND WEAKNESS SINCE CHILDHOOD AND A WES SURPRISE

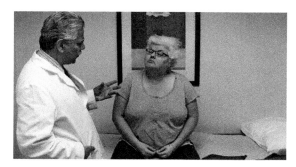

VIDEO 13.14

A 55-year-old woman presented with proximal weakness in the legs since childhood and extreme fatigue that has gradually progressed as she grew up. She had to use a wheelchair to walk from the elevator to the clinic (a distance of 200 feet). Her exam revealed proximal leg and arm weakness. The CK level was normal and EMG showed nonirritative myopathy. Because of her fatigue, RST was done on the left SAN and revealed a 12% decrement that repaired and then exhausted after exercise. Forced vital capacity was 1.7 L with moderate restriction. Family history was negative except for frequent falls by the mother. There was no myotonia, scapular winging, or dysphagia. There were no exercise-induced muscle cramps, nor was there calf atrophy or hypertrophy. Muscle biopsy revealed nonspecific, mild myopathic findings. Such a chronic story with extreme fatigue, normal CK, and possibly positive family history suggested a hereditary syndrome. Response to steroids is not specific. The limb girdle muscular dystrophy (LGMD) genetic panel was negative. Decremental response to RST suggested a postsynaptic neuromuscular disorder. Whole-exome sequencing revealed a pathogenic homozygous mutation of the DOK7 protein.

The following is a feature of DOK7 congenital myasthenic syndrome (CMS):

1. It affects a subunit of postsynaptic acetylcholine (ACh) receptors.
2. It responds well to pyridostigmine.
3. It responds well to beta agonists like salbutamol.
4. It is associated with tubular aggregated in muscle biopsy.
5. It is an adult disease.

DIAGNOSIS

- The patient has DOK7 CMS, which is a postsynaptic neuromuscular junction (NMJ) disorder due to mutation of the postsynaptic protein DOK7, which is important for the maintenance of the synaptic structure.
- This kind of CMSa can be worsened by acetylcholinesterase inhibitors.
- Response to 3,4-diaminopyridine is variable.
- Dramatic response to ephedrien and salbutamol is consistently reported.
- Tubular aggregates in the muscle biopsy is not a feature.
- This patient responded very well to salbutamol and did not need to use the wheelchair anymore. Her response to prednisone is interesting.
- The clinical picture of CMS with *DOK7* mutations is highly variable.
  - The age of onset may vary between birth and the third decade.
  - Most patients display a characteristic "limb-girdle" pattern of weakness, with a waddling gait and ptosis, but without ophthalmoparesis.
  - Respiratory problems are frequent.

SUGGESTED READINGS

Burke G, Hiscock A, Klein A, Niks EH, Main M, Manzur AY, Ng J, de Vile C, Muntoni F, Beeson D, Robb S. Salbutamol benefits children with CMS due to DOK7 mutations. *Neuromuscul Disord* (2013) 23(2): 170–175.

Müller JS. Phenotypical spectrum of *DOK7* mutations in congenital myasthenic syndromes. *Brain* (2007); 130(6): 1497–1506.

CASE 13.15: TOE WALKING SINCE CHILDHOOD

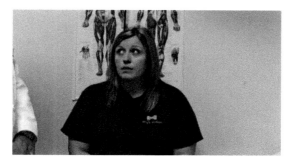

VIDEO 13.15

A 31-year-old woman presented who has had difficulty walking since childhood. She walked on her toes and had surgical lengthening of the Achilles tendons. Over the last 10 years, she has developed progressive myalgia and painless proximal and distal weakness in the legs and proximal weakness in the arms. Hypertrophy of extensor digitorum brevis (EDB) suggests myopathic foot drop. EMG revealed generalized, nonirritative myopathic process with no myotonic discharges or fibrillations in the TPS muscles or neuropathy. She had no scapular or facial involvement. She has no myotonia or facial wasting to suggest myotonic dystrophy. The CPK level was 1,062 IU/L. Muscle biopsy findings are shown in Figure 13.15.1. She has two daughters, 10 and 14 years old; one of them complained of muscle cramps during activity similar to what her mother had when she was a child. Patient's grandfather was wheelchair bound. No more information was available. She was not sure of her ancestry.

The following muscle disease is the least likely to fit this description:

1. A carrier case of dystrophinopathy
2. Dysferlinopathy
3. Titinopathy
4. FSHD
5. Myofibrillar myopathy (MFM)

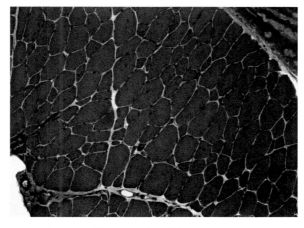

FIGURE 13.15.1 left bicep muscle biopsy. H&E stain (100X)

DIAGNOSIS

- Muscle biopsy showed chronic nonspecific myopathy.
- Statistically, a carrier case of dystrophinopathy is the most common possibility. The high CK reading supports this. The lack of family history is not atypical, as sporadic mutations of the dystrophin gene explain 30% of cases. The disease of her grandfather, if related to her myopathy, would be exclusive of dystrophinopathy.
- MFM is suggested by bilateral foot drop. However, there is no family history to support this AD disease. There is no indication of cardiac involvement. There are no spontaneous discharges in the EMG.
- Dysferlinopathy is suggested by distal weakness and high CK. Although Miyoshi myopathy usually is posterior, tibial syndrome is also described.
- FSHD is suggested by foot drop, but such a symmetrical proximal weakness in the arms and legs and remarkably elevated CK level are atypical of this disease.
- Genetic testing revealed homozygous mutations of the *Titin* gene.
- Heterozygous pathogenic mutations of the *Titin* gene on chromosome 2q31.2 is responsible for Udd myopathy (From Finland), which is late onset and AD.
- Homozygous mutations of the same gene lead to LGMD2J, in early-onset form and with a more severe and generalized myopathy.

SUGGESTED READING

Evilä A, Palmio J, Vihola A, et al. Targeted next-generation sequencing reveals novel TTN mutations causing recessive distal titinopathy. *Mol Neurobiol.*;2016 Oct 29;25(Suppl2):S282–S283.

CASE 13.16: CHRONIC PROXIMAL LEG DENERVATION

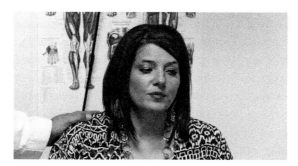

VIDEO 13.16

A 40-year-old woman in the video. The CPK level was 91 IU/L. EMG revealed chronic neurogenic changes [motor unit potential (MUP) amplitude of 9 mv and duration of 15 ms] in the anterior thigh muscles and hip flexors, with normal sensory responses and motor NCS. The MRI of the LS spines revealed no significant pathology.

Differential diagnosis includes all of the following except:

1. Spinal muscular atrophy, proximal type
2. Progressive muscular atrophy
3. Bulbospinal muscular atrophy
4. Adult-onset Tay-Sachs disease
5. Sandhoff disease

DIAGNOSIS

- Bilateral proximal denervation with normal sensory responses and LS spines MRI suggest MND. The chronic course suggests any of the mentioned options. Kennedy disease is X linked and is vanishingly rare in female. The lack of bulbar involvement is very atypical.
- Genetic testing for 5q and non-5q spinal muscular atrophy (SMA) types was negative.
- Whole exome sequencing revealed a compound heterozygous mutation of the *HEXB* gene that is expected to be pathogenic.
  - HEXB enzyme activity in the WBCs was decreased to below 20%, confirming the diagnosis of Hexsosaminidase B deficiency (Sandhoff disease). The *HEXA* gene was normal.
- Sandhoff disease is a rare disease and even more rare in adults than in children.
  - It is a progressive neurodegenerative disorder characterized by an accumulation of GM2 gangliosides, particularly in neurons.
  - It is clinically indistinguishable from Tay-Sachs disease.
  - In infants, it causes weakness, intellectual impairment, deafness, cherry red spot in the retina, and organomegaly.
  - In adults, it causes spinocerebellar ataxia (SCA), MND, and sensorimotor neuropathy. Increased risk of dementia is reported.
- The patient enrolled in a National Institutes of Health (NIH) clinical trial.
- Classification of hereditary MNDs is beyond the scope of this book.
- Chronic proximal symmetrical MND of genetic etiology is usually caused by mutation of:
  - *SMN* gene: 5q; recessive,
  - Androgen receptor mutation (Bulbospinal muscular atrophy or Kennedy disease)
  - The Hexsosaminidase A or B gene

SUGGESTED READINGS

Frey, LC, Ringel SP, Filley CM. Natural history of cognitive dysfunction in late-onset GM2 gangliosidosis. *Arch. Neurol.* 62:989–994, 2005.

Jamkozik Z, Lugowska A, Maczewska J, et al. Late onset GM2 gangliosides mimicking spinal muscular atrophy. *Gene.* 2013;527:679–682.

CASE 13.17: CHRONIC LEG WEAKNESS

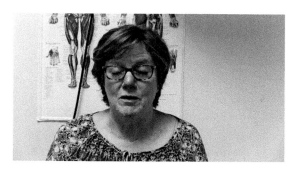

VIDEO 13.17

A 54-year-old woman presented with a 15-year history of weakness of the legs in the demonstrated fashion. She had no dysphagia, dyspnea, muscle cramps, or sensory symptoms. Examination is shown in the video. Her medical history is remarkable for hyperparathyroidism treated with para-thyroidectomy. She had three healthy brothers and two healthy daughters. The CK level was 340 IU/L. EMG revealed high amplitude (9–10 MV) unites with long duration and increased firing frequency in all extremities, proximally and distally. Genetic testing for *SMN* gene mutations was negative.

The most likely diagnosis is:

1. ALS
2. Postpolio syndrome.
3. SMA
4. Progressive muscular atrophy
5. West Nile virus (WNV)–associated, poliolike syndrome.

DIAGNOSIS

- Chronic symmetrical purely motor proximal weakness in adults is usually myopathic.
  - Mild CK elevation does not distinguish neurogenic from myopathic weakness, but EMG does.
  - Needle EMG clearly demonstrates high-amplitude, long-duration, fast-firing units, usually diffusely.
- SMA is a group of disorders characterized by accelerated genetically programmed death of motor neurons.
  - Most of the cases are due to mutations of *SMN* located in 5q13.
  - No 5q13 types of SMA are diagnostically challenging.
    - They can be AD, AR, or X linked. They may start at any age, and they may start in the arms or the legs.
    - An adult-onset, non-5q form of SMA characterized by proximal AD disease is caused by mutation of vesicle-associated membrane protein/synaptobrevin-associated membrane protein B (VABP).
      - It is located on chromosome 20q 13.32. Average age of onset is 49 years.
- The other given diagnostic options are not compatible with such a gradual onset and slow progression.

SUGGESTED READING

Nishimura, AL, Mitne-Neto M, Silva HCA, et al. A mutation in the vesicle-trafficking protein VAPB causes late-onset spinal muscular atrophy and amyotrophic lateral sclerosis. *Am. J. Hum. Genet.* 2004;75:822–831.

CASE 13.18: MUSCLE WEAKNESS AND CONSANGUINEOUS MARRIAGE OF THE PARENTS

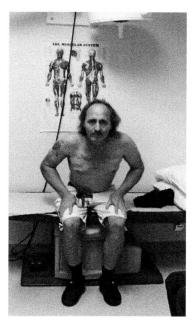

VIDEO 13.18

A 55-year-old man with a 25-year history of difficulty climbing stairs and standing up from a chair. Gradually, he developed difficulty lifting his arms. He denied dysphagia. In his 20s, he had testicular cancer, which was treated with cisplatinum. He developed congestive cardiac failure (CCF) and cardiac arrhythmias 15 years later. He had a pacemaker and then cardiac transplantation, and 5 years later, he developed diabetes mellitus (DM) type 2. He had 2 sisters; one died in her 50s from similar symptoms of progressive muscle weakness. Consanguineous marriage of his parents was reported. Examination is shown in the video. The CK level was 1,100 IU/L. EMG revealed sensorimotor neuropathy and nonirritative myopathy.

This is most likely a case of which of the following:

1. LGMD 2B
2. LGMD 2A
3. LGMD 2E
4. BMD
5. FSHD

DIAGNOSIS

- The chronic course, family history, and limb girdle distribution suggest LGMD. Despite scapular winging and family history, the lack of facial weakness and the presence of cardiac involvement argue against FSHD.
- Despite significant hyperCKemia and cardiac involvement, the involvement of the sister argues against DMD.
- LGMD 2A and 2B do not cause cardiomyopathy. LGMD2B starts at an earlier age.
- Homozygous pathogenic mutation was found in the *SGCB* gene (LGMD2E).
- Sarcoglycanopathies are AR LGMDs and represent 20%–25% of all LGMDs.
  - Clinical picture varies from DMD-like dystrophy to mild weakness.
  - LGMD2E is a rare form of sarcoglycanopathy.
    - In the vast majority of cases, weakness is proximal, with the legs affected more severely.
    - Axial and distal weakness occurs as the disease progresses.
    - Contractures of tendons is common.
    - Cardiac involvement occurs in 50% of cases, usually in a form of dilated cardiomyopathy; and 28% of patients develop arrhythmias and conduction abnormalities.
    - Severe respiratory involvement occurs in 19% of cases.

SUGGESTED READING

Semplicini, C, Vissing J, Dahlqvist JR, et al. Clinical and genetic spectrum in limb-girdle muscular dystrophy type 2E. *Neurol.* 2015;84(17):1772–1781.

CHAPTER 14

QUADRICEPS WEAKNESS

CASE 14.1: SEVERE THIGH PAIN AND WEAKNESS

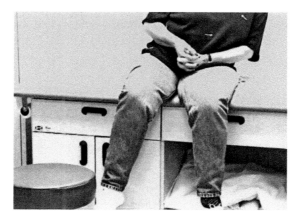

VIDEO 14.1

A 43-year-old nondiabetic woman had woken up with severe, burning pain in the left thigh that mandated an emergency room visit. The pain was barely responsive to hydrocodone every 4 hours. She started losing her balance 2 weeks later. A few weeks later, she had weakness of the right leg. Examination is shown in the video. She also had absent knee jerks. Lumbar spine magnetic resonance imaging (LS MRI) was not remarkable. HbA1c was 5.5%. Electromyography (EMG) showed active denervation of the bilateral anterior and medial thigh muscles and glutei. Lumbosacral (LS) paraspinal muscles also showed fibrillation and positive, sharp waves. Nerve conduction study (NCS) revealed a mild sensory neuropathy.

The features suggest:

1. Nondiabetic LS radiculoplexus neuropathy (LSRPN)
2. Compressive LS polyradiculopathy
3. Diabetic polyneuropathy
4. Herpes zoster radiculitis
5. Paraneoplastic syndrome

DIAGNOSIS

- Nondiabetic LSRPN is pathologically and clinically similar to its diabetic counterpart, diabetic amyotrophy (diabetic LS radiculoplexus neuropathy [DLSRPN]) (Table 14.1.1). It is due to microvasculitis of the LS plexus.
- The pain is usually severe and is caused by nerve infarction, and it may need high doses of potent analgesics for control.
- As the pain subsides, atrophy appears in the affected areas, mostly the anterior thigh muscles.
- While most cases are represented by a mild, unilateral, self-limiting thigh pain, in one-third of cases, it spreads to the other side, and in 15% of cases, it spreads distally, leading to unilateral or bilateral foot drop.
- In 12% of cases, weakness spreads to the arms.
- A total of 15% of cases are associated with severe, intercostal pain (thoracoabdominal radiculopathy).
- Denervation detected by EMG is usually more diffuse and severe than expected clinically.
- The presence of some demyelinating features in NCS may lead to diagnostic confusion with chronic inflammatory demyelinating polyneuropathy (CIDP).
- Steroids may reduce pain and enhance cooperation with physical therapy, especially early in the disease course, but they do not change the natural history.
- Management relies on pain control and rehabilitation.
- Weakness usually resolves spontaneously, but it may take 2 years for maximum recovery to happen, and some residual deficit is common.

TABLE 14.1.1 COMPARISON BETWEEN DLSRPN AND NONDIABETIC LSRPN

Mean Value	DLSRPN	LSRPN
Age (years)	65	69
Sex (male-to-female %)	60%	51%
Onset to bilateral (years)	3.0	3.0
Weight change (pounds)	−30	−15
CSF protein (mg/ml)	89	66
Pain at onset	81%	85%
Foot weakness	36%	36%
Thigh weakness	54%	57%
Wheelchair dependence	48%	49%
Walker or cane usage	42%	49%
Multifocal degeneration	57%	65%
Perivascular inflammation	100%	100%
Mural inflammation	45%	51%
Hemosiderin in macrophages	57%	53%

CASE 14.2: THIGH WEAKNESS AND BIG CALVES

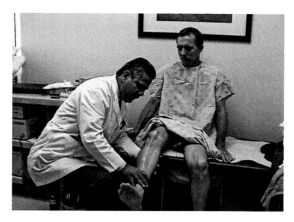

VIDEO 14.2

A 40-year-old man presented with slowly progressive weakness of the legs and frequent falls. Examination is shown in the video. Sensation was normal and knee reflexes were absent. The creatine kinase (CK) level was 4,500 U/L. Electrocardiography (ECG) revealed second-degree heart block. EMG revealed many small polyphasic units in the proximal muscles with early recruitment. Family history was negative. A muscle biopsy revealed remarkable variation of fiber size, with features of regeneration.

Quadriceps atrophy and calf hypertrophy are typically seen in:

1. Inclusion body myositis (IBM)
2. Becker muscular dystrophy (BMD)
3. Myofibrillar myopathy
4. Myotonic dystrophy
5. Facioscapulohumeral muscular dystrophy (FSHD)

DIAGNOSIS

- BMD is a mild form of dystrophinopathy inherited as an X-linked, recessive disease.
- A total of 10% of cases are due to spontaneous mutation.
- While most cases present with a limb girdle pattern of weakness, some cases show a predilection to the quadriceps muscles.
- Calf hypertrophy helps to differentiate BMD from other causes of quadriceps atrophy, like IBM.
- Late onset and slow progression differentiate BMD from Duchenne muscular dystrophy (DMD).
- In some cases, the only presentation is cardiomyopathy, myoglobinurea, myalgia, or asymptomatic hyperCKemia.
- Cardiac involvement is common.
- CK is usually elevated by 20–200.
- Immunostaining with antibodies against carboxy terminal of dystrophin is positive (unlike with DMD).
- Mothers or daughters of patients are obligate carriers.
- CK level is not sensitive for carrier state detection (50% normal CK). Genetic testing is the most reliable method for carrier detection.
- Stem cell replacement therapy is being evaluated in animals.
- Unlike with DMD, steroids are not routinely recommended to treat BMD.

CASE 14.3A: THIGH WEAKNESS

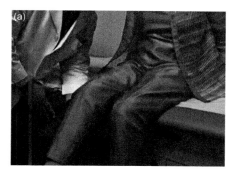

VIDEO 14.3A

A 61-year-old nurse presented with a 7-year history of poor balance and frequent falls and dysphagia. Examination is shown in the video. Knee reflexes were absent. There was no scapular winging. The CK level was 630 U/L. EMG revealed long and short duration motor unit potentials (MUPs) in the proximal leg and arm muscles. NCS was normal. LS MRI was normal for the patient's age.

The most relevant finding in the muscle biopsy would be:

1. Abnormal dystrophin staining
2. Chronic denervation of the quadriceps
3. Red-rimmed vacuoles
4. Lobulated fibers
5. Periodic acid–Schiff (PAS)–positive vacuoles

DIAGNOSIS

- The muscle biopsy shows red-rimmed vacuoles (Fig. 14.3.1).
- IBM is the most common myopathy after age 50 years.
- Insidious onset: A typical case is diagnosed 5 years after the onset of symptoms.
- The most common presentation is loss of balance due to buckling of the knees from quadriceps weakness.
- Patients tend to modify their physical activities to accommodate weakness for years before seeking medical advice.
- Weakness of hand grip is common and could be asymmetrical. Weakness of the finger flexors and poor hand grip may lead to diagnostic confusion with myotonic dystrophy.
- Dysphagia occurs in two-thirds of cases, and facial weakness in half of cases, leading to confusion with FSHD.
- Different patterns of presentations exist, and some patients present with only distal arm weakness, while others present with mainly quadriceps weakness.
- CK is usually mildly elevated.
- EMG can be confusing due to the presence of long- and short-duration units together (mixed potentials), which need some experience to sort out. Otherwise, a diffuse denervation will be erroneously diagnosed, adding more to the clinical suspicions of amyotrophic lateral sclerosis (ALS) on the basis of hand weakness and dysphagia.
- As opposed to ALS, the weakness of the finger flexors leads to atrophy of the muscles in the volar aspect of the forearms instead of the intrinsic muscles of the hands.
- IBM is characterized pathologically by red-rimmed vacuoles (Fig. 14.3.1) and eosinophilic cytoplasmic inclusion bodies (ECIBs), along with chronic myopathic and inflammatory features.
- Early in the course of the disease, inflammatory features in the muscle biopsy predominate; therefore, the diagnosis of polymyositis is erroneously and commonly made. In the later stages of the disease, degenerative features such as red-rimmed vacuoles and ECIB predominate.

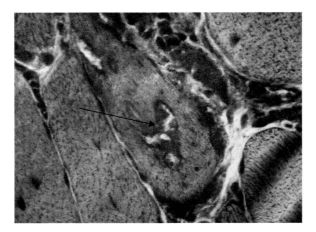

FIGURE 14.3.1 Modified Gomori trichrome stain (400X).

CASE 14.3B: IBM DIAGNOSTIC CRITERIA WERE MET 15 YEARS LATER

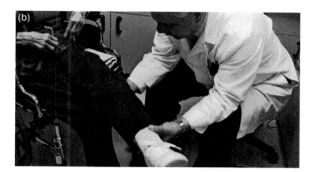

VIDEO 14.3B

A 76-year-old nurse had been diagnosed with IBM 15 years earlier. Diagnosis was based on chronic progressive quadriceps weakness and finding of cytoplasmic eosinophilic inclusion bodies (Fig. 14.3.2), red-rimmed vacuoles, and congophilic material on muscle biopsy. Initially, her phenotype was not typical, but gradually she evolved into a typical IBM phenotype.

The following muscles are commonly affected in typical IBM, except:

1. Facial muscles
2. Pharyngeal muscles
3. Quadriceps
4. Finger flexors
5. Cardiac muscle

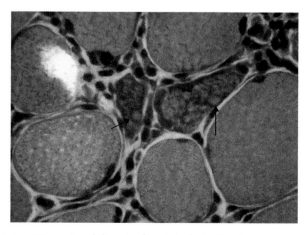

FIGURE 14.3.2 H&E stain. 400x. eosinophilic cytoplasmic inclusion bodies.

DIAGNOSIS

- The typical case of IBM presents with several years' history of loss of balance and falls due to quadriceps weakness, and it usually affects white males after age 50 years.
- Simultaneously, there is weakness of the finger flexors, and sometimes bilateral foot drop.
- A typical pattern of weakness affects quadriceps more than iliopsoas, and biceps more than deltoids.
- Facial weakness occurs in 30% of cases, and dysphagia occurs in the majority of cases at some point, although it can be the presenting feature.
- CK is usually mildly elevated, and EMG shows mixed short- and long-duration potentials, indicating chronicity.
- Muscle biopsy usually shows chronic myopathic findings with eosinophilic cytoplasmic inclusions (ECIs), red-rimmed vacuoles, congophilia, and endomysial inflammation in variable proportions and to variable degrees.
- The following atypical features are not uncommon, at least at the time of presentation, but eventually, most of the diagnostic criteria are met:
  - Polymyositis-like phenotype
  - Isolated quadriceps weakness
  - Isolated finger flexor weakness
  - Severe dysphagia at presentation
  - CK higher than 10 times normal
  - Polymyositislike pathology (leading to misdiagnosis of polymyositis)
- It seems that the initial inflammatory phase is associated with high CK levels and severe endomysial inflammation, but a few years later, a degenerative phase supervenes and is characterized by mild CK elevation and the presence of vacuoles and inclusions in the biopsy.
- The most common cause of refractory "polymyositis" is IBM.
- No clinical trial has demonstrated the efficacy of steroids, IVIG, chemotherapeutic agents, or interferon in IBM.

CASE 14.4: BIG BUT WEAK CALVES

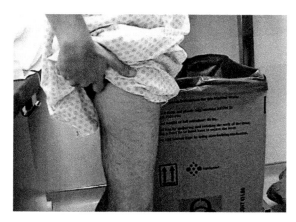

VIDEO 14.4

A 26-year-old man presented with gradually evolving difficulty climbing stairs. Examination is shown in the video. The CPK level was 5,000 U/L. EMG revealed many short-duration polyphasic units in the proximal and distal arm and leg muscles. None of his three brothers were affected.

Calf hypertrophy is a feature of all the following except:

1. BMD
2. Amyloid myopathy
3. Charcot-Marie-Tooth disease (CMT) type 1A
4. Miyoshi myopathy
5. Neuromyotonia

DIAGNOSIS

Hypertrophy of the calves is commonly seen in neuromuscular clinics.

It is clinically useful to differentiate between several types of calf hypertrophy, as follows:

- Hypertrophy due to replacement of muscle by other tissue (pseudohypertrophy). Depending on the type of tissue, the following subtypes are recognized:
  - Fatty tissue replacement, such as in dystrophinopathies
  - Amyloid structure replacement, such as in systemic amyloidosis
  - Glycosaminoglycans, such as in hypothyroidism. In this condition, there is also an increase in the endomysial connective tissue.
  - D-glycogen deposition: debrancher enzyme deficiency
- Reinnervation: Chronic denervating conditions usually are associated with significant reinnervation and sometimes hypertrophy, such as CMT and S1 radiculopathy.
- Due to hyperactivity of muscle fibers such as in neuromyotonia
- Myotonic disorders such as myotonia congenita (MC)
- Sarcoglycanopathy (LGMD 2C-F), telethoninopathy (LGMD 2G), and LGMD 2I (fukutin-related protein)
- Focal enlargement: neoplasm, inflammation

Muscle sonography provides an objective measurement of calf girth and can determine the type of hypertrophy. Calf hypertrophy and thigh weakness are typically seen in dystrophinopathies.

Miyoshi myopathy is characterized by calf atrophy.

SUGGESTED READINGS

Praveen K, Aslam S, Dutta TK. Hoffmann's syndrome: a rare neurological presentation of hypothyroidism. *Int J Nutr Pharmacol Neurol Dis.* 2011;1:201–203.

Reimers CD, Schlotter B, Eicke BM, Witt TN. Calf enlargement in neuromuscular diseases: a quantitative ultrasound study in 350 patients and review of the literature. *J Neurol Sci.* 1996 Nov;143(1–2):46–56.

CASE 14.5: PROGRESSIVE WEAKNESS AND DIFFUSE DENERVATION

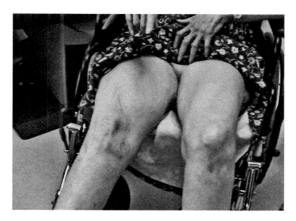

VIDEO 14.5

A 70-year-old woman presented with a 6-month history of difficulty walking and falls. She became wheelchair bound. Examination revealed weakness and atrophy of the anterior thighs and forelegs and mild proximal arm weakness. Sensation was normal. Deep tendon reflexes (DTRs) were 3+ in the legs and arms. The CK level was 340 U/L. MRI of the entire spine was normal. EMG revealed fibrillation and positive, sharp waves in the proximal and distal leg muscles bilaterally and TPS muscles and few fibrillations in the proximal arm muscles.

The most likely cause of thigh weakness in this case is:

1. Limb girdle muscular dystrophy (LGMD)
2. ALS
3. BMD
4. Diabetic amyotrophy
5. LS radiculopathy

DIAGNOSIS

- Thoracic paraspinal (TPS) muscles play a very important role in the neuromuscular diagnostic process for the following reasons:
  - They are rarely affected by spondylosis, which usually affects the cervical and LS spine due to their curvatures and weight-bearing properties.
  - They are affected early in denervating conditions due to their proximity to the motor neurons, to which they are connected by short posterior spinal rami.
- TPS muscle involvement in ALS provides an affected segment to three of the four required segments (cranial, cervical, thoracic, and LS) for the diagnosis of ALS according to El Escorial criteria (EEC).
- TPS muscles are also affected early in inflammatory and metabolic myopathies, as they show evidence of increased irritability in a form of fibrillation and positive, sharp waves.
- The most appropriate way to test TPS muscles is to insert the needle right adjacent to the corresponding spinous process until resistance is met due to the transverse processes; then the needle is pulled back a few millimeters.
- It is important to remember that the myotome level does not correspond to the spine levels because the spinal cord is shorter that the spinal column.
- Poor relaxation is the most important hurdle in examination of the TPS muscle. This can be minimized by optimizing room temperature, explaining the procedure to the patient, and positioning the patient on the side and flexing the hips and head.
- In the presented case, the progressive course, atrophy, hyperreflexia, normal sensation, and diffuse denervation argued for ALS.

CASE 14.6: PROGRESSIVE CALF ATROPHY AND ELEVATED CREATINE KINASE (CK)

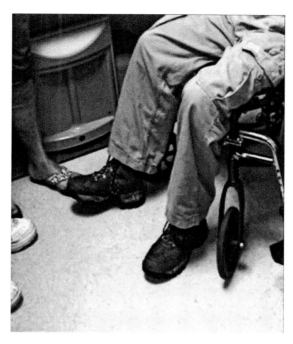

VIDEO 14.6

A 27-year-old man had noticed 10 years earlier an inability to stand on his toes, but he did not seek medical advice. He had difficulty climbing stairs 2 years later. He moved his apartment to the ground floor. Another 2 years later, he could not arise from a chair without help. His examination revealed atrophy of the calves and proximal weakness. The CPK level was 4,350 U/L. EMG revealed 40% short-duration units in the proximal and distal leg muscles and 2+ fibrillations and positive, sharp waves in the TPS muscles.

The most appropriate next test is:

1. A blood sample for dysferlin mutation
2. A muscle biopsy for dysferlin staining
3. A blood sample for calpain mutation
4. A muscle biopsy for calpain staining
5. A dry blood spot for acid alpha glucosidase activity

DIAGNOSIS

- Dysferlin gene mutation accounts for 1% of unclassified LGMD cases and 60% of distal myopathies.
- It is allelic to LGMD 2B.
- Western blot (WB) analysis on white blood cells (WBCs) correlates well with WB on muscle tissue and is the test of choice in the suspected cases.
- With muscle biopsy, absent dysferlin is more significant than patchy staining for achieving an accurate diagnosis.
- Patients with absent dysferlin also show abnormal calpain staining, and caution should be taken to avoid erroneous diagnosis of calpainopathy.
- Endomysial inflammation is common in muscle biopsies, leading to erroneous diagnosis of polymyositis.
- Dysferlinopathy may also present as LGMD, or even as asymptomatic rhabdomyolysis. Rarely, it presents with bilateral foot drop.
- Asymmetry is very common in Miyoshi myopathy, and that can be a source of confusion with S1 radiculopathy.
- No cardiac involvement is expected in Miyoshi myopathy.

CASE 14.7: DANCING DIFFICULTY

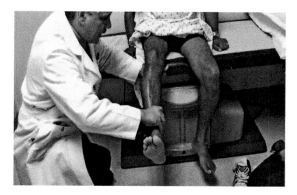

VIDEO 14.7

A 41-year-old man presented with a 10-year history of difficulty holding up his arms and dancing. The quadriceps atrophy in this case is likely due to:

1. BMD
2. IBM
3. FSHD
4. Diabetic amyotrophy
5. Scapuloperoneal syndrome

DIAGNOSIS

The demonstrated clinical findings are typically seen in FSHD, except quadriceps weakness.
Atypical features of FSHD include:

- Quadriceps weakness
- Respiratory involvement (which occurs in 1% of cases of FSHD)
- Extraocular muscle weakness

Typical features include:

- Asymmetry can be so striking that facial nerve palsy is erroneously diagnosed.
- Endomysial inflammation in the muscle biopsy may lead to diagnostic confusion with polymyositis.
- Hearing loss and retinal telangiectasia occur in two-thirds of cases.
- Distal weakness is common, leading to asymmetrical foot drop and weakness of wrist extensors. Hypertrophy of the extensor digitorum brevis (EDB) indicates myopathic rather than neurogenic foot drop.

Quadriceps: selective weakness.

- Hereditary myopathies include:
  - BMD
  - LGMD: 1B; 2B; 2H; 2L
  - Emery-Dreifuss muscular dystrophy: Lamin A and C
  - Hereditary inclusion body myopathy 3 (HIBM3)
- Inflammatory myopathies include:
  - IBM
  - Polymyositis with mitochondrial pathology
  - Focal myositis
- Myopathy with ring fibers
- Nerve disorders:
  - Spinal muscular atrophy (SMA)
    - 5q: Type III and IV
    - Lower extremity dominant
  - Femoral neuropathy
  - Diabetic amyotrophy
  - L3–L4 radiculopathy
  - LS plexopathies: especially neoplastic

SUGGESTED READING

Tawil R. Facioscapulohumeral muscular dystrophy. *Neurotherapeut.* 2008 Oct;5(4):601–606.

CASE 14.8A: LEG WEAKNESS AND AREFLEXIA

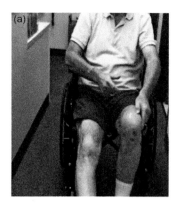

VIDEO 14.8A

A 55-year-old man presented with a 6-month history of progressive gait instability and foot numbness. In addition to what is shown in the video, he had diffuse areflexia. Cerebrospinal fluid (CSF) protein was 160 mg/dl. Immunofixation protein electrophoresis (IFPE) revealed IgM spikes. He had severe motor slowing and prolonged distal latencies. He responded to IVIG. A few months later, he had a flulike illness, followed by severe weakness (shown in Video 14.8A). His sulfatide antibody titer was 1:100,000.

The deterioration was likely:

1. An exacerbation of CIDP
2. Due to the appearance of sulfatide antibodies
3. Triggered by a viral illness
4. Due to an unrelated disease
5. Due to monoclonal gammopathy

DIAGNOSIS

- The case meets inflammatory neuropathy cause and treatment (INCAT) diagnostic criteria of CIDP.
- A total of 80% of CIDP cases respond to initial therapy, but less than 30% achieve remission off medication.
- The natural course of CIDP is as follows:
  - Chronic monophasic: 15%
  - Chronic relapsing-remitting: 34%
  - Stepwise progressive: 15%
  - Steady progressive: 15%
- Monoclonal gammopathy is present in 25% of cases.
  - Unlike Guillain-Barré syndrome (GBS), only a small number of patients have autoantibodies against myelin protein. IgM is more likely to be pathogenic than IgG, and IFPE needs to be monitored for malignant transformation.
- IVIG and plasma exchange (PLEX) are equally effective in CIDP.
- IVIG has become the treatment of choice, mostly due to convenience and low side effects.
- After induction with 2g/kg/bw divided over 2 days, booster doses and frequency will need to be individualized according to the clinical response and side effects. We use 1 g/kg/bw every month times three, and then reduce the dose and frequency, if tolerated, until completely off. Some cases, like this one, need more frequent infusions.
- Exacerbations of CIDP are usually triggered by viral infection, emotional stress, surgery, trauma, and vaccination, but frequently, no clear precipitating factors are found.
- The significance of sulfatide antibodies that appear in a minority of CIDP cases is controversial. These cases are difficult to differentiate from regular CIDP cases. They may have more sensory ataxia and tremor and may be less responsive to IVIG.
- Therefore, the presence of these antibodies should not affect the way that these cases are treated and should not warrant splitting these cases from CIDP.
- The answers are 1 and 3.

SUGGESTED READING

Querol L, Rojas-Garcia R, Casasnovas C, et al. Long-term outcome in chronic inflammatory demyelinating polyneuropathy patients treated with intravenous immunoglobulin: A retrospective study. *Muscl Nerve*. 2013 Dec;48(6):870–876.

CASE 14.8B: IMPROVED BUT DEVELOPED SWOLLEN LEGS AFTER INTRAVENOUS IMMUNOGLOBIN (IVIG)

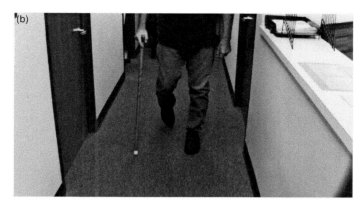

VIDEO 14.8B

The patient in Case 14.8A responded again to IVIG but could not tolerate less frequency of infusions than weekly. A few months later, he developed deep vein thrombosis (DVT).

Complications of IVIG include all of the following except:

1. DVT
2. Renal impairment
3. Myeloproliferative disorder
4. Aseptic meningitis
5. Flulike reaction

DIAGNOSIS

- IVIG has become a common modality of treatment of many autoimmune disorders in neuromuscular clinics.
- Side effects occur in 20% of cases. Only 5% are serious.
- Side effects are more common in first users and in the elderly, diabetics, dehydrated patients, and in patients with renal impairment.
- Flulike reaction and headache due to aseptic meningitis usually respond to premedication with antihistamines and steroids.
- While infection is not a contraindication, it increases the risk of flulike reaction due to the release of cytokines from dead bacteria. Treatment of infections before IVIG is recommended.
- DVT and renal failure are also reported.
- Changing products may help some of the side effects, especially acute reactions.
- Severe skin rash, hyponatremia, leucopenia, and anaphylaxis are uncommon.
- Myeloproliferative disorder is not a known complication of IVIG therapy

CASE 14.9: SEVERE THIGH PAIN IN A NONDIABETIC PATIENT

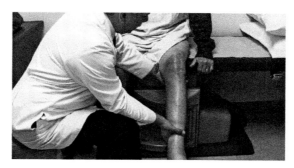

VIDEO 14.9

A 76-year-old nondiabetic man developed acute, severe, lancinating left anterior thigh pain, followed 3 weeks later by leg weakness. Examination is shown in the video. MRI of the LS spine and plexi revealed mild degenerative changes. EMG revealed active denervation of the left hamstrings, quadriceps, tibialis anterior and posterior, gastrocnemius, glutei, and normal LS paraspinal muscles. Sural responses were absent, and motor amplitudes were low in the legs. CSF examination revealed a protein of 80 mg/dl and normal cells. HbA1C was 6% and ESR was 25 mm/hour.

The most likely diagnosis is:

1. Nondiabetic LSRPN
2. Systemic vasculitis
3. Diabetic amyotrophy
4. Inflammatory myopathy
5. LS polyradiculopathy

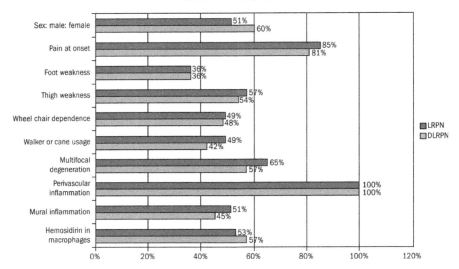

FIGURE 14.9.1 Comparison between lumbosacral radiculoplexus neuropathy (LSRPN) and diabetic lumbosacral radiculoplexus neuropathy (DLSRPN).

Permission from Nerve and Muscle Center of Texas

DIAGNOSIS

- Nondiabetic LSRPN is a syndrome similar to diabetic amyotrophy that affects nondiabetic patients. Symptoms are due to vascular inflammation of LS plexus and consist of severe unilateral thigh pain followed by atrophy.
- Spread of symptoms to the other leg occurs in 30% of cases and to the arms in about 15% of cases. EMG reveals denervation that is more severe and extensive than clinically suspected. There may be some subtle demyelinating features, but the predominant picture is that of axonal neuropathy. CSF protein is slightly elevated.
- This syndrome may be triggered by viral infections.
- The symptoms progress for a few months, then stabilize for a few months, and then improvement follows. It may take up to 2 years for maximum improvement to occur, and some residual deficit is common. Many of these patients undergo lumbar surgery due to the presence of incidental spondylotic findings.
- Pathologically, microvasculitis is the predominant finding. However, steroids did not change the natural history of the disease in at least one double-blind clinical trial.
- Effective pain management and early initiation of a rehabilitation program are crucial.
- Similarities with its diabetic counterpart are so amazing that diabetes is considered a risk factor rather than the cause of diabetic LSRPN.
- This syndrome should be differentiated from CIDP and necrotizing vasculitis.

SUGGESTED READING

Dyck PJB, Norell JE. Non-diabetic lumbosacral radiculoplexus neuropathy: Natural history, outcome and comparison with the diabetic variety. *Brain.* 2001;124:1197–1207.

CASE 14.10: WEAKNESS AND ATROPHY
OF QUADRICEPS AND HAMSTRINGS

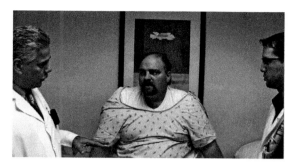

VIDEO 14.10

A 48-year-old man presented with a 2-year history of progressive inability to climb stairs and arise out of a chair. He had no back pain or sensory symptoms. He had no symptoms in the arms. There was no significant family history. Examination is shown in the video. Sensation was normal. The CK level was 320 U/L. The demonstrated EMG activity was detected in all the tested muscles proximally and distally in the legs.

The most likely diagnosis is:

1. SMA
2. IBM
3. BMD
4. ALS
5. Progressive muscular atrophy

DIAGNOSIS

- Such severe painless symmetrical quadriceps atrophy could be myopathic (IBM, dystrophi-nopathy, etc.) or neurogenic (radiculopathy, plexopathy, motor neuronopathy, etc.).
- Mild CK elevation is common in both scenarios.
- The loss of knee reflexes can occur in both, but loss of ankle reflexes is more in favor of a neurogenic cause.
- The pattern of weakness with involvement of the hamstrings, hip flexors, and knee extensors is also more consistent with motor neuron dysfunction, as opposed to myopathy.
- EMG confirms the neurogenic etiology by showing high-amplitude MUPs and high firing frequency.
- The lack of hyperreflexia argues against ALS. The progressive nature, over a year or two, argues against SMA.
- PMA is the most likely diagnosis. It is a variant of motor neuron disease that affects only the LMNs. It is less aggressive than ALS.

CASE 14.11: BIG CALVES AND WASTED THIGHS

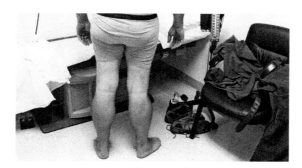

VIDEO 14.11

A 29-year-old gentleman with a 9-year history of difficulty climbing stairs and frequent buckling of the knees and falls. As a child, he walked on tiptoes. In middle school and high school, he had a mild problem playing basketball and baseball. He denied pain in the thigh muscles or weakness in the arms or swallowing or speech difficulty. MRI of the LS spine revealed mild degenerative changes. He denied exercise-induced muscle cramps or change in the color of the urine anytime in the past. He denied weakness of hand grips or sensory symptoms except for mild nocturnal tingling in the hands. The CPK level was 340 IU/L. EMG revealed nonirritative quadriceps myopathy with normal finger flexors. The TPS muscles displayed no spontaneous activity.

The most likely diagnosis is:

1. IBM
2. BMD
3. Diabetic amyotrophy
4. DMD
5. Bilateral L4 radiculopathy

DIAGNOSIS

- Genetic testing revealed pathogenic mutation of exons 45 through 47 of the dystrophin gene
- Quadriceps weakness and atrophy in adults may be due to:
  - MNDs
  - LS plexopathy (e.g., diabetic amyotrophy)
  - Femoral neuropathy
  - L4 radiculopathy
  - Myopathy. The most important myopathic causes are:
    - IBM, which typically appears after age 50 years and is associated with weakness of the finger flexors
    - Dystrophinopathy, whose phenotypes include:
      - DMD (starting between 3 and 5 years of age).
      - BMD, which may present as a limb girdle myopathy or quadriceps myopathy
        - BMD starts as late as 30 years of age.
        - Cardiomyopathy is common.
        - Calf hypertrophy and musculoskeletal abnormalities are common.
        - Calf muscles are replaced by fat (pseduohypertrophy).
      - Dilated cardiomyopathy.
      - Rhabdomyolysis.
      - Muscle cramps.
- The dystrophin gene is the only gene whose pathogenic variants are known to cause DMD and BMD.
- The best diagnostic strategy for the diagnosis of BMD is to test the DMD gene for duplications/deletions and if this is negative, obtain gene sequence analysis, and if this is negative, obtain muscle biopsy for WB analysis.

SUGGESTED READING

Flanigan KM. Duchenne and Becker muscular dystrophies. *Neurol Clin*. 2014 Aug;32(3):671–688.

CASE 14.12: UNUSUAL CAUSE OF QUADRICEPS ATROPHY

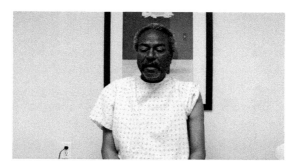

VIDEO 14.12

A 58-year-old man with history of seizure disorder treated with Dilantin. History and exam were shown in the video. The CPK level was 732 IU/L, and EMG revealed irritative myopathy.

Preferential biceps weakness is a feature of all of the following except:

1. IBM
2. FSDH
3. Polymyositis
4. Dysferlinopathy
5. Anoctaminopathy (*ANO5* mutation)

DIAGNOSIS

- The first look suggested IBM because it is the most common myopathy after age 50 years and typically presents with chronic weakness of the quadriceps and biceps.
- 30 years duration and weakness of the hamstrings are atypical.
- When he was undressed, he had horizontal clavicles and inverted axillary folds with mild scapular winging. Although facial weakness is a feature of IBM, in the context, the diagnosis of FSHD was raised.
- All the mentioned diagnoses are associated with more weakness of biceps than triceps except typical polymyositis cases which cause more or equal deltoid than biceps weakness.
- It is very important to undress patients in the neuromuscular clinic to determine the pattern of muscle involvement which is essential for the diagnostic process. Many findings can be otherwise missed such as fascicualtions of the chest and upper back muscles, skin lesions such as Café Au lait spots, scapular winging, horizontal clavicles, inverted axillary folds, rippling muscle disease, etc.).
- Such a preferential quadriceps weakness is atypical of FSHD and polymyositis, but is common in the other options.
- Genetic testing confirmed FSHD. To avoid misdiagnosis, one should not totally rely on phenotype to diagnose myopathies

SUGGESTED READING

Tawil R, Kissel JT, Heatwole C, et al. Evidence-based guideline summary: evaluation, diagnosis, and management of FSHD. *Neurol.* 2015;85:357–364.

CASE 14.13: PAINFUL CRAMPS AND ATROPHY OF THE QUADRICEPS MUSCLES

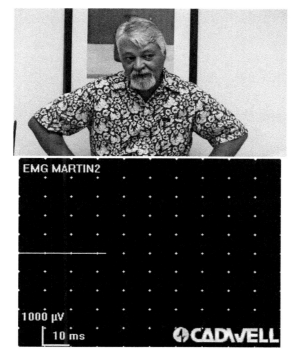

VIDEO 14.13

A 49-year-old mechanic presented with symptoms that started 18 years earlier and got much worse over the last 3 years. His main symptom was painful muscle cramps in the lower extremities, frequent falls, and difficulty climbing stairs and dancing. There were no numbness, bowel or bladder disturbance, or weakness in the arms. He denies dysphagia, dysarthria, diplopia, or radicular symptoms. He had chronic lower back pain attributed to an old accident. He had 2 sisters and 2 siblings with no family history of muscle weakness. Sensory and motor NCSs were normal. Needle EMG of the quadriceps muscles, iliopsoas, and tibialis anterior and posterior muscles revealed the findings demonstrated in Video 14.13.2. TPS muscles and glutei were normal. The CPK level was 122 IU/L. MRI of the lumbar and the thoracic spine revealed mild degenerative changes. MRI of the thighs revealed atrophy and fatty replacement of the medial and anterior thigh muscles and flexors.

The cause of quadriceps weakness in this case is most likely:

1. IBM
2. Chronic bilateral L4 radiculopathy
3. SMA
4. ALS
5. Postpolio syndrome

The firing frequency of the MUPs in Video 14.13.2 was:

1. 10 Hz
2. 20 Hz
3. 30 Hz
4. 40 Hz
5. 50 Hz

DIAGNOSIS

- The wasting, weakness, resting muscle cramps, and fasciculation of the affected proximal muscles with normal sural responses suggested a neurogenic etiology.
- Needle EMG confirmed chronic denervation and showed 10-mv amplitude MUPs with large duration and increased firing frequency to 20 Hz (1,000 divided by the interspike time of 50 milliseconds).
- The chronicity and diffuse bilateral proximal denervation and loss of DTRs suggest SMA.
- Genetic testing of SMN revealed no mutations. Whole-exome sequencing revealed DYNC1H1 pathogenic mutation.
- There is a variant of SMA that predominantly affects the lower extremities and is characterized by predominant quadriceps weakness. This is due to mutation of dynein, cytoplasmic 1, heavy chain 1 (DYNC1H1) on chromosome 14q32.31. it is an autosomal-dominant (AD) disease.
- ALS is excluded by the chronic course.
- Muscular causes of quadriceps atrophy, such as BMD and some types of LGMD and IBM, are ruled out by neurogenic EMG.
- Bilateral L4 radiculopathy without pain is very atypical. MRI of the lumbar spine revealed no compressive insult at these levels.

SUGGESTED READING

Scoto M., Rosso AM, Harms MB, et al. Novel mutations expand the clinical spectrum of DYNC1H1-associated spinal muscular atrophy. *Neurol.* 2015 Feb 17;84(7):668–679.

CASE 14.14: QUADRICEPS MITOCHONDRIAL MYOPATHY

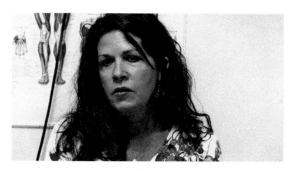

VIDEO 14.14

Symptoms started 10 years earlier with knee buckling, poor balance, and difficulty climbing stairs. There were no pain or muscle cramps. Gradually, she had difficulty holding her arms up to style her hair. She denies dysphagia, dysarthria, or dyspnea. She denies symptoms earlier in life when she was in high school. She did not physically lag behind her peers. She quit dancing 5 years ago because her knees would buckle and she would fall. Gradually, she lost mass from the quadriceps muscles. The CK level was 600 IU/L. EMG revealed irritative myopathy. Right quadriceps muscle biopsy revealed nonspecific mitochondrial changes. LS spine MRI revealed mild degenerative changes. She has 2 children, 23- and 20-year-old males, and a sister and a brother with no similar symptoms. Her parents had no weakness. She was otherwise healthy except for breast augmentation that happened several years ago. She was referred to our center 8 years after the symptoms started due to continuation of progression. EMG revealed short- and long-duration units in the quads, glutei and hip flexors, with early recruitment suggestive of a chronic myopathic process. Fibrillation was also noticed in these muscles and in TPS muscles, suggestive of irritative myopathy. Similar changes were found in the left biceps muscle. Another muscle biopsy from the left biceps showed abnormalities (Fig. 14.14. 1–5).

The most likely diagnosis is:

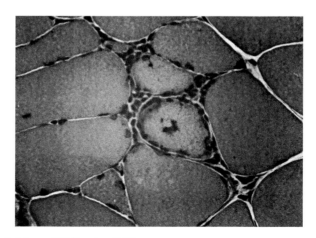

FIGURE 14.14.1 muscle biopsy. H&E stain; 400X

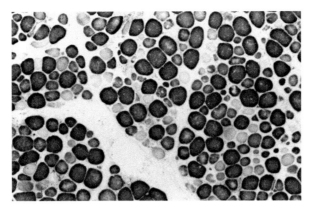

FIGURE 14.14.2 NSE reaction, 400x

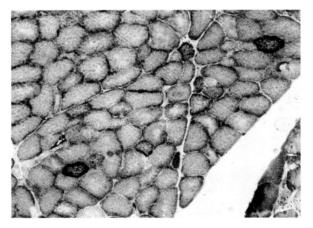

FIGURE 14.14.3 SDH reaction. 100X

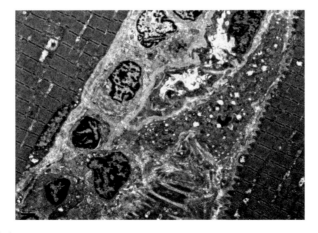

FIGURE 14.14.4 EM picture

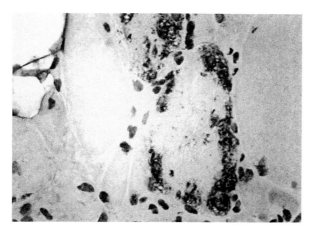

FIGURE 14.14.5 P62 IHC.

1. Polymyositis
2. Mitochondrial myopathy
3. IBM
4. LGMD
5. BMD

DIAGNOSIS

IBM:

- Chronic, progressive, painless proximal weakness, mostly affecting the quadriceps more than the hip flexors and the biceps more than the deltoid, is highly suggestive of IBM.
- The muscle biopsy showed endomysial inflammation with invasion of nonnecrotic fibers by mononuclear inflammatory cells (Fig. 14.14.1), which is seen in inflammatory myopathies.
- A cytochrome oxidase (COX) stain showed many negative fibers (Fig. 14.14.2) that stained positive, with succinate dehydrogenase (SDH) stain (ragged blue fibers) (Fig. 14.14.3) suggestive of mitochondrial myopathy. An electron microscopy (EM) exam confirmed the presence of aggregates of large, swollen mitochondria (Fig. 14.14.4).
- Mitochondrial dysfunction with inflammatory features is highly suggestive of IBM despite the lack of red-rimmed vacuoles and cytoplasmic inclusions, especially with quadriceps weakness. Positive P62 antibody reaction is very specific for IBM, and it was positive (Fig. 14.14.5). An NT5C1A antibody titer was also used to confirm IBM, but it was negative.
- Laminopathy, LGMD 2B (dysferlinopathy), and LGMD 2L (ANO5) are other possible causes of differential quads weakness and pathological inflammation, but there are no dystrophic changes in the biopsy to support any of these myopathies.
- BMD is unlikely due to the lack of significant CK elevation and the sex of the patient.
- Proximal neurogenic disorders such as SMA may lead to mixed MUPs, However, muscle pathology was not neurogenic.
- This entity is called polymyositis-mitochondrial myopathy. However, availability of more specific histopathological antibodies for IBM made most experts consider this entity as a form of IBM.
- In summary, this is a case of IBM variant. The age is earlier than typical. This form of IBM is slower-progressing than classical IBM.

SUGGESTED READINGS

Brady, S, Squier W, Sewry C. A retrospective cohort study identifying the principal pathological features useful in the diagnosis of inclusion body myositis. *BMJ*. 2014 Apr 28;4(4).

Temiz, P, Weihl CC, Pestronik A. Inflammatory myopathies with mitochondrial pathology and protein aggregates. *J Neurol Sci*. 2009 Mar 15;278(1–2):25–29.

Shaibani, Medlink neurology.

http://www.medlink.com.

CHAPTER 15

DISTAL ARM WEAKNESS

CASE 15.1: FOREARM PAIN AND FINGER WEAKNESS

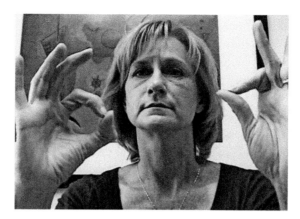

VIDEO 15.1

A 45-year-old woman presented with acute, severe left shoulder and forearm burning pain, followed a week later by the inability to hold a pen. A few weeks later, the pain resolved, but the weakness continued, and she developed atrophy of the volar left forearm muscles. She had no tingling or numbness in the fingers or forearm.

Electromyography (EMG) is expected to show denervation of the following muscles:

1. Flexor digitorum profundus (FDP)
2. Pronator quadratus (PQ)
3. Flexor pollicis longus (FPL)
4. Flexor carpi radialis (FCR)
5. Flexor carpi ulnaris (FCU)

DIAGNOSIS

- The anterior interosseus nerve (AIN) is a pure motor nerve that branches off the median nerve proximally in the forearm; it supplies the FDP I, II, FPL, and PQ.
- AIN can be affected by multiple factors, the most common of which is idiopathic brachial plexitis [Parsonage-Turner syndrome (PTS)]. As a matter of fact, it can be the only feature of brachial plexitis.
- No sensory symptoms are expected, but deep forearm pain is common, which can be very severe and may last days or weeks.
- Characteristically, patients cannot pinch or form the letter *O* with their thumb and index finger, as there is weakness of flexion of the distal phalanges of these fingers, which are flexed by the FDP and FPL (the flexor digitorum superficialis (FDS), which supplies the middle interphalangeal joint, is supplied by the median nerve before the branching of the AIN).
- When the AIN is affected, along with other nerves such as the long thoracic nerve, spinal accessory nerve (SAN), and suprascapular nerve, the diagnosis of PTS is not hard to make, but when it is the only feature, other causes should be considered, and an attempt to explore and look for a compression is reasonable after 6 months of conservative treatment.
- Other causes include:
  - Fibrous band within pronator teres
  - Compartmental syndrome
  - Soft tissue and peripheral nerve tumors
  - Ischemia from arteriovenous fistula, or vasculitis
  - Multifocal motor neuropathy
  - Trauma
- The presence of sensory symptoms in the fingers should suggest a more proximal median neuropathy, which has a different set of causes.

CASE 15.2: HAND AND FINGER FLEXOR WEAKNESS AND MYOPATHIC ELECTROMYOGRAPHY (EMG)

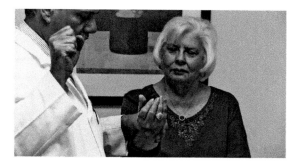

VIDEO 15.2

A 65-year-old woman presented with a 15-year history of slowly progressive weakness of the arms and legs, as demonstrated in Video 15.2. She had normal quadriceps strength and no dysphagia. The creatine kinase (CK) level was normal, and EMG revealed mixed long- and short-duration potentials in the bilateral distal arm and leg muscles. The left biceps biopsy is shown in Figures 15.2.1 and 15.2.2.

The most likely diagnosis is:

1. Inclusion body myositis (IBM)
2. Polymyositis
3. Granulomatous myositis
4. Spinal muscular atrophy (SMA)
5. Charcot-Marie-Tooth (CMT)

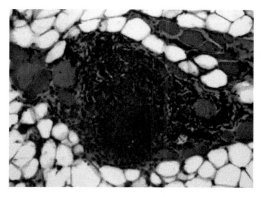

FIGURE 15.2.1 H & E stain (100x).

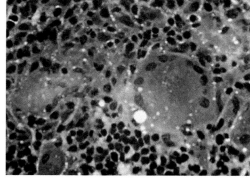

FIGURE 15.2.2 H & E stain (1000x).

DIAGNOSIS

- Muscle biopsy revealed multiple noncaseating granulomata that contained many multinucleated giant cells.
- Patients with chronic distal hand weakness are usually given various diagnoses, such as carpal tunnel syndrome (CTS), cervical radiculopathy, arthritis, and others, and it may take years before they see a neuromuscular specialist.
- The lack of sensory symptoms and the diffuse nature of the weakness suggested the following:
  - Myopathy
  - Motor neuron disease (MND)
  - Hirayama disease
  - Myasthenia gravis (MG)
- CK elevation and myopathic EMG confirmed the diagnosis of distal myopathy and raised the following possibilities:
  - Hereditary myopathies
  - IBM
  - Myofibrillar myopathy
- Muscle biopsy revealed an unexpected findings of several noncaseating granulomas and endomyseal inflammation.
- Granulomatous myopathy is a rare form of inflammatory muscle disease.
  - It may present as progressive proximal weakness, along with MG and thymoma.
  - Alternatively, it may present as a chronic distal weakness as a manifestation of sarcoidosis.
  - Frequently, the search for sarcoidosis is not productive and the diagnosis of idiopathic granulomatous myopathy is given.
  - The prognosis is not good; unfortunately, response to immunosupression or modulation is poor in the distal form.
  - Unlike the proximal variant, the distal idiopathic type of granulomatous myopathy does not affect the heart, but it may extend to the proximal muscles.

SUGGESTED READING

Jasim S, Shaibani A. Nonsarcoid granulomatous myopathy: two cases and a review of literature. *Int J Neurosci.* 2013 Jul;123(7):516–520.

CASE 15.3: A POLICE OFFICER WHO COULD NOT PULL THE TRIGGER

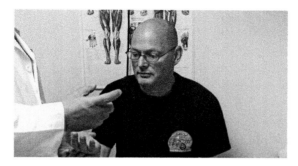

VIDEO 15.3

A 50-year-old police officer noticed difficulty pulling the trigger 3 years earlier. Gradually, he developed difficulty dancing and swallowing. His mother was diagnosed with facioscapulohumeral muscular dystrophy (FSHD) due to facial and leg weakness. Two aunts and two cousins were diagnosed with limb girdle muscular dystrophy (LGMD). One of them had congestive heart failure. The CPK level was 124 U/L, and EMG revealed mixed short- and long-duration potentials in the distal and proximal muscles of all extremities. Left biceps biopsy revealed chronic myopathic changes with no inflammation. Desmin staining was normal. Rare red-rimmed vacuoles were noted.

The following gene mutation analysis would be most appropriate:

1. *GNE*
2. Myosin
3. Desmin
4. *PABPN1*
5. *FSHD*

DIAGNOSIS

- The pattern of weakness (quadriceps, finger flexors, and foot extensor weakness), chronicity, and red-rimmed vacuoles suggested IBM. The age of the patient and the family history suggested hereditary IBM (hIBM).
- Rimmed vacuoles are not specific and can be seen in:
  - IBM: both sporadic IBM (sIBM) and hereditary types
  - Oculopharyngeal muscular dystrophy (OPMD)
  - Including OPMD
  - Hereditary distal myopathies:
    - Welander myopathy
    - Finnish-Markesbery myopathy
    - Distal myopathy with vocal cord weakness (MPD2)
- IBM subtypes:
  - sIBM
  - IBM1 (myofibrillar myopathy)
  - IBM2 (*GNG* mutation)
  - IBM3: Joint contractures and ophthalmoplegia
  - IBM and paget dementia
- hIBM type 1:
  - Desminopathy, chromosome 2q35, dominant
  - Onset: 25–40 years
  - Quadriceps weakness and foot dorsiflexion weakness
  - Slow progression
  - Normal or mildly elevated CK
  - Red-rimmed vacuole and myopathic changes
- IBM2 (*GNE*) mutation is autosomal recessive (AR) and causes high CK, and it usually spares the quadriceps.
- Even sIBM has a genetic component. Polymorphism in the TOMM40 gene modifies the risk of sIBM and the age of onset.

SUGGESTED READINGS

Dalakas MD, Park KY, Semino-Mora C, et al. Desmin myopathy, a skeletal myopathy with cardiomyopathy caused by mutations in the desmin gene. *NEJM*. 2000 Mar 16;342(11):770–780.

Mastaglia FL, Rojana-udomsart A, James I, et al. Polymorphism in the TOMM40 gene modifies the risk of developing sporadic inclusion body myositis and the age of onset of symptoms. *Neuromuscul Disord*. 2013 Dec;23(12):969–974.

CASE 15.4: "FISH MOUTH" HANDSHAKE AND FACIAL WEAKNESS

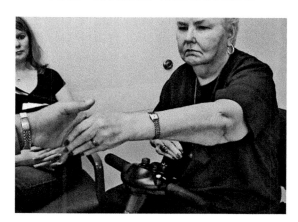

VIDEO 15.4

A 67-year-old woman presented with a 5-year history of gait imbalance and dysphagia. Examination is shown in the video. CPK was 800 U/L, and EMG revealed mixed short- and long-duration potentials in the proximal and distal arm and leg muscles bilaterally. Discontinuation of atorvastatin and treatment with oral steroids reduced the CK to 300 and led to improvement of the stamina for a couple of months. No objective changes in the muscle strength were noted.

Regarding this case, which of the following statements is true?

1. CK reduction with steroids argues against IBM.
2. The disease is due to statins.
3. Statins may have worsened the weakness produced by IBM.
4. She is a good candidate for intravenous immunoglobulin (IVIG).
5. The pattern of weakness is not typical for IBM.

DIAGNOSIS

- The practice of adjusting the dose of prednisone based on the CK level is not recommended, as steroids stabilize the cell membrane and reduce the CK level regardless of the cause.
  - Strength measurement is the most valid outcome measure in monitoring recovery of myopathies. The 6-min walk test has been the standard for assessing function in clinical trials.
- Statins can cause different kinds of myopathies, including necrotizing myopathy and autoimmune inflammatory myopathy, with positive antibodies against 3-hydroxy-3-methyl-glutaryl-CoA (HMG-Co A) reductase.
- Also, statins may unmask an underlying metabolic or mitochondrial myopathy, as 30% of statin-induced myopathies showed evidence of an underlying metabolic defect, such as carnitine palmitoyltransferase II (CPT II), myoadenylate deaminase (MAD), and phosphorylase deficiency.
- Some of these myopathies may improve after discontinuation of the statins, but it may take several months for maximum recovery. Others need to be treated with steroids, other immunosuppressive agents, or both.
- An IBM phenotype is not reported in association with statin therapy. Myopathies may be worsened by statins, which therefore are not recommended in patients with muscle disease.
- The pattern of weakness in this case was very typical for IBM, which should be highly suspected just after shaking hands with the patient ("fish mouth" handshake appearance due to weakness of the finger flexors).
- Neither IVIG nor prednisone, azathioprine, or any other immunomodulatory agents have proved to be effective in treating IBM.
  - Some authorities advocate 3 months of steroid therapy to patients who show a CK level of more than 20,000 and intense endomysial inflammation. In our experience, improvement, if it happens, is transient, and steroids do not change the natural history of the disease.

CASE 15.5: A FISHERMAN WHO COULD NOT PEEL SHRIMP ANYMORE

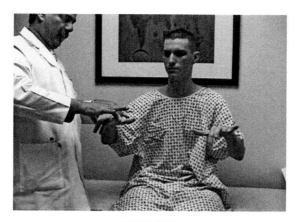

VIDEO 15.5

A 21-year-old shrimp peeler had developed weakness in his fingers 5 years earlier, which has progressed to a degree that was not compatible with his job. He had no neck pain, arm numbness, dysphagia, or muscle twitching. Family history was irrelevant. Examination is shown in the video. The CPK was 530 U/L, and EMG revealed chronic diffuse denervation of the arm muscles, with normal sensory and motor responses. EMG of the legs was normal.

The most likely diagnosis is:

1. Amyotrophic lateral sclerosis (ALS)
2. Hirayama disease
3. IBM
4. West Nile virus (WNV) infection
5. Cervical radiculopathy

DIAGNOSIS

- Chronic unilateral or bilateral pure motor weakness of the hand muscles in a young patient is not common. Differential diagnosis:
  - Cervical cord pathology such as syringomyelia: Dissociated sensory loss is typically present.
  - Brachial plexus pathology: Sensory findings are usually present.
  - MND: ALS, SMA.
  - Distal myopathies.
- The cervical spine is usually investigated before neuromuscular referrals are made.
- The lack of pain, radicular or sensory symptoms, and normal sensory nerve action potentials (SNAPs), as well as cervical magnetic resonance imaging (MRI), ruled out most of the abovementioned possibilities except:
  - Distal myopathy (usually not unilateral) and SMA.
- EMG/NCS (electromyogram/nerve conduction study) demonstration of chronic distal denervation with normal sensory responses and no demyelinating features limited the diagnosis to MND.
- Segmental denervation pattern further narrowed the diagnosis to Hirayama disease.
- Hirayama disease is a sporadic and focal form of SMA that affects predominantly males at age 15–25 years.
  - Weakness and atrophy usually start unilaterally in the C8–T1 muscles of the hand and forearm, typically in the dominant hand.
  - In a third of cases, the other hand is affected, and weakness may spread to the proximal muscles.
  - Deep tenson reflexes (DTRs) are normal or brisk, unlike most SMA cases, where the reflexes are decreased or absent.
  - After a progressive course of 6 years or less, the progression plateaus.
  - Extreme exacerbation of weakness in the cold and focal hyperhidrosis are reported.
  - The disease is more common in India.
  - Hypothesis: Radiological forward displacement of the cervical dural sac and compressive flattening of the cervical cord during flexion suggest that this is a form of cervical myelopathy. The resulting ischemia leads to preferential damage of the motor neurons. Decompressive surgery is unlikely to be effective due to the chronic nature of the neurological insult.

SUGGESTED READING

Hirayama K, Tokumaru Y. Cervical dural sac and spinal cord in juvenile muscular atrophy of distal upper extremity. *Neurol.* 2000;54:1922–1926.

CASE 15.6: A WRIST DROP AFTER A LONG FLIGHT

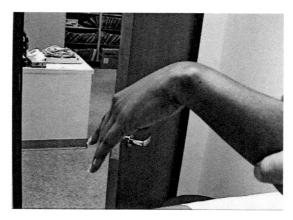

VIDEO 15.6

A 25-year-old woman presented with painless left wrist drop, which occurred after a 22-hour flight. She was stressed because she had never lived away from her family, and she was crying during the examination.

The preservation of extension at the distal interphalangeal joints:

1. Suggests a psychogenic etiology
2. Is typically seen in radial neuropathy
3. Suggests brachial plexopathy
4. Rules out C7 radiculopathy
5. Suggests distal myopathy (Welander type)

DIAGNOSIS

Wrist drop is due to weakness of the wrist extensors, which are supplied by the radial nerve. Problems with the innervation of the wrist extensors [the extensor carpi radialis (ECR) and extensor carpi ulnaris (ECU)] may result from an injury to the wrists' nerve supply anywhere between the forearm and the brain. We will not discuss here the central causes of wrist drop, such as cerebral ischemia, but these causes should be kept in mind, especially when exaggeration of the brachioradialis and triceps reflexes is evident.

- From the neuromuscular standpoint, the following levels of involvement should be considered:
  - The radial nerve or one of its branches, such as the posterior interosseus nerve
  - Brachial plexus, especially the posterior cord
  - C7 nerve root
  - Motor neurons
- There is a wide spectrum of pathology that can cause any of the abovementioned levels of involvement, including trauma, immune related, ischemia, are different pathologies.
  - The most common cause of wrist drop is radial nerve palsy:
    - It is due to prolonged compression of the nerve in the spiral groove due to faulty sleeping position during intoxication or long travel, or by an anomalous muscle or severe triceps contraction.
  - Diabetics are prone to compression, even with minimal pressure, as are hereditary neuropathy with liability to pressure palsy (HNPP) patients.
  - Clinically, radial muscles below the branch to the triceps are affected, including wrist and finger extensors and brachioradialis.
  - While anatomic charts show radial sensory supply to cover the dorsum of the hand and forearm, practically and due to overlap, only the skin overlying the snuffbox is affected.
  - Superficial radial SNAP and radial compound muscle action potential (CMAP) are decreased.
  - EMG shows denervation of the radial muscles distal to the triceps.
  - Recovery occurs in most cases with no residual deficit, but it may take months for axonal injury to recover.
  - Progressive deficit or even lack of improvement within 3 months should lead to a search for other causes, like tumors along the course of the nerve.
  - Preservation of extension at the distal interphalangeal (DIP) joints differentiates radial palsy from psychogenic weakness.
  - Radial nerve palsy preserves extension at the DIP joints subserved by the median- and ulnar-innervated lumbricals.

CASE 15.7: WEAK HANDS AND CONGENITAL CATARACT

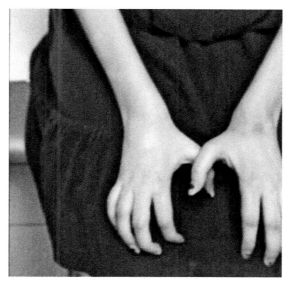

VIDEO 15.7

A 21-year-old woman who was diagnosed with congenital cataract at age 1 year, and ovarian agenesis a few years later, developed severe hand weakness at age 3, which gradually progressed to severe wasting and weakness of the distal arm, leg, and facial muscles. She was areflexic in the arms and normo-reflexic in the legs. At age 18, she had had one generalized seizure. Brain MRI was normal. There was no ocular or bulbar weakness. CK level and NCS were normal, including sural responses. EMG revealed mixed short- and long-duration motor unit potentials (MUPs) in the distal arm muscles. Tibialis anterior muscle biopsy revealed end-stage muscle disease. There was no significant family history (Fig. 15.7.1).

Such widespread and multisystemic abnormalities should raise suspicion of:

1. Muscular dystrophy (MD)
2. Mitochondrial cytopathy
3. Endocrinopathy
4. Motor neuronopathy
5. Fatty acid oxidation abnormalities

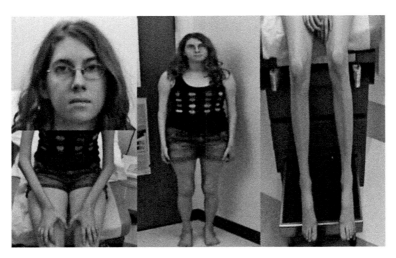

FIGURE 15.7.1 Patients photos showing wasting of the distal arm and leg muscles.

DIAGNOSIS

Severe hand weakness with cataract and ovarian agenesis:

Neuromuscular clinics sometimes receive enigmatic cases that defy diagnosis by the available tests. These cases are opportunities for the neuromuscular specialist to think creatively, looking for explanations.

- Involvement of multiple systems is seen in amyloidosis, vasculitis, and mitochondrial disorders.
- Cataract, ovarian agenesis, and seizures suggested a chromosomal disorder, but the chromosomal microarray was normal.
- In this case, the EMG suggested a chronic myopathic process, although MNDs could not be excluded. Muscle biopsy was not helpful due to the end-stage nature of the disease process.
- Urine organic acid analysis revealed a high level of 3-methylglutaconic acid, with normal level of 3-hydroxyisovaleric acid.
- Mitochondrial genetic studies detected abnormal *POLG. POLG* sequencing revealed a heterozygous variant, c.2851T>A (p.Y951N), which was predicted to be deleterious.
- *POLG* mutations are heterogenous genetically and clinically. Neuromuscular manifestations of *POLG* mutations include:
  - Progressive external ophthalmoplegia
  - Neuropathy, ataxia, and retinitis pigmentosa (NARP)
  - Myoclonic epilepsy, myopathy sensory ataxia (MEMSA)
  - Mitochondrial spinocerebellar ataxia and epilepsy (MSCAE)

SUGGESTED READING

Bekheirina MR, Zhang W, Eble T, et al. POLG mutation in a patient with cataracts, early-onset distal muscle weakness and atrophy, ovarian dysgenesis and 3-methylglutaconic aciduria. *Gene.* 2012;499(1):209–212.

CASE 15.8: FINGER FLEXOR WEAKNESS AND QUADRICEPS SPARING

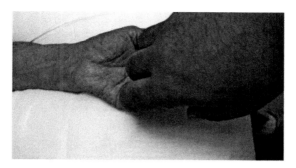

VIDEO 15.8

A 71-year-old woman presented with a 4-year history of gradually increasing inability to twist off jar lids and difficulty swallowing water. Her quadriceps and facial muscles were normal. The CK level was 283 U/L. EMG revealed evidence of irritative myopathy. A left biceps biopsy is shown in Figures 15.8.A and 15.8.B.

According to the IBM diagnostic criteria, this case qualifies for the diagnosis of:

1. Definite IBM
2. Probable IBM
3. Possible IBM
4. No IBM
5. hIBM

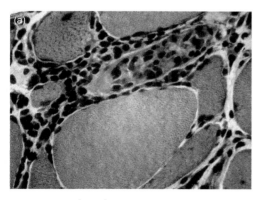

FIGURE 15.8A (400x).

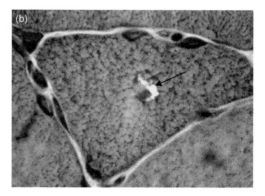

FIGURE 15.8B (100x).

DIAGNOSIS

- Muscle biopsy showed evidence of inflammatory myopathy (A) with red-rimmed vacuoles (B).
- There are at least 12 sets of diagnostic criteria for IBM; none of them is validated for sensitivity and specificity. At best, the most liberal of these criteria identifies 75% of cases clinically and 25% pathologically at the time of diagnosis. The most commonly used of these are the Griggs criteria.
- The presented case did not fulfill all the pathological criteria. However, it did show invasion of nonnecrotic fibers with mononuclear cells and red-rimmed vacuoles, but Congo red staining and EM examination were not done to look for congophilic material and nuclear or cytoplasmic inclusions.
  - The clinical criteria were met, including disease duration, the presence of proximal and distal weakness, and slightly elevated CK.
  - Quadriceps weakness is not required, so long as there is finger flexor weakness or wrist flexor weakness.
  - There is no category for "probable IBM" in Griggs criteria (see supplement on page XXX).
  - This is a case of possible IBM.

SUGGESTED READING

Griggs RC, Askanas V, DiMauro S, et al. Inclusion body myositis and myopathies. *Ann Neurol.* 1995;38:705.

CASE 15.9: DYSPHAGIA AND HAND GRIP WEAKNESS

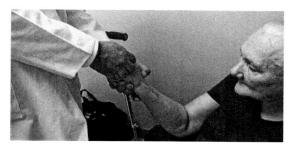

VIDEO 15.9

A 70-year-old woman presented with a 5-year history of right hand grip weakness that spread to the left hand after 2 years. She then developed dysphagia and weight loss. Leg muscle strength was normal. The CK level was 450 U/L. EMG showed many short- and long-duration units in the biceps and wrist flexors.

The combination of chronic facial weakness, dysphagia, and distal arm weakness is typically seen in:

1. IBM
2. FSHD
3. Dystrophia myotonica (DM)
4. Polymyositis
5. ALS

DIAGNOSIS

- Chronic dysphagia and facial weakness are seen in DM, IBM, polymyositis, FSHD, and some congenital myopathies and MG.
- If weakness of finger flexors is added, IBM and DM are the only qualified disorders.
- IBM has many phenotypes. Quadriceps sparing occurs in 5%–10% of cases.
- Mild CK elevation is common in all the above mentioned possibilities.
- A careful examination for percussion and grip myotonia and for waxing and waning EMG discharges is important; if found, a blood test for *DMPK* mutation would be more appropriate than a muscle biopsy. Otherwise, a muscle biopsy would be indicated to look for red-rimmed vacuoles and cytoplasmic inclusion bodies, which are the pathological hallmark of IBM.
- MG may cause distal weakness, but it almost always affects wrist extensors, not finger flexors.
- FSHD is more likely to cause distal leg weakness (foot extensors) than hand weakness. Dysphagia is not common.
- Sometimes, although the clinical picture is suggestive of IBM, the muscle biopsy shows endomysial inflammation without red-rimmed vacuoles or inclusions (polymyositis picture). Some experts tend to treat these cases as polymyositis, particularly if the CK is significantly elevated. Almost always, these cases behave like IBM, and lack of degenerative features in the biopsy is common in the initial inflammatory phase of the disease.
- The NT5C1A antibody titer is elevated in 72% of IBM cases and helps confirm the diagnosis of questionable cases.
- Immunohistochemistry with P62 provide very specific diagnostic information about IBM.

SUGGESTED READING

Nakano S, Oki M, Kusaka H. The role of p62/SQSTM1 in sporadic inclusion body myositis. *Neuromuscul Disord.* 2017 Apr;27(4):363–369.

CASE 15.10: HAND MUSCLE ATROPHY
AND MILD CREATINE KINASE (CK) ELEVATION

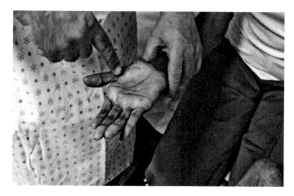

VIDEO 15.10

A 64-year-old woman presented with a 1-year history of bilateral hand muscle weakness. The CK level was 420 U/L, and cervical MRI was normal. EMG revealed diffuse denervation of the distal arms muscles. NCS was normal.

Most likely, this is a case of:

1. Bilateral C8 radiculopathy
2. MND
3. Distal myopathy
4. MG
5. SMA

DIAGNOSIS

- Progressive, painless weakness and atrophy are the diagnostic hallmarks of ALS. However, early in the course of the disease, weakness and atrophy may be focal, and the diagnosis can be challenging.
- Onset of the disease may be marked by upper motor neuron (UMN) symptoms, lower motor neuron (LMN) symptoms, or both, in the following regions:
  1. Bulbar weakness: occurs in one-third of cases and is characterized by dysarthria and, less commonly, dysphagia. It is more common in the elderly and has the worst prognosis.
  2. Proximal muscles: LMN type in the arms (brachial atrophic diplegia) or legs (lumbar atrophic diplegia).
  3. Distal onset in the legs (foot drop) or arms (as in this case).
  4. A total of 1% of cases present with ventilatory weakness.
- ALS is also classified according to the predominance of motor neurons affected:
  - UMNs: primary lateral sclerosis
  - LMNs: progressive muscular atrophy
  - Both: ALS proper
- The farther the initial deficit is from the head, the better the prognosis.
- Cervical MRI is needed to rule out cervical myeloradiculopathy.
- Mild CK elevation is common and should not sway the diagnosis toward myopathy.
- EMG is crucial to confirm the diagnosis and determine the extent of denervation.
- Progression of the disease within a few months is a required criterion for the diagnosis of ALS.
- Some benign MND variants, like monomelic amyotrophy and SMA, are differentiated by being chronic and less progressive.

CASE 15.11: RIGHT HAND WEAKNESS

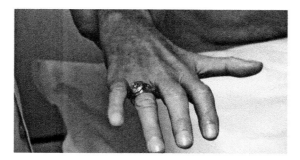

VIDEO 15.11

A 47-year-old man presented with a 13-year history of weakness of the right hand, causing inability to write. He was diagnosed with thoracic outlet syndrome (TOS), but surgery did not help. He progressed for 5 years and then plateaued. EMG revealed chronic denervation of the distal right arm flexors and extensors. Erb's point stimulation revealed no conduction block. Sensory responses were normal. Cervical MRI and CPK were both normal.

The level of insult is likely:

1. Motor neurons
2. Nerve roots
3. Peripheral nerves
4. Brachial plexus
5. Spinal cord

DIAGNOSIS

- Chronic progressive weakness and atrophy of distal arm muscles unilaterally is a diagnostic challenge.
- Most distal myopathies are bilateral from the beginning. Lower cervical radiculopathies are usually painful and are associated with sensory symptoms such as tingling that radiates along the C7 and C8 distribution (i.e., the back of the arm and the ulnar side of the hand). Nevertheless, it is an important differential that needs to be ruled out by a good EMG and cervical MRI. EMG usually shows denervation that can be traced along the myotomes of the affected nerve roots.
- In this case, the chronic denervation involved the distal hand muscles that are supplied by all three hand nerves, with no proximal denervation. These were all C7 (wrist flexors and extensors and long finger flexors and extensors) and C8–T1 (intrinsic hand muscles). The lesion is most likely at the level of motor neurons.
- Multifocal motor neuropathy with conduction block is an important consideration for this purely motor distal weakness and areflexia. However, there is no conduction block or motor slowing; instead, there is diffuse distal denervation.
- There are many chronic MNDs; most of them are genetic.
  - Monomelic amyotrophy is a sporadic disease that predominantly affects young males. After a few years of progression, the disease stabilizes. DTRs are usually absent but can be normal or brisk. ALS may be suspected initially, but the lack of spread and progression rules it out. Brachial plexitis is usually acute, painful, and self-limiting.

CASE 15.12: CHRONIC DYSPHAGIA AND HAND STIFFNESS

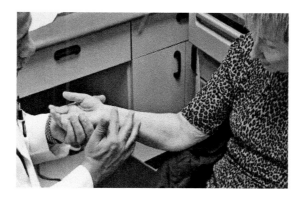

VIDEO 15.12

A 65-year-old woman presented with a 10-year history of frequent falls and slowly progressive dysphagia and facial weakness. She had several syncopal episodes a few years earlier, and a pacemaker was inserted. She had no significant family history. The CK level was 95 U/L. The examination is shown in the video.

Which of the following features does not favor IBM, but does favor DM?

1. Female patient
2. Caucasian race
3. Quadriceps weakness
4. Facial weakness
5. Syncope

DIAGNOSIS

- The picture was very suggestive of IBM, including chronic course, weakness of the finger flexors and quadriceps muscles, facial weakness, dysphagia, and mild CK elevation. Syncope could be incidental or due to a cardiac conduction abnormality that is associated with DM, one of the mimicking conditions.
- EMG revealed diffuse waxing and waning 150-Hz discharges and myopathic units. Reexamination revealed mild percussion myotonia. Muscle biopsy was canceled; instead, mutation analysis for DM type 1 was requested, which revealed a cytosine-thymine-guanine (CTG) repeat expansion to 1,200 repeats in the *DMPK* gene, confirming the diagnosis of DM1.
- Examination for percussion and grip myotonia is often left out of the evaluation, even though it can provide very relevant (and sometimes unexpected) information.
- IBM is the most common myopathy after age 50, and DM is the most common MD in adults. Although DM is an autosomal-dominant (AD) disease, symptoms in the parents can be very subtle (unreported) compared to their offspring, due to the genetic phenomenon of anticipation.
- Cardiac conduction abnormalities are very common in DM, and they contribute to mortality. Most patients will need a pacemaker by age 50 years, and therefore serial monitoring of electrocardiography (ECG) for detection of conduction defects is important.
- Sometimes syncope due to heart block is the presenting feature of DM.

CASE 15.13: CHRONIC BILATERAL WRIST EXTENSOR WEAKNESS

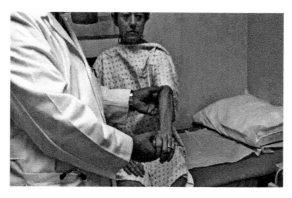

VIDEO 15.13

A 61-year-old woman presented with a 10-year history of slowly progressive arm weakness. She had a normal CK and myopathic EMG. Muscle biopsy revealed chronic myopathic findings.

The history and examination suggests that this could be a case of:

1. FSHD
2. Dysferlinopathy
3. Calpainopathy
4. Dystrophinopathy
5. Cavuolinopathy

DIAGNOSIS

- Chronic and slowly progressive weakness of the wrist extensors and scapular winging with normal CK and nonirritable myopathic EMG are not seen in many diseases.
  1. FSHD: Facial sparing occurs in less than 10% of cases. Wrist extensor weakness occurs late in the disease. Leg weakness is usually distal (asymmetrical foot drop). In this case, normal D4Z4 size ruled out type 1 FSHD.
     - With a FSHD phenotype and normal D4Z4 repeat size, one has to think of FSHD2, which is associated with mutation of the *SMCHD1* gene on chromosome 18P. As in FSHD, a permissive distal A allele is required for the diagnosis. FSHD2 is an AD disease identical to the FSHD1 phenotype, and a positive family history is expected in 50% of cases. Beside chronic myopathic pathological findings, muscle inflammation is not uncommon.
  2. LGMD2B (calpainopathy): Scapular winging and weakness of the wrist extensors and flexors are recognized features. It is AR. Many lobulated fibers are usually seen in muscle biopsy.
  3. This combination of findings (particularly the normal CK) is not a feature of dystrophinopathy, Miyoshi myopathy (again, normal CK is very atypical), or caveolinopathy (rippling muscle disease).
  4. Wrist extensor weakness is common in many hereditary distal myopathies (especially Welander myopathy), but scapular wingging is exceedingly rare.

SUGGESTED READING

Lemmers, RJ, Tawil R, Petek LM, et al. Digenic inheritance of an SMCHD1 mutation and an FSHD-permissive D4Z4 allele causes facioscapulohumeral muscular dystrophy type 2. *Nature Genet.* 2012;44:1370–1374.

CASE 15.14: SEVERE CHRONIC DYSPHAGIA AND FACIAL WEAKNESS

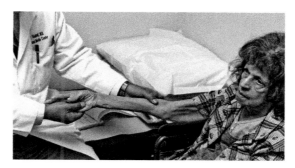

VIDEO 15.14

A 70-year-old woman presented with a 10-year history of dysphagia and arm weakness. Her quadriceps muscles were 3/5, and she had bilateral foot drop and severe weakness of the finger flexors. The CK level was 400 U/L. EMG revealed long- and short-duration MUPs in the arms, with no spontaneous activity. Sensory responses and motor conduction studies were normal. Muscle biopsy is shown in Figures 15.14.1 and 15.14.2.

The most likely diagnosis is:

1. Polymyositis
2. IBM
3. Vasculitis
4. MD
5. Necrotizing myopathy

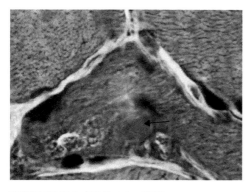

FIGURE 15.14.1 H&E stain: 1000x.

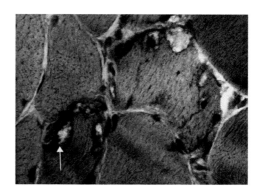

FIGURE 15.14.2 Modified Gomori trichrome stain: 400x.

DIAGNOSIS

- The clinical picture is classical of sIBM, and muscle pathology confirmed the diagnosis by showing red-rimmed vacuoles and cytoplasmic eosinophilic inclusion body.
- IBM remains a dismal disease.
- The response to treatment is poor. Progressive weakness is the rule. The older the age of onset, the more rapid the loss of strength and function is. Within 10 years of the diagnosis, most people become wheelchair bound. Patients lose 5% of strength per year.

Complications of IBM and causes of death:

- Loss of ambulation due to severe weakness of the legs
- Aspiration pneumonia due to severe dysphagia
- Exposure keratitis from facial weakness
- Malnutrition due to dysphagia and depression
- Immobility complications, such as deep vein thrombosis (DVT) and skin ulceration
  - Life expectancy is normal, but morbidity rate is high.
  - There is no increase in the risk of systemic diseases or malignancy.

CASE 15.15: LOSS OF "PINCH" AND SCAPULAR WINGING

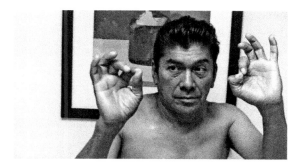

VIDEO 15.15

A 43-year-old man presented with acute burning pain and tingling in the right shoulder and forearm that mandated the use of hydrocodone. He had weakness of the fingers of his right hand 3 weeks later, as shown in the video and winging of the right scapula. MRI of the neck was normal. The pain subsided 6 weeks later, but the weakness and atrophy continued.

NCS/EMG will likely show dysfunction of the following nerves on the right side:

1. AIN
2. Phrenic nerve
3. Long thoracic nerve
4. Radial nerve
5. SAN

DIAGNOSIS

- The pain of PTS is usually poorly defined, burning, deep, and severe, and it affects the neck and deep tissue around the shoulder. Diagnosis is usually not made until weakness appears 2–3 weeks later. The pain initially is considered musculoskeletal or psychogenic.
- Such a severe neuropathic pain is produced by inflammation of the sensory branches of the brachial plexus.
- Weakness appears 2–3 weeks later, as previously noted, and it affects the muscles supplied by the affected nerves or nerve trunks or cords.
  - The upper and/or middle trunk with involvement of the long thoracic nerve, suprascapular nerve, or both occurs in 70% of cases.
  - A total of 30% of cases are bilateral from the beginning or sequentially.
  - Individual nerves may be affected, such as median and radial nerves and the AIN.
  - In a minority of patients, nerves outside the brachial plexus are affected, such as the phrenic nerve, lingual nerve, recurrent laryngeal nerve, and lumbar plexus.
  - In 10% of cases, pain is not prominent, and the diagnosis of multifocal motor neuropathy with conduction block (MMNCB) is suspected, but NCS with stimulation at Erb's point fails to show conduction block.
  - Recurrence occurs in 25% of cases within 6 years. These cases can be difficult to differentiate from hereditary neuralgic amyotrophy (HNA), which tends to occur in a younger age group with more involvement of nerves outside the brachial plexus and with more serve residual weakness.

SUGGESTED READING

van Alfen N, van Engelen BG. The clinical spectrum of neuralgic amyotrophy in 246 cases. *Brain*. 2006 Feb;129(Pt 2):438–450. Epub 2005 Dec 21.

CASE 15.16: CHRONIC FACIAL AND HAND GRIP WEAKNESS

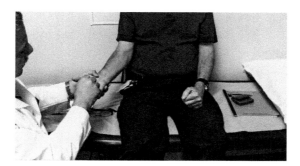

VIDEO 15.16

A 50-year-old man presented with chronic, progressive weakness of the bilateral hand grip and facial muscles.

Weak finger flexors and facial muscles are typically observed in:

1. IBM
2. Polymyositis
3. DM
4. Facial onset sensorimotor neuropathy (FOSMN)
5. FSHD

DIAGNOSIS

- Patients with chronic progressive weakness of hand grip without sensory symptoms usually belong to one of the following categories:
  - Distal myopathy: purely distal, or part of a more generalized myopathy
  - SMA: distal type or part of a more generalized type
  - Lower cervical radiculopathy: pain and numbness possibly minimal
  - Lower cord or trunk brachial plexopathy: pain and numbness possibly minimal
  - Motor neuropathy, such as MMNCB
- Unlike SMA, in myopathic weakness, usually there is no atrophy of the intrinsic hand muscles, but rather weakness of the finger flexors and atrophy of the volar forearm muscles.
- Facial weakness limits the diagnosis to the first two categories.
- Mild CK elevation is common in both, but more than 10 times normal would be more in favor of a myopathic condition.
- A good EMG can sort out the myopathic from the neurogenic type (diffuse high-firing frequency is commonly seen in SMA, and low-amplitude, short-duration units with early recruitment are features of myopathy), although in chronic cases, mixed MUPs are difficult to sort out. A muscle biopsy in these cases is useful.
- Among the chronic myopathic ailments, the ones that cause facial weakness, finger flexor weakness, and dysphagia are IBM and DM. It is crucial to look for clinical percussion myotonia, the typical facies of the DM, and the appropriate family history.
- However, due to the phenomenon of anticipation, other family members may be only minimally affected and did not seek medical advice.
- Patients with IBM may get temporalis atrophy, leading to a thin face, and even they may show paraspinal myotonic discharges, or more often pseudomyotonic discharges.
- In these cases, a muscle biopsy is crucial. Red-rimmed vacuoles and intracytoplasmic eosinophilic inclusion bodies of IBM could be easily differentiated from the atrophy and sarcoplasmic masses of DM type 1.

CASE 15.17: DAMN GOOD

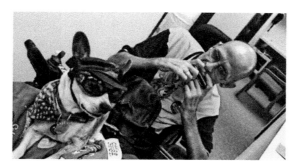

VIDEO 15.17

A 43-year-old man, a Vietnam War veteran with an old spinal cord injury, presented with numbness and weakness of the hands. He was found to have severe bilateral focal ulnar nerve entrapment at the elbows, thought to be related to wheelchair use. He made a living by showing his funny dog to people.

Ulnar nerve entrapment at the elbows:

1. Is more common in wheelchair users
2. Is more common in diabetics with neuropathy
3. Shares some features with C8 radiculopathy
4. Is a typical feature of PTS
5. Is routinely surgically treated

DIAGNOSIS

- Despite the hectic schedule of neuromuscular clinics, there is time for fun. Some patients have a good sense of humor and turn their frustration into hope, while others find the time to celebrate their improvement by showing some funny talents.
- This Vietnam veteran had traumatic paraplegia and had been wheelchair bound for years. He developed compression of the bilateral ulnar nerves at the elbows from excessive use of the arms to propel himself. He tried to show appreciation of our service by showing us a talent that he and his dog, Damn Good, mastered over the years and that had become their main source of income.
- Ulnar nerve is vulnerable to compression at the elbow because it travels through a narrow space (cubital tunnel) with little support. C8 radiculopathy also causes pain along the ulnar side of the arm and atrophy of First dorsal interosseous (FDI). Atrophy of thenar muscles and denervation of nonulnar C8 muscles are not features of ulnar neuropathy.
- Arthritis and repetitive elbow flexion are the main risk factors, but in the majority of cases, no clear cause is found for compression. It is more common in diabetics with neuropathy due to increased vulnerability of nerves to pressure. PTS typically affect the upper trunk.
- Avoidance of pressure on the elbows and elbow support are to be tried first.
- Surgery is indicated if there is wasting of the intrinsic hand muscles or if the compression is severe.
- Cubital tunnel release and medial nerve transposition are the main surgical techniques. They are equally effective.

SUGGESTED READING

Calliandro P, La Torre G, Padua R, Giannini F, Padua L. Treatment for ulnar neuropathy at the elbow. *Coch Database Sys Rev*. 2011 Feb;16(2): CD006839.

CASE 15.18: DECLINING GOLF PERFORMANCE

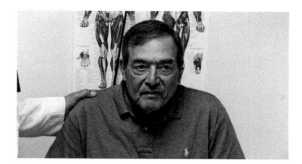

VIDEO 15.18

A 68-year-old man presented whose clinical findings are shown in the video. The CPK level was 433 IU/L. EMG showed mixed short- and long-duration units in the FDP of the hand grips. Muscle biopsy is shown in Figure 15.18.1. There were no red-rimmed vacuoles or cytoplasmic inclusion bodies. The NT5C1A antibody titer was negative.

The case is most likely due to:

1. Polymyositis
2. Mitochondrial myopathy.
3. IBM
4. Granulomatous myopathy
5. MD

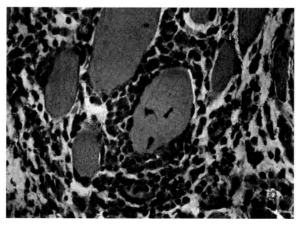

FIGURE 15.18.1 Left biceps muscle biopsy. H&E stain; 400X.

DIAGNOSIS

- The age, sex, slow progression, weakness of finger flexors and facial muscles, dysphagia, high CPK, and mixed MUPs in the EMG are very suggestive of IBM.
- Lack of quadriceps weakness is atypical, seen in only 15% of cases.
- Early facial weakness, the lack of dysarthria, and weakness of the FDP as opposed to the intrinsic hand muscles are atypical of ALS.
- Muscle biopsy shows only inflammatory myopathy in about 10%–15% of IBM cases, especially early in the course of the disease before the degenerative phase starts.
- An NT5C1A antibody titer is obtained in atypical IBM cases to confirm IBM, as it is positive in 40%–60% of cases (with false positives in 30% of cases).
- Regarding an IBM diagnosis, when there is inflammatory myopathy lacking red-rimmed vacuoles:
  - The presence of mitochondrial changes is 100% sensitive and 73% specific for IBM.
  - Characteristic p62 aggregates are specific (91%) but lacked sensitivity (44%).
- Alternatively, another muscle biopsy a year or more later will likely show the typical red-rimmed vacuoles and inclusion bodies. However, this is rarely necessary, as the clinical picture, the time course, and the exclusion of other causes (such as granulomatous myositis) by muscle biopsy are enough to make the diagnosis unless more evidence is needed for clinical trials.

SUGGESTED READING

Brady S, Squier W, Sewry C, Hanna M, Hilton-Jones D, Holton JL. A retrospective cohort study identifying the principal pathological features useful in the diagnosis of inclusion body myositis. *BMJ Open.* 2014;4:e004552.

CASE 15.19: PROGRESSIVE HAND WEAKNESS AND GRANULOMA IN MUSCLE BIOPSY

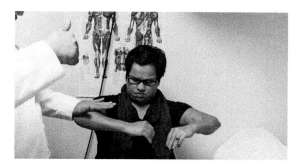

VIDEO 15.19

A 38-year-old woman with history of rheumatoid arthritis (RA) treated with abatacept and hydroxychloroquine presented with progressive, painless weakness of hand grips over a year and difficulty climbing stairs. Examination is shown in the video. The CK level was 1,600 IU/L, but it came down to 800 after she discontinued atorvastatin. SR was 80 mm/hour. EMG revealed irritative myopathy. A left biceps muscle biopsy showed granulomatous myopathy (Fig. 15.19.1). Computed tomography (CT) scan of the chest was negative.

Predominantly distal weakness with inflammatory myopathy in the muscle biopsy is typically seen in all of the following except:

1. IBM
2. Granulomatous myopathy
3. Sarcoidosis
4. Statin autoimmune inflammatory myopathy
5. Miyoshi myopathy

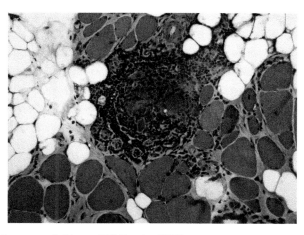

FIGURE 15.19.1 Left biceps muscle biopsy. H&E stain. 400X

DIAGNOSIS

- Statin autoimmune inflammatory myopathy typically does not present with distal weakness.
- The rest of the choices do present with distal weakness and show inflammatory myopathy in the muscle biopsy.
- IBM usually shows cytoplasmic inclusion bodies and red-rimmed vacuoles. Rare cases of granuloma formation are reported.
  - However, besides finger flexor weakness, quadriceps and facial weakness with dysphagia and onset after age 50 years are typically present.
  - Clinical and pathological features of IBM with granuloma are not different than those without it.
- Granulomatous myopathy may be related to sarcoidosis, but the angiotensin-converting enzyme (ACE) level and CT scan of chest were normal.
- Increased SR may be due to RA, muscle inflammation, or both.
- Miyoshi myopathy (dysferlinopathy) is associated with distal weakness and muscle inflammation, with more than 10 times the normal CK elevation. Granuloma is not a feature.
- Granulomatous myopathy is a rare form of inflammatory muscle disease.
  - It may present as progressive proximal weakness along with MG and thymoma, or as a chronic distal weakness as a manifestation of sarcoidosis.
  - Frequently, the search for sarcoidosis is not productive and the diagnosis of idiopathic granulomatous myopathy is given.
  - CK level is normal to 5 times the normal level.
  - EMG shows chronic myopathic findings (mixed short- and long-duration MUPs and early recruitment).
  - Prognosis is poor, and unfortunately, response to immunosuppression or modulation is poor in the distal form.
  - Unlike the proximal variant, the distal idiopathic type does not affect the heart, but it may extend to the proximal muscles.

SUGGESTED READINGS

Jasim S, Shaibani A. Nonsarcoid granulomatous myopathy: two cases and a review of literature. *Int J Neurosci C*. 2013 Jul;123(7A):516–520.

Sakai K, Ikeda Y, Ishida C, et al. Inclusion body myositis with granuloma formation in muscle tissue. *Neuromusc Disord*. 2015 Sep;25(9):706–712.

CHAPTER 16

DISTAL LEG WEAKNESS

CASE 16.1: FOOT PAIN AND POSTURAL SYNCOPE

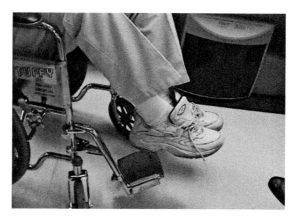

VIDEO 16.1

A 66-year-old man presented with a 3-year history of severe burning sensation in the feet and loss of balance. He then developed hand numbness and postural lightheadedness. He fainted once when he stood up fast. A year later, he lost weight due to diarrhea. His examination revealed moderate proximal and distal weakness, right foot drop, distal sensory impairment, and diffuse areflexia. His older brother and father had similar symptoms. Electromyography (EMG) revealed mixed axonal and demyelinating neuropathy. Also, he had moderate bilateral focal median nerve lesion at the wrists. Cerebrospinal fluid (CSF) protein was normal. Due to the progression of the illness and the lack of the clinical findings, he had a left sural nerve biopsy.

Which of the following stains or preparations would be most useful for the diagnosis?

1. Modified trichrome
2. Congo red stain viewed under polarized light
3. Hematoxylin and eosin (H&E) stain
4. Semithin sections
5. Teased nerve fiber preparation

What diagnosis is suggested by the combination of the following findings?

1. Family history
2. Dysautonomia features
3. Bilateral carpal tunnel syndrome (CTS)
4. Painful neuropathy
5. Progressive course

DIAGNOSIS

Familial amyloid polyneuropathy (FAP):

- Nerve biopsy revealed green birefringent deposits when Congo red–stained tissue was visualized under polarized light. Mutation analysis revealed transthyretin (TTR) mutation diagnostic of a form of FAP.
- Amyloid is a misfolded, insoluble protein that cannot be digested and degraded; therefore, it accumulates in the tissue and damages it. It can be systemic or localized to certain organs.
- The most vulnerable tissues are the nerves, autonomic ganglia, kidneys, gastrointestinal (GI) tract, and heart.
  - Familial amyloidosis is usually autosomal dominant (AD) and is caused by mutation of TTR, apolipoprotein A1, or gelsoline.
  - Primary amyloidosis (AL amyloidosis) is caused by the deposition of immunoglobin G (IgG) light chains. It could be part of lymphoma, multiple myeloma, or other lymphoproliferative disorders, or it could lack a clear cause.
- The triad of dysautonomia (which usually presents as postural hypotension), severe CTS (hand numbness), and painful feet (polyneuropathy) is highly suspicious of FAP, especially if there is a family history or nerve conduction study (NCS) evidence of axonal polyneuropathy.
- Diagnosis is made by the finding of apple green birefringent deposits in the nerve tissue, abdominal fat, or rectal biopsy. These deposits do not react to antibodies to light chains (unlike AL amyloidosis), but rather to antibodies to TTR, gelsoline, or apolipoprotein A1.
- TTR mutation is the most common FAP, and it occurs in two phenotypes:
  - FAP I: develops in the third to fourth decades. CTS is not severe, but foot pain and hypotension are severe. Renal and cardiac involvement is common.
  - FAP II: the milder form, with more severe CTS and less severe dysautonomia and renal/cardiac involvement. It appears in the 70s, and the patients have long survival.
- Abdominal fat aspiration, if done from at least two sites, is probably as sensitive as nerve biopsy to detect amyloid deposits.
- Blood test for mutations of TTR, apolipoprotine A1, and gelsoline is advised to characterize this familial disorder further.

CASE 16.2: ASYMMETRIC PAINFUL FOOT DROP

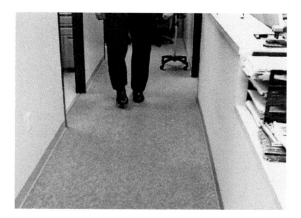

VIDEO 16.2

A 54-year-old man with a 3-month history of severe foot pain that started on the left side. He then developed hand numbness and proximal leg weakness and weight loss. The erythrocyte sedimentation rate (ESR) rate was 25 mm/hour, and antinuclear antibodies (ANA) were negative. EMG revealed axonal polyneuropathy. CSF protein was 75 mg/dl. Nerve biopsy pictures are shown in Figures 16.2.1 and 16.2.2.

The pathological picture confirms the diagnosis of:

1. Amyloidosis
2. Vasculitis of the peripheral nervous system (PNS)
3. Sarcoidosis
4. Chronic inflammatory demyelinating polyneuropathy (CIDP)
5. Leprosy

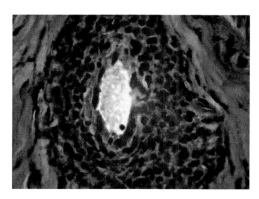

FIGURE 16.2.1 H&E stain: 400x.

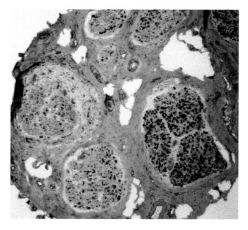

FIGURE 16.2.2 Modified Gromori Trichorme stain: 100x.

DIAGNOSIS

- Foot drop is commonly seen in neuromuscular clinics. It can be caused by polyneuropathy, peroneal neuropathy, L5 radiculopathy, lumbosacral (LS) plexopathy, and certain myopathies and myasthenia gravis (MG).
- Painful neuropathy is commonly seen in amyloidosis, vasculitis, familial autonomic and sensory neuropathy, and diabetes mellitus (DM).
- Progressive, asymmetrical, painful neuropathy with asymmetrical foot drop should always raise the possibility of vasculitis, which could be systemic in the context of viral infections, connective tissue disease, malignancy, etc, or isolated to the PNS (nonsystemic vasculitis). In these cases, a nerve biopsy is indicated, as it would be the only way to confirm the diagnosis.
- Nerve biopsy findings diagnostic of vasculitis are reported in 50% of cases, but partial findings can be useful in the right clinical context.
- There are no clinical trials on the treatment of isolated PNS vasculitis, but the standard therapy is a combination of steroids and intravenous (IV) or oral cyclophosphamide. The response rate is high, but 30% of cases relapse, and some develop chronic foot pain, even after resolution of vasculitis.
- Nerve biopsy findings of vasculitis:
  - Endoneurial and perineurial inflammation and mural infiltration with mononuclear inflammatory cells (Figure 16.2)
  - Eosinophils may predominate the inflammatory infiltrate in some cases of systemic vasculitis (i.e., Churg-Strauss syndrome and Wagner granulomatosis)
  - Fibrinoid necrosis of the small endoneurial blood vessels
  - Thrombosis, obliteration of lumen
  - Differential fascicular degeneration (Figure 16.2.2) and recanalization (chronic cases)
- Combined nerve and muscle (and maybe skin) biopsy increases the diagnostic yield. In patients with foot drop, superficial peroneal nerve and peroneus brevis muscle biopsy is appropriate. In other cases, sural nerve and gastrocnemius muscle biopsy is equally productive.

CASE 16.3: FAMILIAL DISTAL WEAKNESS

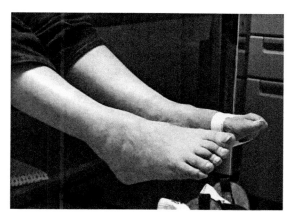

VIDEO 16.3

A 66-year-old woman presented with bilateral foot drop and wrist extensor weakness that evolved over 5 years with no sensory symptoms or signs. Deep tendon reflexes (DTRs) were absent diffusely, and proximal strength was normal. There was no facial weakness. She had three children with similar symptoms. Sural responses were normal. EMG revealed chronic distal denervation of the lower and upper extremities and low compound muscle action potential (CMAP) diffusely.

The most likely diagnosis is:

1. Charcot-Marie-Tooth (CMT) disease
2. Spinal muscular atrophy (SMA)
3. Lead poisoning
4. Diphtheria
5. Vasculitis

DIAGNOSIS

- The pure motor nature of the symptoms and the normal sural responses suggested a motor neuropathy or neuronopathy. Areflexia and chronic denervation by EMG support this notion.

- The chronicity and family history suggest distal SMA. Some of these cases are confused with neuronal CMT, but the preservation of the sensation and sural responses suggest that this is a motor neuronopathy. Distal myopathies are also to be ruled out before embarking on the diagnosis of distal SMA.

- There are many types of SMA, depending on the age of onset, mode of inheritance, first affected region, and type of genetic defect, but all share degeneration of motor neurons for genetic etiology. High foot arches are common.

- Distal SMA does not affect longevity. It is rare. It may start in the legs or arms. It can be autosomal recessive (AR) or AD. Mutations in the *BSCL2* and *GARS* genes explain some cases of distal SMA.

- A fatal form is reported in infants associated with respiratory distress (spinal muscular atrophy with respiratory distress syndrome, or SMARD1) due to mutation of the *IGHMBP2* gene.

- Other than ankle braces, fall precautions, and rehabilitation programs, not much can be offered to help these cases, and there is no drug in the pipeline to treat this genetically determined neurodegenerative disorder.

SUGGESTED READING

Harding AE, Thomas PK. Hereditary SMA: a report of 14 cases and a review of the literature. *J Neurol Sci.* 1980;45:337–348.

CASE 16.4: A RECLINER AND FOOT DROP

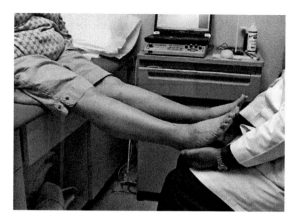

VIDEO 16.4

A 53-year-old diabetic woman presented with painless left foot drop developed over a few months (which spread to the right foot a month later) and a shocklike sensation from the knees to the shins. There was no foot numbness or proximal weakness. Lumbar spine magnetic resonance imaging (LS MRI) was nonrevealing, and EMG revealed conduction block of both peroneal motor nerves at the fibular heads and denervation of the tibialis anterior, but not the tibialis posterior. She gave a history of using a recliner 13 hours a day due to poor mobility from arthritis.

The cause of this bilateral peroneal compressive neuropathy is likely:

1. Vasculitis
2. Compression
3. CIDP
4. CMT disease
5. Factitious disorder

DIAGNOSIS

- As in other branches of medicine, careful observation and sound reasoning are crucial for the right diagnosis and to save patients unnecessary procedures.
- Sequential foot drop in this patient suggested vasculitis, but the lack of foot pain and the preservation of the sural responses and ankle reflexes and the focal conduction block of the peroneal nerves at the fibular heads suggested compressive lesions at the knees.
- The patient was not aware of the importance of the recliner in causing her symptoms, and therefore she did not volunteer to mention it. Only when she was questioned did she gave that part of the history. She was advised to quit using the recliner, and her peroneal neuropathy recovered completely within 6 weeks.
- Compression of the peroneal nerves is common in patients with polyneuropathy, especially diabetic neuropathy and alcoholic neuropathy, but in this case, there is no evidence of polyneuropathy.
- L5 radiculopathy is ruled out by having normal tibialis posterior EMG and nonremarkable LS MRI.
- If conduction block was seen in other sites, especially in not-at-risk patients, one had to look for hereditary neuropathy with liability to pressure palsy (HNPP).

CASE 16.5: RIGHT FOOT DROP AND INFLAMMATORY MUSCLE BIOPSY

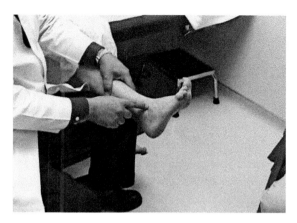

VIDEO 16.5

A 61-year-old woman presented with the shown findings. The CK level was 650 U/L.
The most appropriate next testing is:

1. Muscle biopsy
2. FSHD mutation analysis
3. LS MRI
4. Emerin gene mutation analysis
5. NCS

What diagnosis is suggested by the combination of the following findings?

1. Asymmetric onset
2. Distal weakness
3. Scapular winging
4. Facial weakness
5. Inflammatory pathology

DIAGNOSIS

Myopathic foot drop:

- Painless, asymmetrical foot drop, scapular winging, and myopathic EMG suggest FSHD. Neurogenic and myopathic scapuloperoneal syndrome is also possible. This patient had contraction of the *D4Z4* allele, confirming the diagnosis of FSHD.
- Unilateral or bilateral foot drop may be caused by muscle disease.
- Factors that would suggest a myopathic etiology include:
  - Preserved bulk or even compensatory hypertrophy of the extensor digitorum brevis (EDB) due to the lack of involvement of the intrinsic foot muscles, unlike neurogenic etiology, when these muscles are affected early.
  - The lack of sensory symptoms or signs.
  - The lack of foot pain.
  - Preservation of sural responses.
  - Lack of denervation of the tibialis anterior; spontaneous activity may be seen as a part of irritative myopathy.
  - The presence of other features of muscle disease, like proximal weakness and scapular winging.
- FSHD is a common inherited muscle disease where the tibialis anterior muscles are affected early, leading to unilateral or bilateral foot drop, usually in association with scapular winging and facial weakness. A total of 20% of cases do not show facial weakness.
- Foot drop can be the presenting symptom of FSHD, which may lead to diagnostic confusion with peroneal neuropathy and L5 radiculopathy, and sometimes amyotrophic lateral sclerosis (ALS).
- Affected family members may not be aware of their myopathic features, and their examination is usually helpful.
- Asymmetry can be striking, leading to unilateral foot drop or facial weakness.
- Inflammation in the muscle biopsy is characteristic, leading to misdiagnosis as polymyositis. Muscle biopsy is not required for the diagnosis, which can be made from a blood sample.
- A total of 20% of patients end up in a wheelchair.

CASE 16.6: CALF ATROPHY AND MODERATELY HIGH CREATINE KINASE (CK) LEVEL

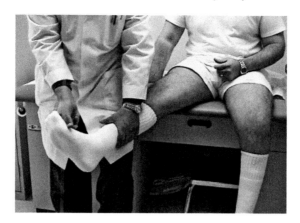

VIDEO 16.6

A 30-year-old man presented who had difficulty walking on his toes at age 15 years. At that time, he was found to have a CK level of 2,800 U/L, and EMG revealed fibrillations in the bilateral calf muscles. He was diagnosed with axonal neuropathy. Gradually, he developed more atrophy of the calves, proximal leg and arm weakness, and weakness of the finger flexors. The CK level was 3,000–4,000 U/L, and NCS were normal. EMG revealed irritative myopathy involving the proximal and distal muscles of the arms and legs. There was no family history of muscle disease. He started using a walker 7 years after the onset of the symptoms. A left biceps biopsy revealed chronic inflammatory myopathic changes.

The most appropriate immunohistochemical testing on the muscle biopsy is:

1. CD4/CD8 antibodies
2. Dysferlin antibodies
3. Dystrophin antibodies
4. Sarcoglycan antibodies
5. Calpain antibodies

DIAGNOSIS

- Distal myopathy is a feature of many myopathic disorders; most of them are hereditary.
- Among the sporadic disorders, inclusion body myositis (IBM) is the most common myopathy with distal involvement.
- Dystrophic myopathies like myotonic dystrophy usually cause distal weakness, along with facial and proximal weakness.
- There is a group of hereditary myopathies characterized only by distal weakness, at least in the beginning of the disease. These disorders lack molecular understanding, and they are classified according to the region affected, mode of inheritance, and age of onset. Many of them are allelic to specific limb girdle muscular dystrophies (LGMDs). More molecular understanding will likely change the classification in the future.
- Miyoshi myopathy is one of the better-characterized distal hereditary myopathies:
  - It starts in early adult life with calf atrophy and weakness and remarkably elevated CK level and myopathic EMG.
  - It is caused by mutation of the dysferlin gene and is allelic with LGMD 2B.
  - Endomysial inflammation in muscle biopsy may lead to erroneous diagnosis of polymyositis.
- Patients with myopathic calf atrophy do not need a muscle biopsy unless mutation analysis carried on white blood cells (WBCs) fails to reveal absent dysferlin staining.

SUGGESTED READING

Shaibani, A. Distal myopathies: case studies. *Neurol Clin.* 34(2016):547–564.

CASE 16.7: CALF ATROPHY AND MILD CREATINE KINASE (CK) ELEVATION

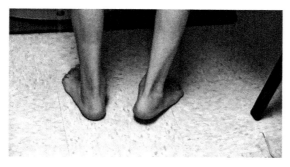

VIDEO 16.7

A 53-year-old man presented with resting painful cramping of the calf muscles that he has had since age 20 years. He noticed the inability to stand on his toes 25 years ago. There was severe atrophy and weakness of the calf muscles. Hip flexors were slightly weak. Arm muscles were 5/5. Reflexes were brisk except for the ankles, which were absent; sensation and sural responses were normal, but CMAPs were low. The CK level was 420 U/L and EMG showed large motor unit potentials (MUPs) with an amplitude of 12–15 mV and a firing frequency of 20–30 Hz in the arms and legs and thoracic paraspinal (TPS) muscles.

The cause of the calf weakness in this case is likely:

1. Miyoshi myopathy
2. SMA
3. ALS
4. Bilateral S1 radiculopathy
5. LS plexopathy

DIAGNOSIS

- Chronic, progressive, distal weakness that starts in the legs is an important scenario in neuromuscular clinics.
- NCS/EMG plays a crucial role in sorting out neurogenic from myopathic conditions.
- Mild CK elevation frequently leads to confusion with myopathy, but it is a common finding in denervating conditions like motor neuron diseases (MNDs).
- In the elderly, it is important to rule out spinal pathology such as severe spondylosis resulting in LS polyradiculopathy, although the lack of pain is atypical.
- Muscle biopsy is not necessary in neurogenic cases; if done, it would show chronic denervation and reinnervation.
- In SMA, loss of DTRs in the affected limbs is expected. Hyperreflexia occurs in 10% of cases. Pes cavus is common.
- Familial ALS (FALS) and neuronal CMT are important considerations.
- Most SMAs manifests themselves during infancy and childhood, but some present in adulthood.
- Some distal SMAs in adults are reported in only one or two families, and their genetic pattern varies from AD to AR, and even X-linked recessive modes. All of them are slowly progressive, and usually they spare the cranial nerves.
- Adult-onset distal SMAs or hereditary motor neuropathies (HMNs):
  - HMN 2A: AD 12q24.3; some with vocal fold and diaphragm weakness
  - HMN 2B AD/AR 7q11.23
  - Distal SMA, X-linked Xq12–q13
  - Distal SMA 3 (DSMA 3): chromosome 11q13.3; recessive

SUGGESTED READING

Wee CD, Kong L, Summer CJ. The genetics of SMA. *Curr Opin Neurol.* 2010 Oct;23:450–458.

CASE 16.8: CHRONIC CALF ATROPHY

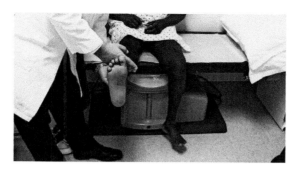

VIDEO 16.8

A 52-year-old man was an avid runner until 18 years earlier, when he had difficulty running, and gradually, he developed atrophy of the distal leg muscles. Examination revealed weakness of plantar flexors and extensors with normal sensation and absent ankle reflexes. The CPK level was 320 IU/L. LS MRI revealed mild degenerative changes. He had seven healthy siblings. EMG revealed diffuse chronic denervation with MUPs of 15 mV amplitude and 20 millisecond duration in all the tested muscles proximally and distally in all extremities.

Mutation that is responsible for non-5q SMA are reported in the following genes except:

1. *CHCHD10*
2. *TRPV4*
3. *DYNC1H1*
4. *BICD2*
5. *SMN1*

DIAGNOSIS

- There has been progress in defining the clinical and genetic features of at least 20 distinct forms of SMA.
- A total of 95% of SMA cases are caused by mutations of the *SMN1* gene on chromosome 5q.
- Only 5% of 5q-related SMA are adult onset. In children, they are the most important cause of floppy baby syndrome.
- Non-5q-related SMA is a genetically and clinically heterogeneous group.
- Non-5q-related, adult-onset SMA, in which the causative gene has been identified, are related to mutations in *AR* (Kennedy disease), *CHCHD10, TRPV4, DYNC1H1,* and *BICD2* genes.
- Genetic testing is now available for many SMAs, providing important diagnostic and prognostic information.
- Distal SMA is associated with mutations on chromosomes 7, 12, and X.
Chromosomes 14 and 22 are associated with mutations that cause proximal SMA.
- Cell and animal models of SMAs have been used to further understand how mutations in SMA-associated genes, which code for proteins involved in diverse functions such as transcriptional regulation, RNA processing, and cytoskeletal dynamics, lead to motor neuron dysfunction and loss.
- Adult-onset SMA often overlaps with HMN.

SUGGESTED READING

Juntas Morales R, Pageot N, Taieb G, Camu W. Adult-onset spinal muscular atrophy: An update. *Rev Neurol (Paris)*. 2017 May;173(5):308–319.

CASE 16.9: MYOPATHIC CALF ATROPHY WITH MILD CREATINE KINASE (CK) ELEVATION

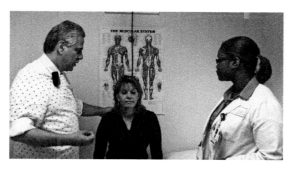

VIDEO 16.9

A 57-year-old woman presented with a 7–10-year history of difficulty running. The CK level was 350 U/L. EMG revealed 40% short-duration polyphasic units and many fibrillations in the calf muscles and normal sural responses. Gastrocnemius muscle biopsy revealed chronic myopathic changes and amorphous cytoplasmic masses. Dysferlin staining was normal. She had no family history of muscle disease. Recent echocardiogram revealed poor ejection fraction.

The next step in evaluation should focus on:

1. Dystrophin staining
2. Calpain Western blot (WB) analysis
3. Desmin staining
4. Repeat dysferlin staining
5. LS MRI

DIAGNOSIS

- Patients with distal weakness are referred to neuromuscular clinics for suspicion of motor neuropathies. Usually, it does not take long for a neuromuscular specialist to diagnose distal myopathies (normal sural responses and myopathic EMG), but sorting out the type of distal myopathy is not easy. Distal myopathy covers a wide spectrum of disorders, such as hereditary inclusion body myopathy, distal hereditary myopathies, and myofibrillar myopathies.

- CK level and muscle biopsy, including electron microscopy (EM) examination, are very useful for categorizing these disorders, but major categories remain unclassified. Genetic studies dissect them further, but most of them remain elusive.

- The lack of red-rimmed vacuoles and the relatively low CK level strongly argued against IBM and Myoshi myopathy, respectively. The appearance of amorphous masses in the cytoplasm of the biopsied muscle tissue deserved further staining. Desmin antibody reaction is an important step. However, desmin accumulation is not specific for myofibrillar myopathy (MFM) and may be seen in SMA, congenital myotonic dystrophies, IBM, and nemalin rode myopathies. Regenerating muscle fibers also may display desmin reaction.

- EM examination to confirm disruption of the Z-disk, which is the hallmark of desmin myopathy, is crucial. MFM is usually AD, but it can be AR and even X-linked. Desmin is a cytoskeletal intermediate filament that binds Z-bands with the sarcolemma and the nucleus. Its presence is not limited to skeletal muscles, but also extends to smooth and cardiac muscle.

- The abnormal desmin is insoluble and causes disruption of the muscle fibers (similar to amyloid, which is another insoluble protein). There are many mutations that lead to abnormal desmin.

- Desminopathies are phenotypically variable and may present as:
  - Scapuloperoneal syndrome
  - LGMD
  - Distal myopathy

- Cardiomyopathy is common.

- Examples of mutations that lead to desmin accumulation are the ones that affect the genes that code for myotilin, B-crystallin, ZASP, and seleno protine.

- The name *myofibrillar myopathy (MFM)* has replaced *desminopathy* to describe this group of distal irritative myopathies with frequent cardiac involvement.

SUGGESTED READING

Selcen D, Engel A. Mutations in myotilin cause myofibrillar myopathy. *Neurol.* 2004;62:1363–1371.

CASE 16.10: PROGRESSIVE CALF ATROPHY AND HYPERREFLEXIA

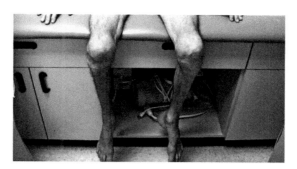

VIDEO 16.10

A 50-year-old man presented with a 9–12-month history of weakness and atrophy of the legs and loss of balance. He developed twitching of the thighs and arms. Examination is shown in the video.

The most likely cause of the distal leg atrophy in this case is:

1. ALS
2. Distal myopathy
3. SMA
4. Neuronal CMT disease
5. None of the above

DIAGNOSIS

- ALS is a progressive degenerative MND. A total of 10% of cases are hereditary, and increasingly, associated mutations are being identified.
- ALS usually starts in the bulbar or upper extremity muscles, leading to dysarthria and hand weakness. In about 10% of cases, weakness starts in the distal leg muscles unilaterally or bilaterally, leading to foot drop, which then may lead to erroneous diagnosis of LS radiculopathy or peroneal neuropathy.
- The following factors should suggest ALS:
  - No sensory symptoms or signs and normal sural responses
  - Atrophy of the affected muscles
  - Fasciculation
  - The presence of proximal weakness and hyperreflexia
  - Progression of weakness within 6 months
- Distal leg onset is more common in hereditary ALS, and the prognosis is better than bulbar-onset ALS.
  - The male-to-female ratio is 1:1, unlike the rest of ALS patients, where the ratio is 1.5:1.
  - Mild elevation of CK is common.
  - The key diagnostic feature is the presence of active denervation in the anterior and posterior leg muscles, which is more widespread than clinically suspected. In this case, denervation was noted up to the thighs.
  - The distal wasting in this case is reminiscent of neuronal CMT, but the progressive course is not for that.
  - Monitoring the clinical course is important since a progressive course is one of the diagnostic criteria.

CASE 16.11: BILATERAL FOOT DROP

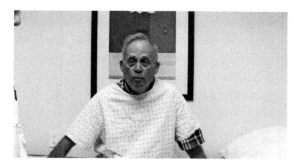

VIDEO 16.11

A 69-year-old man presented. History and examination are demonstrated. He has a 1.5-year history of seizures and treated B_{12} deficiency, and a maternal grandmother died of ALS at age 88. There is no proximal weakness, and there are no sensory or motor deficits in the arms. He has no bulbar symptoms. NCS revealed normal sural responses and nonconductive motor nerves in the legs, with severe distal denervation involving the anterior and posterior compartments below the knees. MRI of the LS spine revealed mild degenerative changes. The CPK level was 760 IU/L.

The most likely diagnosis is:

1. Distal SMA
2. Miyoshi myopathy
3. Anoctamin-5 LGMD
4. ALS with distal onset
5. LS radiculopathy

DIAGNOSIS

- Painless, progressive, asymmetric weakness and atrophy of the anterior and posterior distal leg muscles, absent ankle reflexes (duo to atrophy), brisk knee reflexes, normal sural responses, and severe denervation of the lower extremities with almost normal LS spine MRIs for age suggest MND.
- Family history suggests FALS.
- Elevated CK levels suggested distal myopathy, but EMG was clearly neurogenic.
- ALS may start with distal leg weakness mimicking distal motor neuropathy or LS polyradiculopathy.
- Sensory impairment in the feet in this case may be due to phenytoin therapy and B_{12} deficiency.
- As a rule, denervation extends proximally with time, which would confirm the diagnosis. Therefore, clinical monitoring is very important in questionable cases.
- Short duration is not compatible with SMA.
- The lack of radicular pain and normal LS MRI argue against LS polyradiculopathy.

CASE 16.12: FAMILIAL WEAKNESS
OF PLANTAR FLEXORS

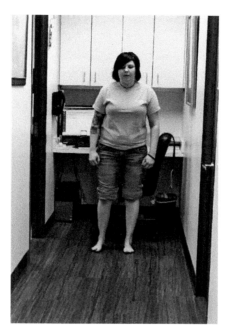

VIDEO 16.12

A 27-year-old woman presented with a 2-year history of difficulty walking and standing on her toes. She was always clumsy and had high foot arches. She denied significant pain or visual or hearing problems. Her mother had had similar symptoms since her 20s. She had a nerve biopsy and she was told she had hereditary neuropathy. Her maternal grandmother had the same symptoms. She had a half-brother with flat foot arches and difficulty with gait. Examination is shown in the video. Sensitivity to vibration was reduced in the feet. NCS revealed mild motor slowing, reduced CMAP amplitudes, and absent sensory responses.

Genetic testing revealed a heterogeneous pathogenic mutation of the *MFN2* gene (CMT2A2). CMT2A2 is characterized by all of the following except:

1. Severe motor slowing
2. Axonal neuropathy
3. Forming 30% of hereditary neuropathies
4. Distal foot weakness
5. AD inheritance

DIAGNOSIS

- CMT affects 1:2,500 of the population and is caused by the mutation of more than 30 genes.
- Identifying the genetic cause is necessary for family planning, prognostication, and inclusion in clinical trials.
- Current genetic testing can identify 70% of cases of hereditary neuropathies.
- CMT2A makes up 4% of genetically identified cases of hereditary neuropathies.
  - It is AD.
  - Characterized by progressive distal leg weakness affecting the plantar flexors and extensors, sensory symptoms, hyporeflexia, and pes cavus.
  - NCS usually reveals axonal neuropathy. Demyelinating features are occasionally seen.
  - Age of onset is 15–55 years.

SUGGESTED READING

Saporta A, Sottile SL, Miller LJ, Feely, SM, Siskind CE, Shy ME. Charcot-Marie-Tooth disease subtype and genetic testing strategies. *Ann Neurol.* 2011 Jan;69(1):22–33.

CASE 16.13: LEG WEAKNESS AND WEIGHT LOSS

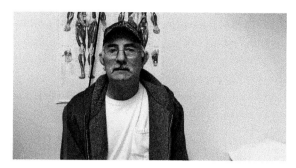

VIDEO 16.13

The findings shown in Video 16.13 are related to antibodies against:

1. Postsynaptic voltage-gated calcium channel (VGCC)
2. Postsynaptic acetylcholine receptor (AChR)
3. Presynaptic VGCC
4. Voltage-gated potassium channel (VGKC)
5. Glutamate acid decarboxylase (GAD)

DIAGNOSIS

- A 58-year-old man with progressive, painless weakness of the arms and legs of 3 months' duration responded to IVIG initially, and then progressed. He also had dry mouth.
- Examination revealed proximal and distal weakness in the arms and legs, with diffuse areflexia and very mild sensory impairment in the feet.
- The weakness of the triceps muscles was clearly facilitated with repeated testing.
- NCS revealed normal sensory responses and decreased CMAP amplitudes diffusely facilitated with exercise.
- Repetitive stimulation testing revealed decremental response to low-frequency stimulation and recovery after rest.
- This picture is very consistent with Eaton-Lambert syndrome.
- The patient is a chronic heavy smoker, and recently he lost weight. Chest X ray revealed hyperinflation of the lungs.

The next step in evaluation should include:

1. Computed tomography (CT) scan of the chest
2. Positron emission tomography (PET) scan
3. CT scan of the abdomen
4. CT scan of the pelvis
5. Paraneoplastic antibodies.
    - The VGCC antibody titer was increased to 670 pmol/L, with an upper limit of normal of 70 pmol/L.
    - CT scan of the chest revealed mediastinal lymphadenopathy. There were no pulmonary lesions.
    - The patient reported mild improvement of the symptoms with pyridostigmine, at 120 mg every 4 hours.
    - Weakness dramatically responded to 3,4-diaminopyridine, at 20 mg every 4 hours.
    - Bronchoscopic biopsy revealed small-cell lung cancer (SCLC), for which he received chemotherapy and radiotherapy.
    - LEMS:
        - A total of 60% of cases are associated with neoplasm (most commonly SCLC). These cases are usually associated with weight loss and rapid progression.
        - Usually presents with proximal leg weakness.
        - Associated features include sensory neuropathy and xerostomia and areflexia (90%).
        - It does not start with ocular symptoms, but these symptoms may appear as the disease evolves.
        - VGCC antibodies are increased in 85% of cases.
        - The chest X-ray is not sensitive. If CT scan of the chest is negative, it should be repeated in 3 months, and then once a year for 5 years.

- Treatment follows the same guidelines as MG; 3,4-diaminopyridine is usually symptomatically effective.

SUGGESTED READING

Motomura M, Nakata R, Shiraishi H. LEMS: clinical review. *Clin Exper Neuroimmun*. 2016 Aug;7(3):238–245.

CASE 16.14: CHRONIC BILATERAL FOOT DROP

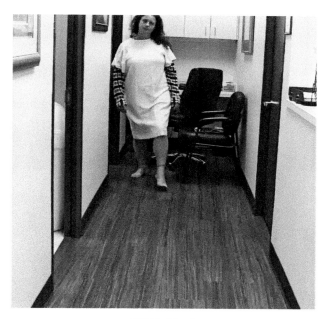

VIDEO 16.14

A 44-year-old woman presented who has had walking difficulty since childhood. Gradually, she developed a high steppage gait to avoid falls. She has difficulty standing up from a deep chair. She has a healthy daughter and son. Her mother and sister were "clumsy". The mother had hammertoes, and the sister had high foot arches. Her father had congestive cardiac failure (CCF). Examination is shown. The CPK level is 210 IU/L. NCS revealed normal sural and peroneal motor responses. EMG of the tibialis anterior revealed chronic irritative myopathy. MRI of the legs showed predominant involvement of the anterior compartment muscles (Figs. 16.14.1 and

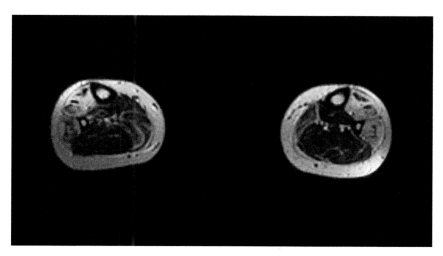

FIGURE 16.14.1 MRI of the legs below the knee: T1.cross section

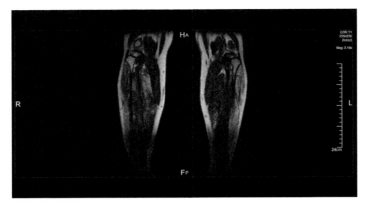

FIGURE 16.14.2 MRI of the legs below the knee, T1. longitudinal section

16.14.2). The other distal muscles were normal. The tibialis anterior muscle biopsy is shown in Figure 16.14.3.

The most likely cause for this chronic distal myopathic foot drop is:

1. IBM
2. Tibial muscular dystrophy
3. Facioscapuloperoneal muscular dystrophy
4. Myotonic dystrophy
5. Miyoshi myopathy

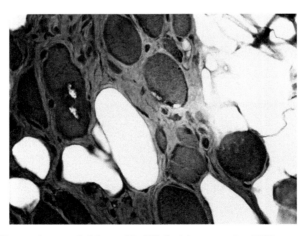

FIGURE 16.14.3 Tibialis anterior muscle biopsy. Modified trichrome stain. 400X.

DIAGNOSIS

- MRI confirmed involvement of the anterior compartment muscles.
- Muscle biopsy showed vacuolar dystrophic myopathy.

- Genetic testing revealed a pathogenic homozygous mutation in the *TTN* gene.
- There are 20 types of hereditary distal myopathy (distal muscular dystrophy, genetically determined distal myopathy).
- Tibial muscular dystrophy (Udd myopathy):
  - This AD disease characterized by gradual bilateral foot drop typically starts after age 40 years.
  - Some degree of proximal weakness may appear later in the course.
  - EDB and hand muscles are preserved.
  - No cardiac/respiratory involvement.
  - CK is mildly elevated.
  - Muscle MRI shows fatty degeneration in the anterior compartment muscles of the distal legs.
  - Muscle biopsy shows rimmed vacuoles and dystrophic myopathy.
  - It is the most common muscle disease in Finland, with prevalence of 20/100,000 in patients with Finnish ancestry.
  - French, Belgian, Spanish, Italian, and Swiss families are also reportedly affected.

SUGGESTED READING

Udd, B. Distal myopathies—new genetic entities expand diagnostic challenge. *Neuromusc. Dis.* 2012 Jan;22(1):5–12.

CHAPTER 17

MUSCLE ATROPHY AND HYPERTROPHY

CASE 17.1: PAINLESS MUSCLE TWITCHING

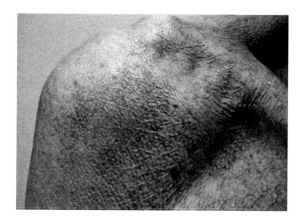

VIDEO 17.1

A 71-year-old man presented with progressive atrophy and twitching of the shown in the video muscles.

The observed abnormal movements represent:

1. Myotonia
2. Fasciculation
3. Myokymia
4. Muscle cramps
5. Rippling muscle disease

DIAGNOSIS

- A fasciculation is a contraction of muscle fibers that belong to a single motor unit due to a brief discharge of its supplying individual axons.
- The discharges may originate from the motor neurons, as in motor neuron diseases (MNDs) such as amyotrophic lateral sclerosis (ALS), poliomyelitis, and spinal muscular atrophy (SMA), or the axons, mostly the terminal axons in peripheral nerve hyperexcitability disorders like benign fasciculation syndrome (BFS).
- The neuronal type is less frequent and more complex (with interspike time of 80 seconds) than the axonal type.
- They are spontaneous and irregular and may be precipitated by muscle percussion.
- Benign fasciculations are part of a spectrum of peripheral nerve hyperexcitability disorders, which is also characterized by lack of weakness, tingling of the feet, frequent fasciculation (mainly in the calves), and no atrophy.
- Malignant fasciculation is less frequent, more complex, is associated with weakness and atrophy, mostly affects proximal muscles, and progresses quickly.
- It is important to distinguish between tremor of the tongue (regular, involving the entire tongue) and fasciculation (random twitching of motor neurons). The tongue is not weak or atrophied in the former.
- Fasciculation worsens with the progression of the disease activity in ALS, but its absence does not exclude the diagnosis.
- Fasciculation of the tongue is a feature of:
  - ALS: bulbar onset or generalized
  - Peripheral nerve hyperexcitability disorder
  - SMA
  - Kennedy disease
  - Organophosphorus poisoning
  - Rarely in MuSK antibody–associated myasthenia gravis (MG)
  - Hypoglossal palsy
- Benign fasciculation usually responds to sodium channel blockers such as oxcarbamazepine.

CASE 17.2: PROGRESSIVE WEAKNESS
AND ABNORMAL DISCHARGES

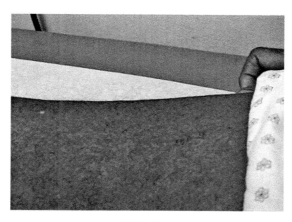

VIDEO 17.2

A 60-year-old man presented with a 6-month history of leg and arm weakness, and the examination revealed atrophy and fasciculations of the upper back muscles and thighs.

The demonstrated in the video electromyogram (EMG) activity is best described as (screen sweep is 500 milliseconds):

1. High firing frequency
2. Low firing frequency
3. Normal firing frequency
4. Fasciculation
5. None of the above

DIAGNOSIS

- Video 17.2 shows atrophy and fasciculation of the upper back muscles and proximal and distal arm and leg muscles.
- Calculating the firing frequency of motor units provides an objective measurement of motor unit recruitment.
- Normally, a motor unit discharges with voluntary effort, starting at a rate of 5–7 Hz, and as the effort is increased, the firing frequency increases until a new motor unit potential (MUP) appears. The frequency of the first MUP at which another MUP appears is called the *recruitment onset frequency*. It is normally 10 Hz. A frequency of more than 15 Hz is abnormal and indicates decreased recruitment, a sign of denervation. That means that there are not enough motor units, so the existing ones fire at a higher frequency to achieve the same result.
- The recruitment ratio is an alternative method of counting the firing frequency of a motor unit, which is derived from dividing the number of MUPs seen on the screen by the number of individual units activated. For example, if two units are firing and the observed frequency on the screen is 30, the firing ratio is 15 Hz. A frequency of 5 Hz or less is normal, and more than 10 Hz is abnormal.
- Sometimes the recruitment pattern is decreased (the screen shows a smaller number of firing units), but the firing frequency is normal. This is typically seen in central and psychogenic disorders.
- In the video, the screen sweep is 500 milliseconds; there are small and large MUPs on the screen representing different motor units. If we calculate the big ones (representing one unit), at second 00:12, there are 9 MUPs (18 MUP/second). Therefore, this is an increased firing frequency.
- Another way of calculating the firing frequency is by dividing 1,000 by the interspike time (in this case, the interspike time averages 55 milliseconds).

CASE 17.3: CHRONIC BILATERAL FOOT AND WRIST DROP

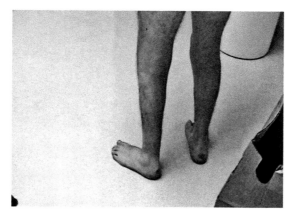

VIDEO 17.3

A 30-year-old man presented with a 10-year history of gradually developing, painless, bilateral foot and wrist drop. His examination revealed normal sensation, diffuse areflexia, normal proximal strength, and distal atrophy of all extremities, with no fasciculation or bulbar involvement. He had two similarly affected brothers and mother. The creatine kinase (CK) level was 280 U/L. EMG revealed a firing frequency of 25 Hz in the proximal and distal arm and leg muscles bilaterally.

The most likely diagnosis is:

1. Kennedy disease
2. ALS
3. Distal myopathy
4. Distal SMA
5. Hereditary inclusion body myositis (hIBM)

DIAGNOSIS

- SMA is a group of genetic slowly progressive lower MNDs.
- They affect different age groups (infantile, juvenile, adult onset) and start in different regions (upper extremities, lower extremities, scapuloperoneal) and have different modes of inheritance, such as X-linked recessive, autosomal dominant (AD), autosomal recessive (AR), and mitochondrial.
- Familial ALS (FALS) differs by being more progressive and affecting bulbar neurons and upper motor neurons (UMNs) as well as lower motor neurons (LMNs).
- Progressive muscular atrophy is a variant of ALS that affects only the LMNs.
- Distal SMA:
  - A rare form of SMA that was considered as a motor variant of CMT in the past.
  - It differs from CMT by having no clinical or neurophysiological evidence of sensory involvement.
  - It shares the distal weakness and foot deformities and mode of inheritance of Charcot-Marie-Tooth (CMT) disease, as 30% are AD. The rest are recessive, sporadic, or X-linked.
  - Weakness may start in the hands or feet.
  - There are at least two genotypes:
    - Mutations of the glycyl t-RNA synthetase (*GARS*) gene on chromosome 7 p15
    - The *BSCL2* gene on chromosome 11q12-q14
  - Genetic and clinical heterogeneity is striking. Pyramidal involvement, vocal cord paralysis, and diaphragmatic paralysis are reported in some cases. Tongue tremor and (rarely) fasciculation are reported.
- These patients usually have no survival limitations, but morbidity is high.

CASE 17.4: INABILITY TO STAND ON TOES AND HIGH CREATINE KINASE (CK) LEVEL

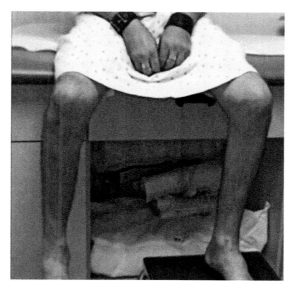

VIDEO 17.4

A 24-year-old man had noticed the inability to stand on his toes since age 15 years. He had atrophy of the calves and hypertrophy of the extensor digitorum brevis (EDB). The CK level was 2,400 U/L, and EMG revealed 40% short-duration units in the proximal and distal arm and leg muscles with fibrillation.

The muscle biopsy is likely to show:

1. Red-Rimmed vacuoles
2. Lack of dystrophin staining
3. Absent dyferlin staining
4. Patchy dysferlin staining
5. Neurogenic atrophy

DIAGNOSIS

- Limb girdle muscular dystrophy (LGMD) comprises a large group of muscle diseases that vary widely clinically and genetically.
- Miyoshi myopathy is one phenotype of dysferlinopathy and has characteristic features.
- The other major phenotype is LGMD2B, which affects proximal muscles initially.
- Presents in late teens or early 20s.
- Early involvement of the calf muscles (atrophy and weakness) and inability to stand on toes since an early age are characteristic.
- Asymmetry.
- Spread of the weakness to the hamstrings and glutei, and then to the distal arms, is common.
- Prominent involvement of anterior tibial muscles is reported in some cases.
- Calf atrophy leads to early loss of ankle reflexes, causing confusion with motor neuropathies.
- Inflammatory foci in muscle biopsy are common, which along with progressive course and elevated CK may lead to diagnostic confusion with polymyositis, but Miyoshi myopathy muscle biopsy shows:
  - No invasion of nonnecrotic fibers.
  - Mycobacteria avium complex (MAC) deposition on the sarcolemma of nonnecrotic fibers is an early finding that is not seen in polymyositis, myotonic dystrophy, or inclusion body myositis (IBM).
- CK is usually elevated to 35–200 times normal.
- Muscle biopsy: dystrophic and inflammatory changes. Vacuoles are rarely reported (Shaibani, Aziz, et al., 1997).
- Western blot (WB) on white cell count (WBC) or muscle tissue reveals the absence of dysferlin.
- Dysferlinopathy constitutes 60% of distal myopathies.
- Dysferlinopathy phenotypes: 80% Miyoshi myopathy, 8% LGMD, 6% asymptomatic hyperCKemia.
- The role of dysferlin is not clear. It may patch defects in sarcolemma, and its deficiency causes defective membrane repair.
- No cardiac involvement is reported.

SUGGESTED READING

Shaibani, A, et al. Miyoshi myopathy with vacuoles. *Neurol.* 48(3 Suppl. 2);1997:A194.

CASE 17.5: FOOT NUMBNESS AND CALF HYPERTROPHY

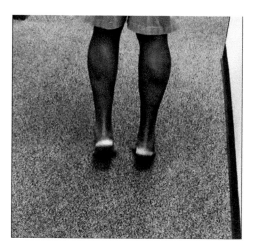

VIDEO 17.5

A 59-year-old man presented with a 1-year history of progressive weakness and hypertrophy of the right calf with minimal numbness of the lateral aspect of the right foot. He had no back pain. Examination showed absent right ankle and decreased right knee jerks. The CK level was 400–800 U/L. Magnetic resonance imaging (MRI) of the claves showed edema of the posterior compartment muscles. EMG revealed the shown in the video abnormal discharges in the right gastrocnemius, hamstrings, gluteus maximus, and lower lumbar paraspinal muscles. Lumbar spine MRI (LS MRI) revealed severe spinal canal stenosis at L5–S1 and severe narrowing of the right L4–S1 foramina. A biopsy of the right gastrocnemius muscle is shown in Figure 17.5.1.

The most likely cause of the patient's right calf hypertrophy is:

1. S1 radiculopathy
2. Becker muscular dystrophy (BMD)
3. Amyloid myopathy
4. Sarcoid myopathy
5. Miyoshi myopathy

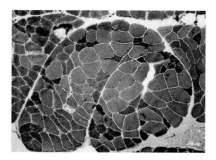

FIGURE 17.5.1 Nonspecific esterase reaction, 400x.

DIAGNOSIS

- The biopsy shows muscle tissues stained with nonspecific esterase, which is used to delineate denervated fibers. There were many small, dark, angulated fibers (moderate denervation).
- Unilateral or bilateral calf hypertrophy or pseudohypertrophy may be caused by:
  - Muscle disease: dystrophinopathy, amyloid myopathy, sarcoid myopathy
  - Nerve hyperexcitability: neuromyotonia
  - Nerve root irritation: S1 radiculopathy
- In this case, because the last possibility is very rare and the CK elevation was more than expected for that cause, a muscle biopsy was necessary to rule out other causes.
- As a rule, radiculopathy causes muscle atrophy, but for poorly understood reasons, hypertrophy can occur. Continuous discharge of the affected nerve root due to irritation is a possible explanation.

SUGGESTED READING

Swartz KR, Fee DB, Trost GR, Waclawik AJ. Unilateral calf hypertrophy seen in lumbosacral stenosis: case report and review of the literature. *Spine (Phila Pa 1976)*. 2002 Sep 15;27(18):E406–E409.

CASE 17.6: CALF ATROPHY

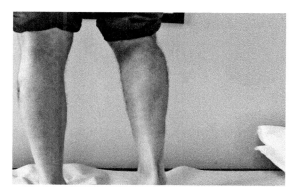

VIDEO 17.6

A 54-year-old man presented with a 15-year history of inability to stand on his toes. He had difficulty buttoning shirts. There was no significant family history. In addition to what is shown in the examination in the video, the rest of the muscles were 5/5. There was calf atrophy. Sensation was intact, and sural responses were normal. The CK level was 390 U/L. EMG revealed mixed short- and long-duration MUPs in the calf muscles with no spontaneous activity. Genetic testing for CMT and SMA were negative. Left gastrocnemius biopsy showed dystrophic, noninflammatory myopathy.

Which of the following typically cause calf atrophy?

1. Dysferlinopathy
2. Telithinopathy (LGMD2G)
3. Desminopathy
4. Calpainopathy
5. Dystrophinopathy

DIAGNOSIS

- Inability to walk on the toes is characteristic of involvement of the posterior compartment muscles of the forelegs. When chronic, patients consider it as normal and not functionally disturbing, and thus do not seek medical advice. They are usually referred due to abnormal CK level.
- The absence of ankle reflexes, in addition to the distal weakness and the presence of family history, may lead to diagnostic confusion with hereditary motor neuropathy and distal SMA.
- Mild CK elevation is not unusual in denervating conditions, so it may not raise a suspicion of myopathy. Mixed (short- and long-duration) MUPs can occur in chronic denervation and in chronic myopathies and may add to the confusion.
- Muscle biopsy is useful in early stages by showing denervation changes (group atrophy in chronic cases) in neurogenic disease and chronic myopathic or dystrophic changes in myopathic disease.
- In severe cases, end-stage pathology does not help this differentiation. Immunostaining on even a few remaining fibers may help to sort out cases of dysferlinopathy and desminopathy. Genetic testing for these disorders in the blood or muscle is becoming the leading diagnostic modality.
- In this case, the CK level was too low for dysferlinopathy, and desmin staining should be attempted.
- Myofibrillar myopathy (MFM), with desminopathy as the most common variant, is a heterogeneous group of disorders that usually cause distal weakness (irritative myopathy) and cardiomyopathy.
- Dysferlinopathy and desminopathy typically cause calf atrophy. Dystrophinopathy and LGMD 2G typically cause calf hypertrophy.

SUGGESTED READING

Bushby, KM. Making sense of limb girdle muscular dystrophy. *Brain.* 1999;122(8):1403–1420.

CASE 17.7: BIG CALVES AND REMARKABLY ELEVATED CREATINE KINASE (CK) LEVEL

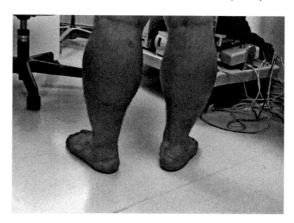

VIDEO 17.7

A 43-year-old man presented with difficulty standing on his toes, noticed 10 years earlier. He had mild quadriceps weakness and a CK level of 3,350 IU/L. EMG showed mixed short- and long-duration potentials.

Calf hypertrophy is a feature of:

1. BMD
2. Amyloid myopathy
3. Sarcoglycanopathy
4. Dysferlinopathy
5. IBM

DIAGNOSIS

- Calf enlargement is an important feature of dystrophinopathies; it is due to fatty replacement rather than actual hypertrophy. It is also observed typically in amyloid myopathy and some sarcoglycanopathies, but not in IBM or dysferlinopathy, where calf atrophy is the rule.
- Dystrophin is a subsarcolemmal protein in the skeletal and cardiac muscles.
  - It stabilizes the membrane during muscle contraction and relaxation.
  - Abnormal level of dystrophin leads to loss of integrity of muscle fibers during contraction and relaxation, leading to membrane damage necrosis.
- The dystrophin gene is a large gene located on Xp21, but less than 1% of the gene codes for dystrophin (exons).
- The phenotype depends on the type of mutation (in frame or out of frame) and the quantity of functional dystrophin in the muscles rather than the site of mutation.
  - Less than 5% of the normal is associated with Duchenne muscular dystrophy (DMD).
  - About 5%–20% of normal correlates with the intermediate phenotype (mild DMD or severe BMD).
  - About 20%–50% of normal is associated with mild to moderate BMD.
- Dystrophin gene mutations:
  - Large deletions: two-thirds of cases
  - Point mutations leading to stop codons: 5%–10%
  - Duplications: 5%
- Out-of-frame mutations lead to complete disruption of translation and result in a total loss of dystrophin: DMD
- In-frame mutations: translation of dysfunctional protein: BMD phenotype
- Phenotypes of dystrophinopathy:
  - DMD
  - BMD
  - Myalgia
  - Myoglobinuria
  - Cardiomyopathy
  - HyperCKemia

CASE 17.8: CHRONIC DISTAL ARM DENERVATION

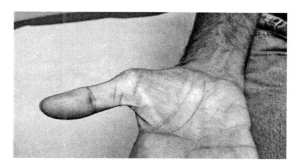

VIDEO 17.8

A 47-year-old man presented with a 13-year history of weakness and atrophy of the right-hand muscles. Thoracic outlet syndrome surgery did not help. The CK level and cerebrospinal fluid (CSF) examination were normal. Cervical MRI was normal. Nerve conduction study (NCS) showed no conduction block. The compound muscle action potentials (CMAPs) of the right median and ulnar nerves were reduced. Sensory responses were normal. EMG revealed diffuse chronic denervation of the right-arm muscles.

The lesion is likely located at the level of:

1. Motor neurons
2. Motor nerves
3. Brachial plexus
4. Axons
5. Myelin

DIAGNOSIS

- The presence of diffuse weakness and denervation that spans multiple nerve roots with preservation of sensory responses and reduced reflexes suggest an LMN lesion.
- Multifocal motor neuropathy with conduction block may present similarly, but the presence of conduction blocks and the lack of diffuse denervation would distinguish these cases. This patient was treated with intravenous immunoglobulin (IVIG), with no improvement before being referred to our center.
- Cervical polyradiculopathy due to an infiltrative lesion of the motor nerve root such as lymphoma is possible, but the long duration and normal cervical MRI ruled out this possibility.
- ALS may start with focal LMN signs, but it usually spreads to other muscles and evolves into a typical picture within a year or two. Distal SMA is usually bilateral and distal.
- A chronic focal lower MND (Hirayama disease, monomelic amyotrophy) is well known.
  - It is sporadic and affects males 10 times more than females. Age of onset is 13–15 years.
  - Starts with distal single limb weakness; the right side is twice as likely affected than the left.
  - Subclinical involvement of the other arm is common, and in 10% of cases, proximal weakness is evident.
  - In 40% of cases, it spreads to the other side. It progresses over 5 years and then plateaus for decades.
  - Most denervation occurs in the C8–T1 muscles, but proximal and even lower extremity muscles may be affected. Cervical MRI: cord atrophy is seen in 30%–50% of cases.
  - It is speculated that posterior epidural venous plexus engorgement during flexion contributes to the pathology, but that does not explain the presence of denervation in the legs.

CHAPTER 18

HYPERREFLEXIA

CASE 18.1: JAW CLONUS

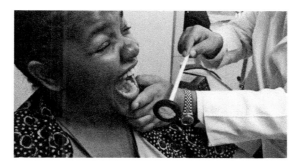

VIDEO 18.1

A 30-year-old woman developed dysarthria, progressive weakness, and hyperreflexia of the arms with normal sensation. Brain magnetic resonance imaging (MRI) was normal. The tongue showed atrophy and fasciculation.

Which of the following disorders is typically associated with jaw clonus?

1. Amyotrophic lateral sclerosis (ALS)
2. Chronic inflammatory demyelinating polyneuropathy (CIDP)
3. Myotonic dystrophy
4. Progressive muscular atrophy
5. Spinal muscular atrophy (SMA)

DIAGNOSIS

- Hyperreflexia is an important sign of upper motor neuron (UMN) dysfunction.
- Hyperreflexia may be present in anxious persons.
- Even normoactive reflexes are considered to be abnormal when they are not expected to be there (e.g., preserved knee reflexes in CIDP or preserved ankle reflexes in the face of severe foot numbness).
- The presence of Babinski and Hoffman signs supports the pathological basis of hyperreflexia.
- The jaw jerk is often omitted from the neurological examination.
  - The jaw jerk is served by the trigeminal nerve for its afferent and efferent connections (unlike the blink and corneal reflexes, which are served by the trigeminal and facial nerves).
  - A brisk jaw jerk indicates a cephalad lesion to mid-pons, where the nerve emerges.
  - A combination of a brisk jaw jerk and tongue fasciculation is characteristic of ALS.
  - Grading of the jaw jerk follows the same medical research council (MRC) grading system that is used to grade other monosynaptic reflexes such as in the knee, biceps, triceps, and ankle.

CASE 18.2: SPASTIC DYSARTHRIA

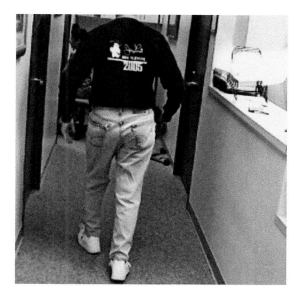

VIDEO 18.2

A 27-year-old man presented with dysarthria and spasticity of the arms and legs that evolved over 5 years to complete disability. He had normal sensation and diffuse hyperreflexia. The tongue was weak but not atrophic. MRI of the brain and spinal cord and cerebrospinal fluid (CSF) examination were normal, and there was no denervation observed by electromyogram (EMG) study.

The most likely diagnosis is:

1. Multiple sclerosis (MS)
2. Primary lateral sclerosis (PLS)
3. Hereditary spastic paraplegia (HSP)
4. Tropical spastic paraplegia
5. Cerebrovascular disease

DIAGNOSIS

- This variant of ALS is the most difficult to diagnosis until later in the course and after other causes of myelopathy are ruled out.
- The most common presentation includes progressive stiffness of the legs and poor balance.
- In some cases, slurring of speech can be subtle and may be confused with myasthenia gravis (MG), especially when some patients report increasing fatigue toward the end of the day.
- Pseudobulbar palsy and hyperreflexia with increased tone in the extremities are common.
- Evolution to ALS occurs in more than 70% of cases, with the appearance of fasciculation and atrophy.
- Other causes of noncompressive myelopathy are to be considered:
  - HSP: The course is more chronic, and family history may be present.
  - Tropical spastic paraplegia: history of living in the tropics, abnormal CSF examination, and positive HTLV-1 antibodies.
  - Adrenomyeloneuropathy: X-linked, abnormal MRI of the brain and spinal cord, increased very-long-chain fatty acids (VLCFAs) in the serum, and *ABCD1* mutation are detected.
  - B_{12} deficiency: presence of sensory symptoms, memory impairment, optic atrophy, macrocytic anemia, and low vitamin B_{12} level.
  - Copper deficiency: Sensory symptoms are common, but cases with purely motor symptoms with fasciculation have been reported. Leucopenia is common, and serum copper level is low. Usually, there is a history of gastrectomy occurring years earlier.

CASE 18.3: INAPPROPRIATE CRYING AND LAUGHTER

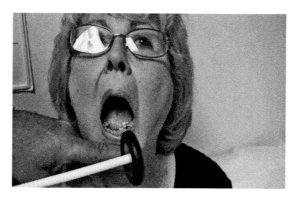

VIDEO 18.3

A 68-year-old woman presented with a 6-month history of inappropriate laughter and crying, cough, and slurring of speech.

Emotional lability or pseudobulbar affect (PBA) can occur in:

1. ALS
2. MS
3. Cerebral multi-infarct state
4. Traumatic brain injury (TBI)
5. All of the above

DIAGNOSIS

- Pathological laughter and crying (emotional incontinence) result from release of the physical components (reflexes) of these emotions from inhibitory cortical control. Therefore, these patients experience outbursts of crying or laughter that are not triggered by appropriate stimuli. Emotions can be paradoxical, such as laughing at bad news.
- Corticobulbar tracts or their cortical neurons are the targets of pathological process leading to PBA.
- The most common causes of PBA are ALS, MS, multi-infarct state, Alzheimer disease, brainstem tumors, and TBI.
- In this case, jaw hyperreflexia and the presence of tongue fasciculation suggested ALS.
- In ALS, PBA carries a poor prognosis since it is associated with bulbar dysfunction (dyspnea, dysphagia, sialorrhea, etc.).
- Patients with pure UMN lesions (primary lateral sclerosis) that start in the suprabulbar pathways may impose a diagnostic dilemma until the evolution of a more complete diagnostic picture.
- PBA can be socially devastating.
- Depression commonly occurs, complicating the clinical picture.
- PBA usually responds to tricyclic antidepressants.
  - Dextromethorphan/quinidine treatment is approved by the U.S. Food and Drug Administration (FDA) for this condition.
  - Transaminases and the QT interval should be checked periodically while taking this medication.
- All the above mentioned options can cause PBA.

SUGGESTED READING

Shaibani AT, Sabbagh MN, Doody R. Laughter and crying in neurologic disorders. *Neuropsych Neuropsychol Behav Neurol.* 1994;7:243–250.

CASE 18.4: PATELLAR CLONUS

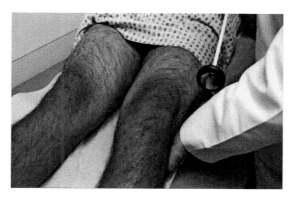

VIDEO 18.4

A 60-year-old man presented with poor balance and spastic gait that started 2 years earlier. He developed atrophy of the thigh muscles and twitching in the arms within a year. The CK level was 350 U/L, and EMG study revealed widespread denervation of the tested legs and thoracic para-spinal (TPS) muscles with normal sensory responses.

The cause of patellar clonus in this case is:

1. Myelopathy
2. ALS
3. MS
4. SMA
5. Myopathy

DIAGNOSIS

- Clonus is a series of involuntary rhythmic muscular contractions. It is usually initiated by tapping a tendon to generate a deep tendon reflex (DTR).
- The self-sustained contractions are due to the lack of central inhibition caused by UMN lesions, such as ALS, MS, stroke, and so on.
- Clonus corresponds to grade 4+ on the DTR grading scale.
- Clonus is usually associated with spasticity.
- A fasciculation is a spontaneous discharge of a motor neuron cell or its axon and is a sign of lower motor neuron (LMN) lesions.
- The presence of myoclonus and fasciculation together is characteristic of ALS.
- Ankle and jaw clonus follow the same rules.
- Myoclonus is totally different from clonus. It is a sudden brief contraction of a muscle or a group of muscles. It is caused by a different group of central nervous system (CNS) diseases, such as encephalopathies or some forms of epilepsy.

CHAPTER 19

MUSCLE TWITCHING

CASE 19.1: PAINLESS MUSCLE TWITCHING

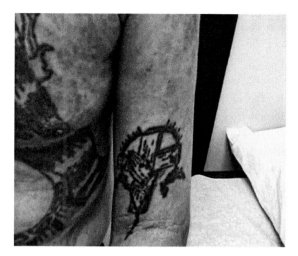

VIDEO 19.1

A 45-year-old man presented with a 1-year history of painless muscle twitching in the arms and chest, painful cramps in the arms, decreased muscle bulk, and weakness of the arms. Deep tendon reflexes (DTRs) were 3/4 and sensation was normal. The creatine kinase (CK) level was 345 U/L.

Comprehensive electromyography (EMG) of this patient is expected to show:

1. Myokymia
2. Focal fasciculation
3. Neuromyotonia
4. Widespread fasciculation
5. Rippling muscle disease

DIAGNOSIS

- A fasciculation is a short-lived irregular spontaneous discharge of individual axons and does both of the following:
  - Causes activation of all or part of muscle fibers that belong to a motor unit
  - Produces visible rippling of the involved muscle
- The old notion that fasciculation is generated only from motor neurons has been challenged. While motor neurons remain a possible origin [in amyotrophic lateral sclerosis (ALS), for example], terminal axons seem to be the source in the majority of fasciculations, such as benign fasciculation syndrome (BFS).
- Fasciculations appear as single motor units in the needle EMG.
- Distal axonal fasciculations are more frequent than more proximal fasciculations (ALS) due to the short refractory period (3–4 milliseconds) and short interspike intervals (5 milliseconds).
- While spontaneous most of the time, fasciculations may be precipitated by percussion, activity, and cold.
- There is no relationship between fasciculation frequency and disease severity.
- Voluntary activity, unlike random fasciculations, is semirhythmic, at an onset frequency of 5–7 Hz.
  - Causes of fasciculation include:
    - Peripheral nerve hyperexcitability disorder
    - Motor neuron diseases (MNDs)
    - Axonal neuropathies
    - Hyperthyroidism and hyperparathyroidism
    - Hypomagnesemia
    - Cholinergic overstimulation (organophosphorus compounds poisoning, pyridostigmine, etc.)
    - Hyperventilation (relative hypocalcaemia)
  - In ALS, besides fasciculation, one may find fibrillations in many muscles, weakness, and hyperreflexia.
  - In BFS, there is no atrophy or weakness.
    - Serial examination is important to look for new onset weakness or atrophy or spread of the fasciculation in ALS.
  - Fasciculation can be confused with tremor, which is regular while fasciculation is random.

CASE 19.2: FACIAL TWITCHING

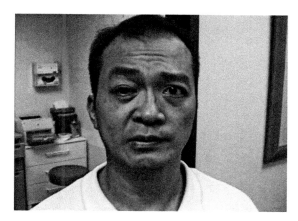

VIDEO 19.2

A 39-year-old man presented with involuntary recurrent blinking of the right eye. There was no facial weakness or numbness. Brain magnetic resonance imaging (MRI) was normal.

The most likely cause of this condition is:

1. Brainstem tumor
2. Aberrant vertebral artery
3. Stroke
4. Neuropathy
5. ALS

DIAGNOSIS

- Involuntary, intermittent twitching of muscles is supplied by the facial nerve (hemifacial spasm).
- Hemifacial spasm is caused by compression of the facial nerve by a branch of the vertebro-basillar system at the base of the brain, or by a tumor.
- Trauma to the nerve (surgery on the facial nerve or previous Bell's palsy) may produce the same effects.
- Periorbital and perioral muscles are affected, and sometimes the spasms spread to the other side.
- A total of 5% of patients have a history of trigeminal neuralgia.
- Periodic botulinum toxin (BT) injections are very effective.
- For refractory cases, microvascular decompression is an option.

CASE 19.3: RHYTHMIC MUSCLE TWITCHING

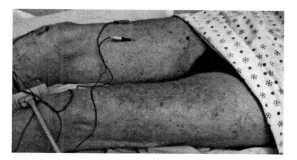

VIDEO 19.3

A 73-year-old man presented with generalized weakness and fatigue of 6 months' duration. His examination revealed resting tremor of the hands, mild shuffling gait, and mild, generalized weakness. The patient was referred to the neuromuscular clinic to be evaluated for "fasciculations of the thighs."

The recorded abnormal twitching shown in the video of the right thing muscles is:

1. Fasciculation
2. Neuromyotonia
3. Voluntary movement
4. Tremor
5. Myoclonus

DIAGNOSIS

- In a progressively weak patient, especially if there is hyperreflexia, neurologists look for fasciculation in order to support the diagnosis of suspected ALS.
- Tremor in these cases is commonly confused with fasciculation. Hyperreflexia is commonly caused by anxiety and nervousness.
- Tongue and limb tremor is common in the normal population. Action tremor is not hard to sort out due to its amelioration at rest. Resting tremor can be more confusing, especially when it occurs in proximal muscles and is not associated with other Parkinsonian features.
- Weakness and atrophy, along with fasciculation, would support the diagnosis of ALS.
- Tremor is rhythmic, while fasciculation is random. However, when fasciculation is frequent, tremor can be mimicked.
- Needle examination often helps to determine the rhythmicity of the discharges and their nature.

CASE 19.4: STRETCHING-INDUCED MUSCLE CONTRACTIONS

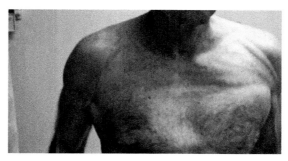

VIDEO 19.4

(courtesy of Michael Weiss, MD)

The patient is a 64-year-old man with a 3-year history of involuntary muscle movement, stiffness, and soreness. His clinical examination demonstrated normal muscle bulk and power. EMG was notable for electrical silence during the induced muscle contractions.

The demonstrated activity is:

1. Fasciculation
2. Myokymia
3. Rippling muscle
4. Tremor
5. Voluntary units

DIAGNOSIS

- Video 19.4 shows rippling of the pectoralis muscles with stretching of the upper chest and shoulders, and percussion-induced muscle contractions.
- Rippling muscle syndrome is a rare disorder with multiple causes.
- The rippling muscles are electrically silent, suggesting that the activity is not generated by the muscle fibers but rather is due to calcium dysregulation by the endoplasmic reticulum.
- Touching or percussing the muscle usually triggers rippling.
- Hereditary rippling muscle syndrome is:
  - Due to caveolin mutations (LGMD 1C).
  - An autosomal-dominant (AD) or autosomal-recessive (AR) muscle disease that presents in the first 2 decades of life with wavelike, painless muscle rippling.
  - Proximal and/or distal weakness and scapular winging.
  - Muscle hypertrophy may happen.
  - CK level is more than 10 times normal.
  - Muscle pathology: nonspecific myopathy with decreased caveolin staining.
- Sporadic rippling muscle syndrome:
  - Is associated with myasthenia gravis (MG) or thymoma and may precede their symptoms.
  - Myalgia and mild CK elevation are common.
  - Worsened by pyridostigmine.
  - May respond to immunosuppression.

CASE 19.5: MUSCLE TWITCHING AND HYPERREFLEXIA

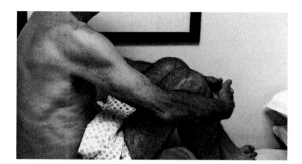

VIDEO 19.5

A 63-year-old man presented with a 6-month history of muscle twitching in the arms and mild weakness in the hand grips. His examination is shown in the video. The EMG in the areas of profuse fasciculations showed only rare fasciculations and neurogenic motor unit potentials (MUPs), with a firing frequency of 25 Hz diffusely. Fibrillations were rare.

On the prognosis of this disease:

1. A total of 20% of patients live 5 years or more.
2. A total of 50% of patients live at least 3 years.
3. A total of 10% of patients survive more than 10 years.
4. A total of 10% of patients live less than 3 years.
5. Bulbar involvement does not change the prognosis.

DIAGNOSIS

- Video 19.5 shows fasciculation in the arms clinically and by EMG and hyperreflexia.
- There are several sets of diagnostic criteria for ALS; all of them suffer from deficiency and miss at least 50% of cases in the time of diagnosis because they are created as a research tool and not for clinical use.
- El Escorial criteria (EEC) are the most commonly used and require the presence of evidence of progressive lower motor neuron (LMN) and upper motor neuron (UMN) degeneration in at least three regions (cranial, cervical, thoracic, and lumbar) for a definite diagnosis.
- Awaji criteria increased the proportion of patients classified as having ALS by 23%, mostly because they recognize fasciculation.
- Sometimes EMG evidence of active denervation lags behind and is replaced by chronic denervation potentials (high-amplitude, long-duration units with high firing frequency) due to reinnervation. Almost always, with disease progression, active denervation appears and becomes widespread.
- Interestingly, needle examination of fasciculation-rich muscles usually shows much less electrical fasciculation than what is noticed clinically, even if the needle is inserted in the fasciculating area itself. The generators of fasciculation may be too deep for the needle to detect.
- Fasciculations are produced by dying motor neurons, and therefore, they are more frequent in the early stages of the disease; as the disease progresses, they are replaced by fibrillations and positive, sharp waves (produced by motor neurons' death). One has to wait for at least 60 seconds with every needled examination before declaring the areas clean of fasciculation.
- A total of 50% of patients with Lou Gehrig's disease (i.e., ALS) live at least three years after diagnosis; 20% live 5 years or more; and up to 10% will survive more than 10 years.
- Bulbar involvement is a bad prognostic sign.

SUGGESTED READING

Costa J, Swash M, de Carvalho M. Awaji criteria for the diagnosis of ALS. A systemic review. *Arch Neurol.* 2012;69(11):1410–1416.

CHAPTER 20

MUSCLE STIFFNESS AND CRAMPS

CASE 20.1A: SEVERE INTERMITTENT MUSCLE SPASMS

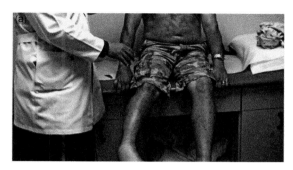

VIDEO 20.1A

A 39-year-old man with progressive stiffness of the back muscles that started a few months earlier, followed by severe, intermittent, sustained painful spasms of the legs and arms, which was triggered by painful stimuli, tapping the patella, or hearing a high-pitched sound. The creatine kinase (CK) level was 300 U/L, and electromyography (EMG) revealed normal but continuous involuntary motor unit potentials (MUPs). The voltage-gated potassium channel (VGKC) antibody titer was normal. Baclofen pumping reduced the cramps by 80%.

Such severe, painful muscle cramps that are triggered by stretching, emotions, and painful stimulation are seen in:

1. Stiff person syndrome (SPS)
2. Tetany
3. Tetanus
4. Myokymia
5. Myotonia

DIAGNOSIS

- Unlike peripheral causes of stiffness and spasms, central causes like SPS and tetanus are provoked by emotions and painful stimuli.
- SPS usually presents with progressive stiffness and gait difficulty. In serious cases, severe, painful cramps may be triggered by sensory stimulation and may produce falling. They are usually bilateral and cause arm, leg, and trunk extension and foot inversion.
- Both agonist and antagonist muscles contract simultaneously. These contractions can be severe enough to cause fractures and disability. Startle response is usually augmented, but trismus is rare. SPS may be associated with seizures, thymoma, and myasthenia gravis (MG). Anti–glutamic acid decarboxylase (GAD) antibodies are very high in 60%–90% of cases.
- Tetanus is caused by a toxin that is produced by clostridium tetani called *tetanospasmin,* which inhibits the release of glycine or gamma aminobutyric acid (GABA).
  - Full immunization against tetanus is 100% protective, but only 10% of Americans complete the series.
  - Acute wound infection is the major source.
  - Severe, painful spasms can be localized or generalized, and the closer the wound is to the head, the worse the prognosis is.
  - Muscle rigidity, trismus, autonomic failure, rhabdomyolysis, and death occur in 15%–30% of cases.
  - Treatment consists of human tetanus immunoglobulin, diazepam, or baclofen and supportive care. Debridement of the infected wound source is crucial.

CASE 20.1B: RESOLUTION WITH BACLOFEN PUMP

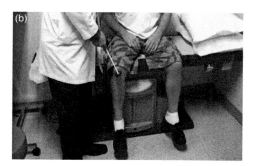

VIDEO 20.1B

The patient in Case 20.1A was treated with intrathecal baclofen. Within a day, the spasms resolved and he was able to walk without a cane, and tapping the patellar tendon did not produce cramping. Deep tendon reflexes (DTRs) are absent due to baclofen.

CASE 20.2: CARPAL SPASMS

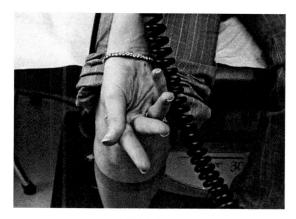

VIDEO 20.2

A 27-year-old woman presented with recurrent painful spasms of the hand and foot muscles. She has had several panic attacks after the recent death of her mother.

The demonstrated in the video signs are:

1. Trousseau sign
2. Babinski sign
3. Chvostek sign
4. Oppenheim sign
5. Chaddock sign

DIAGNOSIS

- *Tetany* is peripheral nerve hyperexcitability due to acute hypocalcemia. Low serum calcium enhances sodium influx to the cells, thus triggering depolarization.
- The most clinical features of hypocalcemia are:
  - Perioral and acral paresthesias
  - Carpopedal spasms: flexion of the writs and metacarpophalangeal joints (MPJs) and extension of the interphalangeal joints (IPJs)
  - Stiffness, myalgia, clumsiness, and fatigue
  - Trousseau sign: Inflation of sphygmomanometer above the systolic blood pressure for 3 minutes leads to carpal spasms due to increased excitability of the nerve trunks by ischemia. Hyperexcitability peaks in 3 minutes and returns to normal afterward, even if ischemia continues.
  - Chovstek sign: Tapping the facial nerve leads to contraction of the ipsilateral facial muscles. It occurs in 10% of normal people.
  - Laryngeal strider
  - Seizures
  - Cardiac involvement: prolonged Q-T interval, hypotension, and arrhythmia
- EMG: Repeated high frequency discharges after a single stimulation are typical. Doublet and triplet fasciculations are common.
- Hyperventilation leads to respiratory alkalosis, which causes the conversion of ionized calcium to protein-bound calcium. Despite preservation of the total serum calcium concentration, the drop in the ionized, physiologically active calcium leads to tetany.
- Other causes of hypocalcemia include chronic renal failure, malabsorption syndrome, hypoparathyroidism, and hypomagnesemia.
- Treatment of hyperventilation is by reassurance and treatment of the underlying anxiety.
- Rebreathing from a plastic bag has not been tested systematically and may cause hypoxia; therefore, it cannot be recommended.

CASE 20.3: CRAMPING AND HYPERTROPHY OF THE CALVES

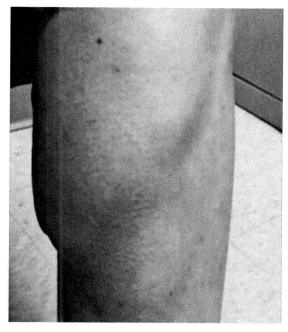

VIDEO 20.3

A 44-year-old woman presented with diffuse muscle pain and episodic, painful cramping of the calf muscles for a 1-year duration. The CPK level was 420 U/L, and EMG revealed high-frequency (120-Hz) discharges.

The following can cause enlargement of the calves:

1. Amyloidosis
2. Hypothyroidism
3. Neuromyotonia
4. Dysferlinopathy
5. Facioscapulohumeral muscular dystrophy (FSHD)

DIAGNOSIS

Calf hypertrophy may be caused by:

- Deposition of nonmuscle tissue:
  - Such as amyloid (amyloidosis)
  - Mucopolysaccharides (hypothyroidism)
  - Fatty tissue (Duchenne muscular dystrophy, or DMD)
- Hypertrophy of muscles due to muscle fiber hyperactivity:
  - Peripheral nerve hyperexcitability such as neuromyotonia
  - Chronic neurogenic insults, such as some cases of chronic inflammatory demyelinating polyneuropathy (CIDP) and S1 radiculopathy
- Ultrasound (US) helps differentiate these two categories.
- EMG shows decreased insertional activity in the first category.
- Dysferlinopathy typically causes calf atrophy.

CASE 20.4A: STIFF BACK MUSCLES

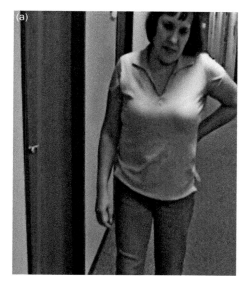

VIDEO 20.4A

A 43-year-old woman presented with intermittent painful cramping of the back muscles that started 3 years earlier. The spasms increased in frequency and severity to a degree that she could not work anymore. She had normal strength and DTRs. CPK was normal and EMG revealed continuous discharges of MUP of normal configuration and frequency. She responded well to diazepam of up to 40 mg a day, with no sleepiness.

What test is likely to be abnormal?

1. GAD antibodies
2. VGKC antibodies
3. S. Ca level
4. S. Mg level
5. Spastin mutation analysis

DIAGNOSIS

- SPS is an autoimmune disorder caused by antibodies against GAD. These antibodies localize to GABAnergic neurons.
- GABA is an important inhibitory neurotransmitter, and its absence causes spasticity.
- GAD also targets pancreatic beta cells, which explains the increased incidence (25% of cases) of diabetes mellitus (DM) type 1 in these patients.
- GAD antibodies are positive in 60% of cases, and the cerebrospinal fluid (CSF) GAD antibodies are more specific than the serum GAD antibodies.
- A total of 70% of DM-1 patients have positive GAD antibodies, but the titer is usually less than 10-fold, while in SPS it is usually 100-fold to 500-fold. In addition, these antibodies recognized deferent epitopes of GAD.
- There are three variants of SPS:
  - Autoimmune
  - Paraneoplastic
  - Idiopathic: negative serology, 30%
- Female-to-male ratio is 3:1; typical age group is 30–70 years.
- Muscle stiffness and rigidity start in the axial muscles, leading to spinal grooving.
- Severe intermittent spasms can be crippling.
- Paroxysmal dysautonomia (hyperpyrexia diaphoresis, tachycardia, mydriasis, and hypertension) may result in sudden death.
- Most people respond to diazepam. Sometimes doses as high as 100 mg/day are needed.
- Interestingly, sleepiness is not a common side effect in patients with SPS.
- Immunomodulation with azathioprine, intravenous immunoglobulin (IVIG), and plasmapheresis are other options in refractory cases.
- A total of 64% of patients remain ambulatory with extended follow-up (up to 23 years).

CASE 20.4B: STIFF PERSON SYNDROME (SPS) AFTER TREATMENT

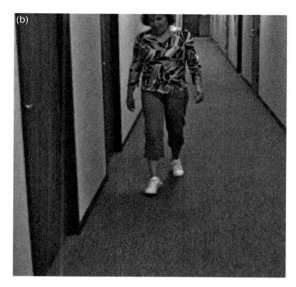

VIDEO 20.4B

DIAGNOSIS

- Diazepam as a GABA agonist is the drug of choice, to which most patients respond at least early in the course of the disease.
- The starting dose is 5 mg TID with gradual titration. Cases are reported to have needed 300 mg/day for symptom control.
- Oral or intravenous (IV) baclofen is also effective in severe cases.
- IV solumedrol and IV gammaglobulin are shown to be effective in refractory cases.
- Plasmapheresis and rituximab are other options.
- Some patients become refractory after an initial response to diazepam.
- The GAD antibody titer does not correlate with severity or improvement.

CASE 20.5: INABILITY TO ROLL OVER IN BED

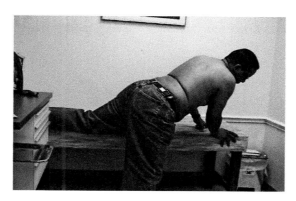

VIDEO 20.5

A 41-year-old man presented with gradually worsening and disabling stiffness of the back muscles, as shown in Video 20.5. He had intermittent stiffness of the leg muscles, worsened by stress. Examination revealed normal DTRs and strength and normal CK level. GAD Ab titer was 70 times the upper limit of normal.

GAD-65 antibodies are reported in 80% of DM type 1 cases, and yet SPS is rare. This is explainable by the following fact:

1. These GAD antibodies recognize different epitopes of the enzyme.
2. Many diabetics have subclinical SPS.
3. GAD antibodies are not pathogenic.
4. The studies that produced these results are not consistent.
5. SPS is genetic.

DIAGNOSIS

- A total of 70%–80% of DM type 1 cases are associated with elevated GAD antibodies, and yet SPS is a rare disease.
- The GAD antibody titer is much higher in SPS than in DM 1 (up to 1,000-fold).
- Sera from SPS but nondiabetic patients recognize a linear NH2 terminal epitope residing within the first eight amino acids of GAD.
- Sera from DM type-1 patients recognize the conformational epitope of GAD.
- T-cells respond to different epitopes: Two regions of GAD molecules produce T-cell proliferative responses in 6 of 8 patients with SPS, but in only 1 out of 17 with type 1 DM.

SUGGESTED READINGS

Kim J, Namchuk M, Bugawan T, et al. Higher autoantibody levels and recognition of a linear NH2-terminal epitope in the autoantigen GAD65, distinguish stiff-man syndrome from insulin-dependent diabetes mellitus. *J Exp Med.* 1994;180(2):595–606.

Lohmann T, Hawa M, Leslie RD, Picard J, Londei M. Immune reactivity to glutamic acid decarboxylase 65 in stiffman syndrome and type 1 diabetes mellitus. *Lancet.* 2000;356(9223):31–35.

CASE 20.6: MUSCLE CRAMPS AND DIARRHEA

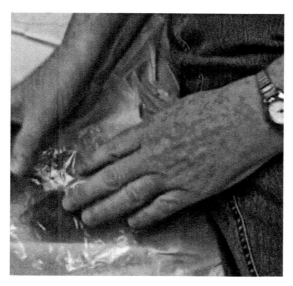

VIDEO 20.6

A 55-year-old woman presented with a several-year history of severe, intermittent, painful spasms of the arm and leg muscles lasting minutes to hours and occurring many times a day. Stool examination showed high fat content. She had no muscle weakness. She had a history of hypothyroidism.

This combination of symptoms suggests:

1. Gluten enteropathy
2. Alopecia universalis
3. Satayoshi syndrome
4. Neuromyotonia
5. Hyperthyroidism

DIAGNOSIS

- Satayoshi syndrome is a triad of diarrhea, alopecia, and muscle cramps.
- It is a multisystemic disease presumed to be autoimmune in nature.
- Adolescents are the main targets, but adult-onset cases are reported.
- It is more common in females.
- The immune nature is supported by:
  - Improvement with steroids
  - Association with other immune diseases
  - Deposition of immune complexes in the muscles
- The spasms can be very severe and progressive, leading to abnormal posturing and problems with speech.
- Malabsorption may lead to nutritional deficiency.
- Sclerosis of the growth plate due to recurrent trauma produced by severe muscle spasms is characteristic.
- Severe spasms may respond to dantrolene, calcium gluconate, or even botulinum toxin (BT).
- The disease usually responds to steroids or IVIG.

SUGGESTED READING

Asherson RA, Giampaolo D, Strimling M. A case of adult-onset Satoyoshi syndrome with gastric ulceration and eosinophilic enteritis. *Nat Clin Pract Rheumatol*. 2008 Aug;4(8):439–444.

CASE 20.7: MUSCLE CRAMPS AFTER BARIATRIC SURGERY

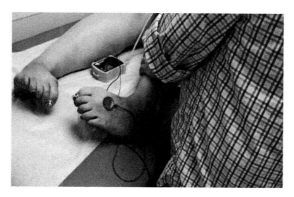

VIDEO 20.7

A 31-year-old woman had developed muscle cramps 3 years after gastric bypass surgery that resulted in a 150-pound weight loss. The cramps were severe enough to dislocate a hip joint and twist her feet violently. She became disabled. She could not tolerate an EMG, and her CK level was 340 U/L. She was taking multivitamins and 500 mg a day of calcium since the surgery. Serum calcium was 5.6 mg/dl (normal 8.5–10.5), and alkaline phosphatase was 500 U/L (20–120). Phosphorus and magnesium levels were normal. She had macrocytic anemia.

Complications of gastric bypass surgery include which of the following?

1. Severe muscle cramps
2. Copper deficiency
3. Polyneuropathy
4. Myopathy
5. All of the above

DIAGNOSIS

- Gastric bypass surgery has become one of the most common surgeries in modern times.
- There are many types of bariatric surgery; all of them are associated with neuromuscular complications, although gastric sleeves have a more benign course.
- Complications can be immediate or remote and may occur up to 20 years after surgery.
- Commonly reported neuromuscular complications are:
  - Peripheral neuropathy:
    - Polyneuropathy, including Guillain-Barré syndrome (GBS)
    - Mononeuropathy, including meralgia paresthetica
  - Myopathy and rhabdomyolysis: Myalgia is common in hypocalcemia due to pseudofractures.
  - Lumbar plexitis.
  - Myeloneuropathy is typically seen in copper deficiency.
- The causes of these complications are not clear:
  - An inflammatory basis has been suggested.
  - Deficiency of vitamins, minerals, and micronutrients (selenium, cadmium, etc.).
- Monitoring of the micronutrient level and prompt recognition can reduce morbidity.
- Most neuromuscular complications are remote and gradually evolving.
- Copper deficiency usually occurs after years and presents with sensory ataxia and hyper-reflexia due to myeloneuropathy.
- Hypocalcemia due to vitamin D deficiency is the most common cause of muscle cramps. Up to 30% of patients develop hypocalcemia.
- Correction of hypocalcemia effectively improves myalgia and muscle cramps in many patients.

CASE 20.8: LEFT LEG STIFFNESS AND FALLS

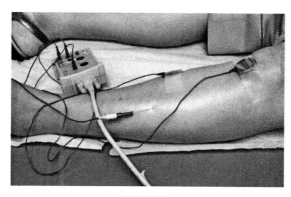

VIDEO 20.8

A 77-year-old woman presented with a 1-year history of intermittent spasms of the left leg muscles with occasional inversion of the foot, leading to falls. She has a history of right S1 radiculopathy. The EMG is shown in the video.

Which test is most appropriate?

1. Acetylcholine receptor (AChR) antibody titer
2. GAD antibody titer
3. VGKC antibody titer
4. SCN4 mutation
5. Voltage-gated calcium channel (VGCC) antibody titer

DIAGNOSIS

- The stiffness of the left leg and continuous EMG activity suggested SPS. The GAD antibody level was 100 nmol/L. Focal SPS is difficult to diagnose.
- Focal SPS usually starts in one leg (stiff leg syndrome) and spares the trunk.
- Onset occurs between 35–60 years.
- Stiffness is provoked by voluntary movement and sensory stimuli, which may cause severe stiffness and torsion of the feet and falls.
- GAD antibody level does not correlate with severity.
- It usually responds partially to diazepam and baclofen. IVIG may lead to temporary improvement.
- Focal SPS is not reported to be paraneoplastic.
- Since isolated leg stiffness is the most common symptom, serologic confirmation is important for the diagnosis.
- It is possible that many seronegative cases are missed.
- In some cases, stiffness generalizes within 2 years, but most cases remain restricted.

SUGGESTED READINGS

McKeon A, Robinson MT, McEvoy KM, et al. Stiff-man syndrome and variants clinical course, treatments, and outcomes. *Arch Neurol.* 2012;69(2):230–238.

Meinck HM, Thompson PD. Stiff man syndrome and related conditions. *Move Dis.* 2002 Sep;17(5):853–866.

CASE 20.9: STIFFNESS AND HYPERTROPHY OF THE THENAR MUSCLES

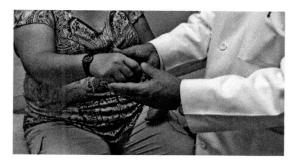

VIDEO 20.9

A 41-year-old woman presented with a several-year history of sweating and intermittent muscle cramps involving the hands. Gradually, the small hand muscles, especially the thenar muscles, became hypertrophic and contracted most of the time, but they were not weak. The EMG is shown in the video.

Which test is most appropriate?

1. AChR Abs
2. GAD Abs
3. VGKC Abs
4. SCN4 mutation
5. VGCC Abs

DIAGNOSIS

- Neuromyotonia is a form of peripheral nerve hyperexcitability in which there are spontaneous irregular bursts of single MUPs at a frequency of 40–300 Hz.
- Age: 9–80 years.
- Muscle twitching, stiffness, and cramping are the main presenting symptoms.
- Distal muscles are affected more than proximal muscles, and stiffness is worsened by exercise, leading to diagnostic confusion with paramyotonia.
- No percussion myotonia is noted.
- Activity persists during sleep but is blocked by neuromuscular blockers.
- Usually, there is no associated weakness of the affected muscles.
- Muscle hypertrophy may occur due to continuous activity.
- No spontaneous remission usually occurs, but fluctuation is common.
- Thymoma, lymphoma, and lung cancer are the most frequently associated neoplasms.
- CK level is elevated in 50% of cases.
- VGKC antibodies are increased in two-thirds of cases.
- Carbamazepine and mexiletine usually help the cramps.
- Steroids and IVIG usually lead to short-term benefits.
- Clinical syndromes with VGKC antibodies include:
  - Neuromyotonia
  - Myokymia
  - Cramp fasciculation syndrome (CFS)
  - Benign fasciculation syndrome (BFS)
  - Morvan's syndrome
  - Limbic encephalitis
  - Painful polyneuropathy

CASE 20.10: SILENT MUSCLE CRAMPS

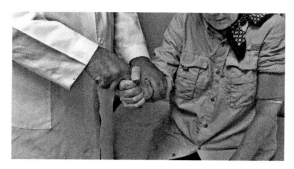

VIDEO 20.10

A 62-year-old woman presented with muscle cramps since childhood. Gradually, the cramps became severe and generalized and were associated with poor relaxation of the contracted muscles. She had mild proximal weakness, and the CK was normal. EMG of the cramping muscles was silent.

The most important causes of electrically silent muscle cramps are:

1. McArdle disease
2. Paramyotonia
3. Brody disease
4. Neuromyotonia
5. SPS

DIAGNOSIS

Brody disease is a rare disorder characterized by impaired skeletal muscle contraction following exercise.

- Activity-induced cramping and stiffness.
- Rapid closure and opening of the fists or eyelids may lead to delayed relaxation.
- There is no percussion myotonia.
- CK level is usually normal.
- EMG usually shows that the muscles that fail to relax are electrically silent, similar to what happens in McArdle disease, but there is a normal rise of serum lactate and ammonia during the forearm ischemic exercise test.
- Muscle biopsy shows type 2 fiber atrophy and reduced Ca-ATPase in type 2 muscle fibers with immunohistochemistry staining.
- It is caused by an autosomal-recessive (AR) mutation of the *ATPA1* gene or autosomal dominant (AD) with the normal *ATPA1* gene.
- This gene encodes sarcoplasmic reticulum calcium-ATPase (SERCA1), a calcium channel present on the smooth endoplasmic reticulum (SR) of type 2 fibers.
- Dantrolene is usually effective.

CASE 20.11: MUSCLE CRAMPS
AND FOOT NUMBNESS

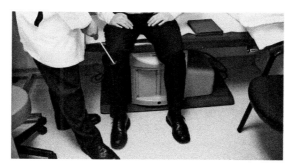

VIDEO 20.11

A 53-year-old man presented with a long history of smoking and daily alcohol drinking who developed painful spasms of the calves, foot numbness, and poor balance over 3 months. Nerve conduction study (NCS) revealed mild axonal neuropathy. The B_{12} level was 250 pg/ml. Examination is shown in Video 20.11.

The next appropriate step is:

1. Magnetic resonance imaging (MRI) of the cervical spine
2. Lumbar spine magnetic resonance imaging (LS MRI)
3. Treating B_{12} deficiency
4. A chest computed tomography (CT) scan
5. CSF examination

DIAGNOSIS

- Sustained painful muscle spasms can be produced by increased muscle tone due to upper motor neuron (UMN) lesions such as myelopathies, hereditary spastic paraplegia, tropical spastic paraplegia, and amyotrophic lateral sclerosis (ALS).
- The sustained spasms are due to loss of central inhibition of the lower motor neurons (LMNs).
- Although the patient had axonal neuropathy (most likely alcohol related), this finding is minor compared to the gait spasticity and hyperreflexia and neurogenic bladder, and it should not preclude further investigation.
- Spinal tap should be avoided before a compressive lesion is ruled out, due to possible worsening of the compression after the procedure.
- A borderline B_{12} level should be verified by measuring methylmalonic acid and homocysteine.
- While myelopathy and neuropathy are features of B_{12} deficiency, sensory ataxia is much more pronounced than spasticity in these cases.
- The history of smoking suggests lung cancer, which can cause cord compression or paraneoplastic neuropathy.
- Involvement of the arms and legs with UMN signs suggest cervical myelopathy. Structural lesions are the most common, particularly cervical spondylosis, Herniated nucleus pulposis, and tumors.
- The rest of the possibilities mentioned here should be investigated and treated as well.
- The most appropriate next step, therefore, is to obtain a cervical spine MRI.

CASE 20.12: FAMILIAL MUSCLE STIFFNESS AND SPASMS

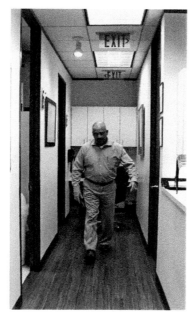

VIDEO 20.12

A 59-year-old man with a 5-year history of pain and stiffness of the left leg and arm with difficulty writing and walking (as demonstrated in the video). Numbness of the feet and painful spasms and (rarely) slurred speech were reported. His mother and 2/5 of his siblings also had stiffness and spasms.

This condition can be caused by mutation of the following genes except:

1. *KIF1A*
2. *KIF5A*
3. *SPG4*
4. *SPG7*
5. *Ataxin-1*

DIAGNOSIS

- Video 20.12 demonstrates spasticity of the legs, especially the left one.
- The familial pattern and chronic progressive spasticity suggest HSP. One-side predominance is well reported.
- Genetic testing revealed a heterozygous pathogenic mutation of the *KIF1A* gene.
  - AR inheritance of a pathogenic gene is associated with hereditary sensory and autonomic neuropathy and, independently, with HSP.
  - AD inheritance is reported to cause a milder and later-onset disease.
- HSP is a large group of clinically and genetically heterogeneous disorders (130 genetic types) with a prevalence of 2–6: 100,000 people; it is characterized by chronic progressive spastic weakness of the legs, with no evidence of other compressive or none compressive myelopathies. Mild distal vibratory impairment is common.
- Other than fall precautions and symptomatic treatment of spasticity (baclofen, botulinum toxin), not much can be offered.
- The *ATAXIN-1* gene mutations are associated with spinocerebellar ataxia (SCA) type 1, not HSP.
- All the mentioned mutations may present with HSP except *Ataxin-1* mutations.

SUGGESTED READING

Ylikallio E, Kim D, Isohanni P, et al. Dominant transmission of de novo KIF1A motor domain variant underlying pure spastic paraplegia. *Eur J Human Genet.*2015 Oct;23:1427–1430.

CHAPTER 21

MYOTONIA

CASE 21.1: A FAMILY WITH MUSCLE STIFFNESS

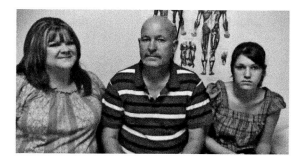

VIDEO 21.1

A 53-year-old man had noticed difficulty relaxing his grip after a handshake at age 35 years. Gradually, he developed stiffness of the leg muscles and cataracts. His asymptomatic daughter's examination revealed grip and percussion myotonia.

The earlier appearance of symptoms in the daughter is due to a phenomenon called:

1. Contraction
2. Anticipation
3. Variable penetrance
4. Heteroplasmy
5. Codominance

DIAGNOSIS

- The phenomenon of earlier-onset and more severe symptoms in successive generations is called *anticipation.*
- This is an interesting genetic phenomenon that was thought to be due to a bias resulting from more attention being given to the disease-related symptoms in the younger generation.
- It is clear now that this phenomenon is due to the instability of a genetic mutation.
- It is mostly noted in genetic disorders that are characterized by the expansion of trinucleotide repeats beyond a certain threshold.
- Triple repeats exist in human genomes' coding and noncoding components; most of the time, though, their expansion is harmless.
- Examples of diseases caused by trinucleotide repeat expansion include:
  - Myotonic dystrophy type 1 (DM 1)
  - Huntington disease
  - Fragile X syndrome
  - Machado-Joseph disease
  - Friedreich's ataxia
- In myotonic dystrophy type 1, the expanded repeat is a Cytosine thymine Guanine (CTG) sequence in the noncoding region of the protein kinase gene on chromosome 19.
  - A normal CTG repeat number is between 5 and 37.
  - A range of 38–49 repeats is called the *permutation range,* and it increases the risk of having affected children.
  - A repeat of more than 50 is almost always symptomatic.
  - Interestingly, the number of CTG repeats positively correlates with an earlier onset and more severe disease.
  - The expanded repeats tend to expand further during meiosis, leading to a larger repeat in successive generations, which explains the phenomenon of anticipation.
  - The cause of instability of the CTG repeat is not clear.
  - More interestingly, CTG repeats expand when they go through a female germline and only rarely through a male germline. This explains the congenital form of the disease.

SUGGESTED READING

Athni S, Shaibani A, Ashizawa T. Anticipation and myotonic dystrophy: Diagnostic and prognostic implications. *Resident and Staff Physician.* 1996;42:57–63.

CASE 21.2: MYALGIA AND MYOTONIA

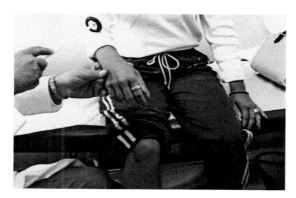

VIDEO 21.2

A 36-year-old woman presented with severe painful spasms of the lower back muscles for 3 years that gradually worsened and spread to the chest muscles, hands, and feet. She did not respond to baclofen, topiramate, and hydromorphone. She became disabled. Her neurologists found diffuse myotonic discharges in the electromyogram (EMG) and therefore referred her for consultation. Mutation analysis revealed no *DMPK* gene mutations.

The most appropriate next test is to look for mutations in the following genes:

1. Sodium channel
2. Chloride channel
3. Cellular nucleic acid-binding protein (CNBP)
4. Potassium channel
5. Mitochondrial

DIAGNOSIS

- Myotonic dystrophy type 2 is caused by mutation of the *CNBP* gene on chromosome 3q21.
- The phenomenon of anticipation is much less common than myotonic dystrophy type 1.
- Congenital form is rare.
- Weakness is more proximal than distal.
- The face is affected in only 12% of cases.
- Calf hypertrophy is reported.
- Myalgia and stiffness occur in 56% of cases and:
  - Are induced by sensory stimuli and palpation or percussion of the affected muscles
  - Increase with cold
  - Are not related to severity of myotonia
  - Affect proximal (including chest) more than distal muscles, leading to suspicion of coronary heart disease, which is enforced by creatine kinase (CK) elevation
- Central nervous system (CNS) involvement is rare.
- Systemic manifestations:
  - Cataracts: 100% over 20 years as visualized with slit lamp examination
  - Cardiac arrhythmias: 20% of cases; conduction defects
  - Diabetes mellitus (DM): 20% of cases
  - Hearing loss: 20% of cases
  - Fertility: normal or reduced
  - Cardiovascular autonomic function: normal
- More benign course than myotonic dystrophy type 1.

SUGGESTED READING

http://neuromuscular.wustl.edu/

CASE 21.3: HAND NUMBNESS AND DIFFUSE ABNORMAL DISCHARGES

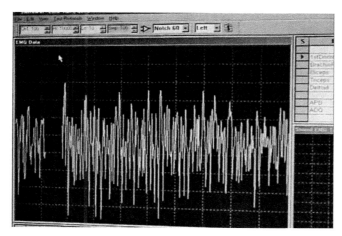

VIDEO 21.3

A 35-year-old woman visited a neurologist for hand numbness. EMG revealed the displayed discharges in many tested muscles in the arms and legs. She also had a mild prolongation of the palmar median sensory latency bilaterally that explained her hand numbness.

These discharges can be seen in the following disorders:

1. Myotonia congenita (MC)
2. Schwartz-Jampel syndrome
3. Myotonic dystrophy
4. Brody syndrome
5. McArdle disease

DIAGNOSIS

- Myotonia is a slow relaxation of skeletal muscles after contraction.
- Muscle fibers are hyperexcitable and they repetitively discharge after a contraction, which results in slow relaxation.
- The contraction is purely myogenic, regardless of motor neuron activity.
- These discharges may be provoked by voluntary contraction (action myotonia), mechanical tapping (percussion myotonia), or needle insertion (electromechanical myotonia).
- Electrically, they appear as waxing and waning positive discharges (fibrillation and positive, sharp waves) in a frequency of 20–80 Hz, similar to accelerating and decelerating motorcycle engine.
- Sometimes patients are referred to neuromuscular clinics because these discharges are discovered during an EMG that is done for a related cause (stiffness, weakness, etc.) or unrelated cause (hand numbness).
- These discharges may be confused with diffuse denervation such as motor neuron disease (MND), neuromyotonia (faster discharges than 150 Hz), or complex repetitive discharges (which end abruptly and do not wax and wane).
- Subclinical myotonia is usually a feature of chloride channelopathy and, to a lesser extent, sodium channelopathy.
- Resting electrical features do not practically distinguish among different myotonic disorders, but short exercise test often does.
- There are disorders that are characterized by muscle stiffness and cramping that sometimes are confused clinically as myotonic disorders, but the EMG is silent. Examples are Brody syndrome and McArdle disease.
- Causes of myotonia include:
  - Myotonic dystrophy
  - Nondystrophic myotonia (chloride and sodium channelopathies)
  - Metabolic myopathies such as acid maltase deficiency
  - Toxic myopathies such as statin myopathy
  - Endocrine myopathy such as hypothyroidism
  - Inflammatory myopathies
  - Myofibrillar myopathies
  - Schwartz-Jampel syndrome

CASE 21.4: PERSISTENT HANDSHAKING

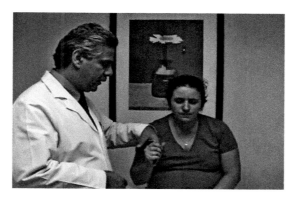

VIDEO 21.4

A 32-year-old woman presented with stiffness of the hand muscles during winter. Shaking hands with patients can be diagnostically useful in:

1. Inclusion body myositis (IBM)
2. Duchenne muscular dystrophy (DMD)
3. Myotonic dystrophy
4. Acid maltase deficiency
5. Mitochondrial myopathy

DIAGNOSIS

- Shaking hands with patients is one of the diagnostic tools in the neuromuscular clinic.
- Parents' advice to their children to look at a person's face while shaking hands applies to the neuromuscular examination as well. The face, along with the hand, is very often a source of diagnostic information.
- A myotonic hand contracts normally but relaxes slowly. A forceful contraction is usually followed by a slow relaxation.
- Repeated handshaking leads to improvement of myotonia (the warming-up phenomenon) in myotonic dystrophy and chloride channelopathies (MC) and worsening of myotonia in sodium channelopathy [paramyotonia congenita (PMC)].
- In patients with IBM, weakness of the long finger flexors and preservation of the finger extensors and intrinsic hand muscles lead to a "fish mouth hand" during shaking, as the fingers cannot be flexed at the interphalangeal joint.
- While myotonic discharges are reported in acid maltase deficiency, it mostly occurs in thoracic paraspinal (TPS) muscles, not in the distal muscles.
- DMD and mitochondrial myopathy do not have special hand features.
- The correct answers are 1 and 2.

CASE 21.5: FAMILIAL SENSITIVITY TO COLD

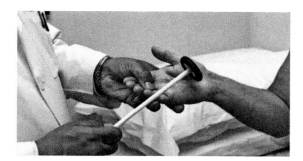

VIDEO 21.5

A 55-year-old woman had moved from Chicago to Houston due to cold-induced muscle stiffness. Her mother had a similar problem. She saw a neurologist in Houston for neck pain radiating to the right arm, and he found her to have diffuse waxing and waning 100-Hz discharges in several tested muscles. There was no mutation in the sodium channel (*SCN4*) gene.

The most appropriate next test is to look for is:

1. CTG repeat expansion at the *DMPK* gene
2. Chloride channel (*CLCN1*) gene mutation
3. Voltage dependent Calcium channel (VDCC) gene mutation
4. Voltage-gated potassium channel (VGKC) gene mutation
5. None of the above

Unlike PMC, MC is usually:

1. An always autosomal-dominant (AD) disorder
2. Often cold-sensitive
3. A syndrome that warms up with repetition
4. A syndrome that does not show a decremental response
5. A syndrome that is associated with hyperkalemic periodic paralysis (HYPP)

DIAGNOSIS

- The most important question when myotonia is clinically or electrically found is whether this is a dystrophic or nondystrophic myotonia (NDM).
  - The phenotype of myotonic dystrophy is characteristic (thin and weak face, temporal wasting, cataract, mental dullness, distal and proximal weakness). Myotonic dystrophy, especially type 2, may present with only myotonia and pain, leading to diagnostic difficulty.
  - It is has been observed that NDM patients sometimes have rounded faces due to occasional hypertrophy of temporalis muscles from myotonic discharges.
- The second question is whether NDM is due to chloride (MC) or sodium channelopathy (PMC).
  - MC is usually a chloride channelopathy and may be recessive or dominant, while PMC is usually due to sodium channelopathy and it is allelic to HYPP. It is an AD disorder.
  - Extreme sensitivity to cold is mostly seen in PMC and is rare in MC.
  - Warming up after repetitive testing is a feature of MC. PMC gets worse with repetition (paradoxical myotonia).
  - Episodic weakness and lid myotonia are seen in PMC but rarely in MC.
  - Warming up and sensitivity to cold can be confirmed neurophysiologically by a long exercise test.
  - Both decrement with a 2-Hz repetitive nerve stimulation (RNS) test. Cooling increased the decrement in PMC.
  - Myotonia caused by *CLCN1* mutations can occasionally be clinically indistinguishable from myotonia caused by sodium channel mutations (*SCN4A* mutations), resulting in PMC (PMC)

SUGGESTED READINGS

Matthews E, Fialho D, Tan SV, et al. The non-dystrophic myotonias: molecular pathogenesis, diagnosis, and treatment. *Brain*. 2010 Jan;133(1):9–22.

Michel P, Sternberg D, Jeannet PY, et al. Comparative efficacy of repetitive nerve simulation, exercise, and cold in differentiating myotonic disorders. *Musc. Nerve*. 2007;36(5):643–650.

CASE 21.6: STIFFNESS THAT GETS BETTER WITH USE

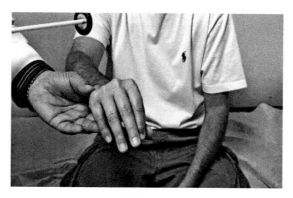

VIDEO 21.6

A 47-year-old man presented with muscle stiffness that started at age 21 years. His parents had premature cataracts, and his sister and three maternal aunts were diagnosed with myotonic dystrophy based on the presence of CTG repeat expansion on chromosome 19.

The demonstrated phenomenon is a cardinal feature of:

1. Sodium channelopathies
2. Chloride channelopathies
3. Calcium channelopathies
4. Myotonic dystrophy
5. Potassium channelopathies

DIAGNOSIS

- The most common sites of demonstrating myotonia clinically are wrist extensors, thenar muscles, tongue, and eyelids.
  - Tapping wrist extensors leads to a slow return of the extended wrist to the baseline.
  - Tapping thenar muscles leads to a slow return of the thumb to its position.
  - Excreting pressure on the tongue leads to grooving due to slow relaxation of the tapped muscles.
  - Lid myotonia is seen more commonly in PMC; it is also seen in hypokalemic periodic paralysis (HypoKPP). It is easy to demonstrate paradoxical myotonia by asking the patient to close his or her eyes repeatedly. With more closure, eye opening becomes more difficult and the eyelids stick to each other longer.
- Warm-up phenomenon was initially reported in MC patients, as they get stiffer in the morning and after a long rest, and their muscle stiffness eases up with exercise and daily muscle use.
- Patients with myotonic dystrophy demonstrate the same phenomenon.
- The molecular biology of this phenomenon is not clear. Mild slowing of sodium channel inactivation is thought to be the cause.
- The correct answers are 2 and 3.

SUGGESTED READING

Lossin C. Nav1.4 slow-inactivation: is it a player in the warm-up phenomenon of myotonic disorders? *Muscl Nerve*. 2013;47(4):483–487.

CASE 21.7: STIFFNESS WORSENED BY ANXIETY

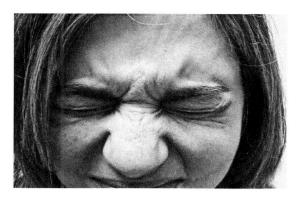

VIDEO 21.7

A 34-year-old woman presented with muscle stiffness worsened by cold temperature and stress. The demonstrated sign can be seen in:

1. PMC
2. MC
3. HypoKPP
4. Polymyositis
5. Oculopharyngeal muscular dystrophy (OPMD)

DIAGNOSIS

- Eyelid myotonia is a feature of PMC and is sometimes observed in HypoKPP, but it is not a feature of MC.
- Worsening of myotonia with repetitive motion (paradoxical myotonia) is a feature of PMC.
- Cold sensitivity is also an important feature of the disease and can be demonstrated neurophysiologically.
- PMC is an AD mutation of the sodium channel Alpha subunit (*SCN4A*) on chromosome 17q23.3. Rarely, paramyotonia is produced by chloride channel mutation.
- PMC is allelic to HYPP, and they can affect the same patient.
- Mutated sodium channels are dysfunctional and abnormally inactivated, leading to continuous leak of sodium into the cell.
- Symptoms usually appear in the first decade of life. During a crying episode, infants may have difficulty opening their eyes due to exercise-induced myotonia.
- Weakness is not prominent, and CK is usually normal or slightly high.
- Mexiletine 150–1,000 mg/day is shown to be effective in a double-blind trial.

SUGGESTED READING

Statland JM, Bundy BN, Wang Y, et al. Mexiletine for symptoms and signs of myotonia in non-dystrophic myotonia. *JAMA*. 2012;308(13):1357–1365.

CASE 21.8: EPISODIC WEAKNESS AND MUSCLE STIFFNESS

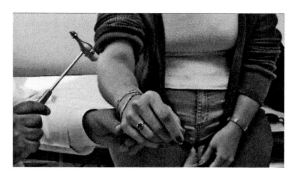

VIDEO 21.8

A 35-year-old woman had developed an episode of paralysis lasting hours after hearing about her father's death at age 15. Since then, she has had milder episodic morning weakness that improves after eating cereal for breakfast. Her examination was shown in Video 21.8.

This condition is typically associated with:

1. *SCN4A* mutation
2. PMC
3. HYPP
4. Myotonic dystrophy
5. MC

DIAGNOSIS

- The examination shows myotonia that gets worse with repetitive testing (paradoxical myotonia). This is typically seen in PMC.
- Recurrent episodic weakness (periodic paralysis) may be familial or nonfamilial (thyrotoxic, hypokalemic, etc.).
- Familial periodic paralysis could be potassium sensitive (hyperkalemic) or hypokalemic.
- HYPP may present without myotonia, present with myotonia, or be associated with full-blown PMC.
- Cooling usually triggers attacks when PMC is present.
- Myotonia is usually subtle and can be elicited by percussing the thenar eminence and finger extensors, and pressing the tongue.
- The attacks usually start in the first decade and occur in the mornings, triggered by rest after exercise, ingestion of potassium-rich food, fasting, and stress.
- The degree of weakness varies, and weakness usually starts in the legs.
- The sphincters, bulbar, and respiratory muscles are usually preserved.
- The frequency of attacks greatly varies from several times a day to once a year; each usually lasts less than 2 hours, and they are rarely profound.
- During the attacks, deep tendon reflexes (DTRs) are usually absent. Between the attacks, eyelid myotonia may be the only finding.
- CK may be slightly elevated and serum potassium is usually normal, but urinary excretion of potassium is high.
- If serum potassium is high, one has to rule out other causes of hyperkalemia.
- Treatment with intravenous (IV) glucose and insulin is needed only in severe attacks. Mild attacks resolve spontaneously.
- Acetazolamide and chlorothiazide may reduce the frequency of attacks.

CASE 21.9: MUSCLE STIFFNESS AND ABORTIONS

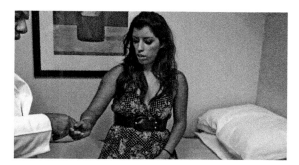

VIDEO 21.9

A 27-year-old woman presented with a 7-year history of muscle stiffness and failure of relaxation of contracted muscles. Her mother was wheelchair bound due to leg weakness, and she had a sister with dropped head and leg weakness. The patient had two abortions.

The following statements are true about the genetics of this condition:

1. Anticipation is associated with a longer CTG repeat.
2. CTG repeats occur in the coding region of the *DMPK* gene.
3. Variable penetrance is a common feature.
4. Permutations are associated with severe disease.
5. Congenital cases occur equally through the father's and mother's lines.

DIAGNOSIS

- Myotonic dystrophy (DM) is the most prevalent neuromuscular disorder in adults.
- A total of 98% of cases are type 1 (DM1). Females and males have equal chances of being affected.
- Penetrance is variable, but it is 100% by age 50 years.
- It is a multisystemic disease. Systemic features include cataract, cardiac conduction abnormalities, DM, hypothyroidism, cognitive abnormalities, and gastrointestinal (GI) motility disorder.
- The disease is caused by a CTG repeat expansion in the noncoding region of dystrophia myotonica protein kinase (DMPK).
- Clinical severity correlates with the size of repeat expansion.
- The mutation is unstable, and the appearance of the disease at an earlier age and in a more severe form in subsequent generations (anticipation) is due to expansion of the CTG repeat during meiosis.
- The repeat size is greater in muscle than blood cells, but it does not correlate with muscle weakness.
- Myotonia is more common in younger age groups, while weakness is more common in older populations.
- Weakness of the finger flexors and face and dysphagia may be confused with IBM.
- An annual electrocardiogram (ECG) to detect conduction abnormalities is recommended.
- Sudden death is mostly due to cardiac arrhythmias or respiratory failure. Tricyclic antidepressants, digoxin, procainamide, propranolol, and quinine are to be avoided.
- If a patient decides to become pregnant, prenatal diagnosis is possible. High-risk perinatal care is recommended.
- The disease is incurable. Progress has been made in animal models to reduce the toxic gain of function that is created by the expanded repeats. Charles Thornton's group used antisense oligonucleotides to target mutant RNA that is retained in the nucleus and exerts a toxic gain of function. They reported the correction of physiological and histopathologic features that were sustained for up to a year after treatment was discontinued.

SUGGESTED READING

Wheeler TM, Leger AJ, Pandey SK, et al. Targeting nuclear RNA for in vivo correction of myotonic dystrophy. *Nature*. 2012 Aug 2;488(7409):111–115.

CASE 21.10: ASYMPTOMATIC PARAMYOTONIA CONGENITA (PMC)

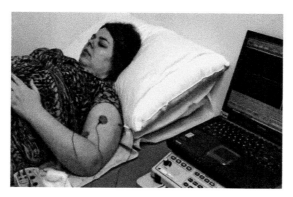

VIDEO 21.10

A 28-year-old woman from Houston was referred by a rheumatologist who found diffuse abnormal discharges during EMG while evaluating her arm numbness. She did not give a history of weakness. She had two vague episodes of muscle stiffness during childhood when she visited her father in Minnesota. Her examination revealed normal strength. Amplitude of compound muscle action potential (CMAP) of the thenar muscles decreased after exercise.

The following diagnostic tests are appropriate:

1. Sodium channel mutation analysis
2. Chloride channel mutation analysis
3. Resting serum potassium concentration
4. Calcium channel mutation analysis
5. Muscle biopsy

The following statements are true about this condition:

1. It is an X-linked recessive disease.
2. Cold exposure increases postexercise decremental response.
3. It is often associated with cardiac involvement.
4. It is associated with HYPP.
5. It is frequently asymptomatic.

DIAGNOSIS

- The lack of EMG findings to explain clinical abnormalities such as weakness, muscle atrophy, or numbness is a common cause of referrals to neuromuscular clinics.
- Nevertheless, unexplained or incidental EMG abnormalities found in general neurology practice are an equally important source of such referrals, although less frequently. Examples of these findings include:
  - Complex repetitive discharges confused with myotonic discharges
  - Myotonic discharges confused with diffuse denervation
  - Positive, sharp wave disease
- Video 21.10 shows percussion thenar myotonia and electrical myotonic discharges.
- Mutation of sodium channel *SCN4A* is confirmed. *SCN4A* is an important cause of myotonia and is found in patients with PMC and HYPP, and in 10% of patients with HypoKPP.
- Chloride channel mutations are usually asymptomatic and can be inherited as AD or autodomal recessive (AR). Myotonia is not as sensitive to cold, and it "warms up."
- Defective sodium channels do not close properly, leading to a continuing influx of sodium molecules into the muscle cells and escape of potassium from these cells. This unwanted depolarization of cell membrane is responsible for myotonia.
- Sodium channelopathy is an AD disease and is rarely asymptomatic. Retrospectively, most patients report cold intolerance and muscle cramping and worsening muscle stiffness during exercise.
- Amplitude of CMAP decreases with exercise and exposure to cold.
- Mexiletine is a potent sodium channel blocker that is shown to be effective in nondystrophic myotonia.

CASE 21.11: FAMILIAL MUSCLE STIFFNESS AND TEMPORAL FULLNESS

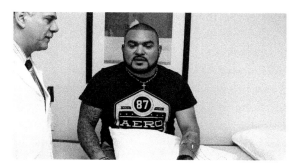

VIDEO 21.11

The shown case most likely represents:

1. Myotonic dystrophy type 1
2. MC, Thomsen disease
3. MC, Becker disease
4. PMC
5. Myotonic dystrophy type 2

DIAGNOSIS

- Muscle stiffness during activity is the main presentation of myotonia (action myotonia).
- This is confirmed by examination, which shows slow relaxation of the tested thenar and wrist extension muscles (percussion myotonia), and by EMG, which shows high-frequency waxing and waning discharges.
- Historically and by examination, myotonia is relieved by activity and repeated use of the affected muscle (warm-up phenomenon), which runs counter to the diagnosis of PMC, which gets worse with exercise.
- There are no dystrophic features (e.g., thin face, frontal baldness) or systemic features (e.g., cataract, heart block, diabetes, testicular atrophy, enteropathy) to suggest myotonic dystrophy.
- Muscle hypertrophy, temporal fullness, age of onset, the mild nature of the symptoms and prevalence in the family support MC, AD type (Thomsen disease). This form is responsible for 37% of cases. Temporal fullness may be due to hypertrophy of the temporalis leading to a rounded face as opposed to the tall, thin face of myotonic dystrophy.
- Becker disease is the AR type, which appears later in life and is causes more severe myotonia.
- Sequence analysis of chloride channels (*CLCN1*) revealed a pathogenic heterozygous mutation, confirming Thomsen disease.
  - This test is positive in 95% of cases, both AD and AR.
- The most cost-effective approach to myotnoia is to order sequencing of a specific gene if one is suspected (CLCN1 gene in this case). However, there is an overlap among different myotonias and atypical presentations are common.
  - If the targeted gene is negative, a multigene panel would be the next step. However, genetic laboratories offer different genetic panels. Some labs offer a panel for myotonia that includes the sodium and chloride channel genes and DM1 and 2 genes. Other genetic labs provide comprehensive neuromuscular panels that include many other genes.
  - The improvement of the whole-exome sequencing technique will make it replace most of these panels because there will be no cost difference in the exchange of broadening diagnostic power.
- A total of 20% of patients suspected of having MC may have mutation of the *SCN4A* gene instead of the *CLCN1* gene. These instances are usually associated with pain, periodic weakness, worsening with cold, sensitivity to potassium, and eyelid myotonia.

SUGGESTED READING

Duno M, Colding-Jorgensen E. Myotonia congenita. *GeneRev*. August 6, 2015.

CASE 21.12: FAMILIAL MYOTONIA AND THE NORMAL *DMPK* GENE

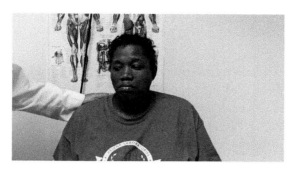

VIDEO 21.12

A 45-year-old woman presented with a 3-year history of muscle stiffness, cramps, difficulty climbing stairs, and difficulty opening her fist after making a hand grip. There was no significant pain. The CPK level was 270 IU/L. EMG showed waxing and waning discharges in all the tested muscles of 80-Hz frequency. She had history of DM type 2, controlled with diet. Her mother, a brother, and a maternal aunt had muscle stiffness. There was no family or personal history of cataract or pacemaker placement, but she did have one miscarriage. The *DMPK* gene was normal.

The following features are typical for DM 2 except:

1. Miscarriage
2. Myalgia
3. Dysmorphic features
4. DM
5. Cataract

DIAGNOSIS

- Miscarriage is not a feature of DM 2, unlike DM 1.
- Severe pain in the proximal myotonic muscles is typical for DM 2 compared to DM 1.
- Dysmorphic and systemic features (cataract, arrhythmias, DM, etc.) are seen in both DM 1 and 2.
- In this case, the lack of pain and dysmorphic and systemic features suggested nondystrophic myotonia (sodium or chloride channelopathy).
- However, the patient had negative testing for chloride and sodium channel gene mutation. Instead, she had CCTG repeat expansion in the *CNBP* gene characteristic of DM 2.
- In the evaluation of myotonia:
  - Absence of systemic features and dystrophic weakness should suggest nondystrophic myotonic disorder. DM2 patients mayalso present initially in this way.
  - If a nondystrophic myotonic disorder is suspected, the next question would be to determine whether the disorder is a chloride channelopathy (Thomsen or Becker disease) or sodium channelopathy (PMC).
    - Warm-up is common in the chloride and some sodium channelopathies, but it is not present in PC, where paradoxical myotonia is often found
    - Eyelid myotonia is uncommon in the chloride channelopathies, but it is often present in the sodium channelopathies;
    - Severe cold sensitivity is a characteristic feature of PMC and some other sodium channelopathies, but it is less common in chloride channelopathies.
    - Obvious potassium sensitivity favors some of the sodium channelopathies over the chloride channelopathies.
    - Transient weakness of short duration (seconds to minutes) is common in Becker disease, but transient weakness of long duration (i.e., measured in hours) is typical of PC and HYPP.
    - Pain can be seen in both chloride and sodium channelopathies, but it is more common in the latter.
- If genetic testing for nondystrophic dystonia is negative, testing for DM 2 is recommended because they may atypically present in a similar fashion.

SUGGESTED READING

Heatwave, CR, Statland JM, Logigian EL. The diagnosis and treatment of myotonic disorders. *Muscl Nerve*. 2013 May;47(5):632–648.

CASE 21.13: STIFFNESS OF THE CHEWING MUSCLES

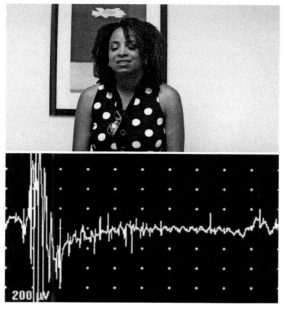

VIDEO 21.13

A 44-year-old woman presented with muscle stiffness as described in Video 21.13.1, which started 20 years earlier and gradually worsened with age. The CK level was 340 IU/L. Left biceps muscle biopsy was reportedly inconclusive. Examination is shown in the video. EMG of the Extensor digitorrum communis (EDC) is shown (Video 21.13.2). Muscle stiffness responded dramatically to mexiletine at 150 mg TID. *DMPK* gene testing revealed no CTG repeat expansion. Sequencing of the chloride and sodium channel genes revealed no significant mutations.

The most appropriate next testing is:

1. Genetic analysis of the *CNBP* gene to look for CCTG repeat expansion
2. Whole-exome sequencing
3. Long exercise test
4. Short exercise test
5. None of the above

DIAGNOSIS

The history and examination raised several important diagnostic points:

- The clinical examination revealed myotonia, which was confirmed by EMG, which showed waxing and waning 50-Hz spontaneous discharges in many muscles.
- Warming upis typical of myotonia, as opposed to paramyotonia (sodium channelopathy)
- The lack of temporal wasting, presence of calf hypertrophy, and family history suggested MC.
- A history of miscarriage is typical of DM 1 (congenital myotonic dystrophy) and is not a feature of DM2.
- The presence of a milder disease in the mother suggested anticipation, which is typical of both DM 1 and DM 2 but is not observed in sodium or chloride channelopathies.
- Response to mexiletine does not differentiate between different myotonia.
- Therefore, the chloride channels were genetically tested first to test for MC, and DM 1 was tested second; both tested negative.
  - Whole exome sequencing is not sensitive for triplet repeat expansion diseases.
  - Long- and short-exercise tests are not useful in myotonic dystrophy.
- Testing for DM 2 was positive for CCTG repeat expansion in the *CNBP* gene.
- This is an atypical case of DM 2 that mimicked MC. It is important to test for DM 2 in atypical myotonia.

SUGGESTED READING

Meola, G, Cardani R. Myotonic dystrophy type 2: an update on clinical aspects, genetic and pathomolecular mechanism. *J Neuromusc Dis*. 2015;2(s2):S59–S71.

PSEUDONEUROLOGIC SYNDROMES

This should go under the discussion above.

Shaibani A, Sabbagh MN. Pseudoneurologic syndromes: recognition and diagnosis. *Am Fam Phys.* 1998 May 15;57(10):2485–2494.

CASE 22.1: MUSCLE SPASMS AND FACIAL NUMBNESS

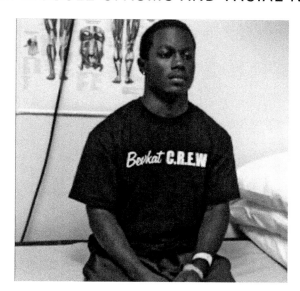

VIDEO 22.1

The patient is an 18-year-old man who is a student-athlete at the University of Missouri. His mother's car was hijacked while his mother was visiting him; accordingly, she decided to move him to Sam Houston University in Houston. Since then, he developed muscle spasms that occurred 20 times a day. He also had foot, hand, and facial numbness and poor balance with normal electromyography (EMG).

The demonstrated in the video signs suggest:

1. Polyminimyoclonus
2. Essential tremor (ET)
3. Ataxic neuropathy
4. Functional tremor (FT)
5. Stiff person syndrome (SPS)

DIAGNOSIS

The following factors suggest the diagnosis of FT:

- Acute onset
- Episodic nature
- Distractibility
- It is a mixture of resting, postural, and action tremor.
- It is irregular.
- The patient was not responsive during the shaking episode. He was coherent right afterward, though, with no postictal confusion to suggest seizure.
- The tremor resolved spontaneously after he settled into the new college.
  - Discussion of pseudoneurologic disorders (PNDs) is beyond the scope of this book. The most common PNDs in neuromuscular clinics are functional gait disorder (FGD) and tremor.
  - FGD may present with monoplegia, hemiplegia, or paraplegia.
  - Hysterical gait can be dramatic, with patients lurching wildly in all directions without falling. Examination of the sensory-motor system, cerebellar system, and extrapyramidal system fails to reveal an explanation.
  - Normal pressure hydrocephalus (NPH) may be misdiagnosed as FGD when dementia and urinary incontinence are not prominent. The presence of normal strength and sensory system enforces this notion.
    - Gait apraxia of NPH tends to be helped by providing cues such as a stick to step over.

CASE 22.2: SPASMS IN A CHRONIC INFLAMMATORY DEMYELINATING POLYNEUROPATHY (CIDP) PATIENT

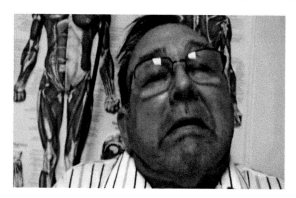

VIDEO 22.2

A 64-year-old man with chronic inflammatory demyelinating polyneuropathy (CIDP) responded to plasmapheresis and azathioprine. He presented with intermittent, painless, short-lived muscle spasms without alteration of consciousness. No triggers were identified. Brain magnetic resonance imaging (MRI) and electroencephalogram (EEG) were normal.

These episodes are:

1. Related to CIDP exacerbation
2. Seizures
3. SPS
4. Pseudoseizures
5. Neuromuscular

DIAGNOSIS

- Patients with legitimate neuromuscular disorders may develop functional symptoms thoroughly out the course of their disease. A neuromuscular specialist, therefore, may be asked to consult to see nonneuromuscular functional disorders in their patients. The first task is to look for any relationship between the new symptoms and their chronic neuromuscular disorder. The second task is to look for an organic explanation for the new symptoms. A good knowledge of psychogenic movement disorders is very helpful to neuromuscular specialists.
- Intermittent posturing and apparent alteration of mental status constitute a common functional disorder that is hard to differentiate from seizures. The preservation of orientation during these episodes is a strong indication that they are not epileptics. Simple partial seizures by definition are not associated with mental status change, but they are not generalized. Frontal lobe seizures may mimic pseudoseizures (pseudopseudoseizures), and only monitoring with depth electrodes can resolve this confusion. Other features that should suggest pseudoseizures are:
  - Tip tongue biting
  - Pelvic thrusting
  - No postictal confusion
  - Situational occurrence
  - Mental coherence during episode
  - Reactive pupils during episodes
  - Postictal whispering
  - Closed mouth during the tonic phase
  - Resisted lid opening
  - Convulsion lasting more than 2 minutes
- Self-injury and urinary incontinence, contrary to common belief, are not very helpful in differentiating seizures from pseudoseizures, as they occur in both.

CASE 22.3: TREMOR AFTER DIVORCE

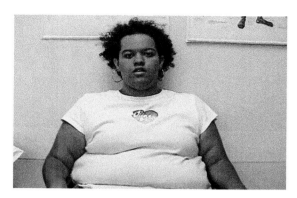

VIDEO 22.3

A 21-year-old woman who was recently divorced was referred for foot numbness, generalized weakness, and shaking. EMG was normal. She had "give way" weakness and hyperreflexia.

This is a case of:

1. ET
2. Parkinson disease (PD)
3. Neuropathy
4. Psychogenic tremor
5. Multiple sclerosis (MS)

DIAGNOSIS

- FT is a common pseudoneurological disorder.
- It usually occurs suddenly and reaches maximum disability quickly, unlike organic tremors (ET, Parkinson disease, cerebellar tremors).
- It ameliorates with distraction and worsens with stress.
- It is constant and not resting, action, or intentional.
- It may affect abdominal muscles.
- Most patients do not have evidence of conversion reaction, but depression seems to be the main associated psychopathology.
- Some patients display other functional symptoms, such as gait disorder.

CASE 22.4: QUADRIPLEGIA WITH NORMAL EMG

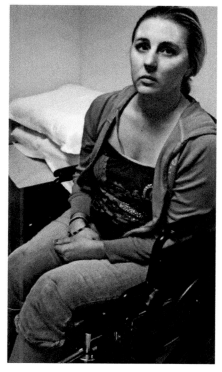

VIDEO 22.4

A 34-year-old woman presented with a 2-year history of subacute quadriplegia and generalized numbness with normal reflexes, creatine kinase (CK) level, cerebrospinal fluid (CSF) examination, brain and spinal cord MRIs, and EMG. Her symptoms were fluctuating and started after she became divorced.

This is a case of:

1. CIDP
2. Myopathy
3. MS
4. Hysterical conversion
5. Myasthenia gravis (MG)

DIAGNOSIS

- According to classical Freudian theory, psychological stress may be converted to physical symptoms such as paralysis, blindness, and deafness, or it may dissociate to cognitive symptoms such as mutism and fugue.
- According to the behaviorist Ivan Pavlov, severe excitation in the frontal region due to stress leads to reciprocal inhibition of other cortical areas, leading to lack of function.
- The term *hysteria* is derived from the Greek word *hystera* (uterus), as the Greeks thought that the uterus wanders in the body and produces symptoms wherever it settles.
- Jean-Martin Charcot rejected this theory; instead, he noted ovarian congestion and tenderness in the victims of so-called hysteria, and accordingly speculated that the ovaries were the source.
- It is not clear how stress is converted to specific physical symptoms in different people, but it is widely thought that by doing so, it provides a defensive mechanism.
- Clinically, pseudoweakness can be challenging, and it may take the form of monoplegia, hemiplegia, paraplegia, or quadriplegia.
- Normal reflexes and sensation and the lack of physiological pattern are clues to the nonorganic nature of the deficit, and a normal EMG of weak muscles indicates that the lesion is central (organic or functional).
- "Give way" weakness is highly suggestive of a functional etiology. It is a stepwise loss of resistance of the weak muscles, unlike the smooth loss of resistance in real weakness.
- Both agonist and antagonist muscles are affected equally, unlike organic weakness.
- Unexpected painful stimulation of the affected extremity may lead to purposeful withdrawal.
- Dropping the paralyzed arm on the face leads to "near miss" slapping of the face.
- Hoover test: the examiner puts his hand under the heel of the weak side and the other arm on the top of the other leg. Pushing the normal leg against resistance leads to pressure felt by the hand under the heel of the weak leg in cases of pseudoweakness. The examiner then switches hands to confirm.
- Adductor sign: Normally, ipsilateral thigh adduction leads to contralateral thigh adduction. The examiner palpates both thigh adductors and asks the patient to adduct the normal side. Contraction of the contralateral (weak) thigh adductors would suggest a functional weakness.
- Some cases of conversion paralysis are chronic, and the benefit of paralysis to draw attention and care unconsciously perpetuates the paralysis.

SUGGESTED READING

Shaibani A, Sabbagh MN. Pseudoneurologic syndromes: recognition and diagnosis. *Am Fam Phys*. 1998 May 15;57(10):2485–2494.

CASE 22.5: "GIVE WAY" WEAKNESS AND LOSS OF BALANCE

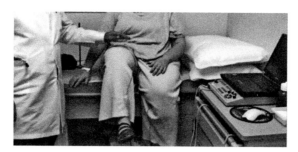

VIDEO 22.5

A 34-year-old woman presented with a 1-month history of tremor, insomnia, generalized fatigue, numbness, and myalgia. She was referred for neuromuscular evaluation of leg weakness. Examination is shown in the video.

The demonstrated proximal weakness is likely due to:

1. Myopathy
2. CIDP
3. Myalgia
4. Psychogenic cause
5. Hip arthritis

DIAGNOSIS

- The term *give way weakness* is used to describe weakness that does not follow a normal smooth yield to resistance; it is mostly functional.
- It can be stepwise, clasp knife, or collapsing weakness (sudden loss of resistance by even touching the weak extremity).
- It takes experience to be able to detect this kind of weakness from the first examination attempt.
- Fortunately, as in this case, there are many clues to the pseudonature of the weakness, including:
  - Multiple other symptoms that do not make sense neurologically, like the inability to open the mouth and the pseudo–right facial weakness.
  - History of depression or current stress.
  - *La belle indifference:* The patient is not much concerned about the symptoms.
- Hyperreflexia is common in this group of patients due to anxiety, and it should not argue against the functional nature of the deficit. Unless it is associated with more objective upper motor neuron (UMN) signs like Babinski sign and spasticity.

CASE 22.6: DYSARTHRIA AFTER A CAR ACCIDENT

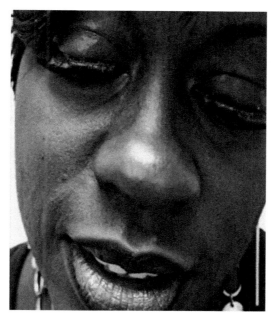

VIDEO 22.6

A 27-year-old woman was referred for neuromuscular evaluation for dysarthria that started 6 weeks earlier, after a car accident. There was no dysphagia, but she had foot numbness, blurred vision, and generalized weakness. She improved minutes after intramuscular injection of normal saline.

This dysarthria is due to:

1. Amyotrophic lateral sclerosis (ALS)
2. Head injury
3. Psychogenic etiology
4. Cerebellar stroke
5. MG

DIAGNOSIS

- Functional speech disorders are common, and some patients are referred to neuromuscular clinics because of suspicion of neuromuscular disorders such as ALS and MG. They include functional mutism, dysphona, and dysarthria.
  - Mutism literally means the inability to speak. Discussing infantile mutism and selective mutism are beyond the scope of this book. In adults, mutism is usually a dissociation hysterical reaction.
  - Dysphonia is a disturbance of phonation and may lead to a whispery voice. Spasmodic dysphonia should not be confused with functional dysphonia. Patients with functional dysphonia may be diagnosed with laryngitis first.
  - Dysarthria also may be psychogenic.
    - The most important features of functional dysarthria are hesitation of pronunciation, especially of sounds in the middle of the words, and being diffuse and involving a combination of lingual, labial, palatal, and laryngeal components.
- Reversal with placebo is typically seen in functional disorders as seen in this case, which responded to normal saline injection. However, the legal and ethical implications of the administration of placebos remain to be worked out.

CASE 22.7: WEAKNESS AFTER FLU SHOT

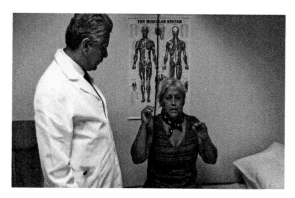

VIDEO 22.7

A 52-year-old woman referred to our neuromuscular clinic due to inability to lift her arms for a year. This started after an inoculation that she believed was a swine flu shot. Deltoid strength was difficult to evaluate due to severe shoulder pain. Her biceps and hip flexors were 5/5, and reflexes were normal. The CK level and EMG of the proximal muscles were normal. MRI of the shoulders showed high-grade tear of supraspinatus tendons bilaterally and severe supraspinatus tendinopathy.

The proximal weakness that occurred after the flu shot was due to:

1. Myopathy
2. Psychogenic etiology
3. Shoulder arthritis
4. Fibromyalgia
5. Antigen in the vaccination

DIAGNOSIS

- Clinical manifestations of organic diseases are often complicated by sickness behavior, which occurs as an unconscious psychological reaction to illness. The patient probably had mild arthritis of the shoulders for a while. The pain of the flu shot may have made shoulder abduction painful for a couple of days, which has augmented the effect of arthritis. Sickness behavior is responsible for the rest.
- Very often, sickness behavior is punctuated by a patient's understanding of his or her condition. A patient with right-hand numbness due to carpal tunnel syndrome (CTS) may develop numbness on the entire right side because of the connection that the patient makes between hand numbness and stroke.
- This patient improved after physical therapy, nonsteroidal anti-inflammatory drugs (NSAIDs), and reassurance. She admitted that she had read a lot of information about the flu shots and their side effects.

CASE 22.8: FACIAL WEAKNESS

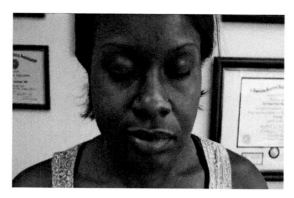

VIDEO 22.8

A 39-year-old woman presented with involuntary movement of the left shoulder and right face, starting after she was fired from work a few weeks earlier. She had facial numbness and pressure like frontal headache. Brain MRI was normal.

The following features suggest psychogenic etiology for facial spasms, as opposed to hemifacial spasms (HFSs):

1. Resolution by distraction
2. Frontal headache and facial numbness
3. Worsened by stress
4. Lack of facial weakness
5. Improvement with botulinum toxin (BT) injection

DIAGNOSIS

- Patients with HFS are referred to neuromuscular clinics due to a suspicion of facial nerve pathology.
- 4% of cases of HFS seen in movement disorders clinics have functional HFS.
- The spasms usually starts in the eyelids and are associated with the tremor of one or more extremities and with psychological disturbances such as anxiety and depression and other symptoms, such as headaches and sensory disturbances.
- Functional HFS usually affects females in their 20s and 30s, while organic HFS affects females in their 40s and 50s.
- The use of MRI and magnetic resonance angiography (MRA) to differentiate these two conditions is not helpful because one-third to one-half of organic HFS cases have normal brain MRIs and 15% of the brain MRA control group shows ectasia of the vertebrobasilar system.
- Depression of the ipsilateral eyebrow, elevation of the contralateral eyebrow, and narrowing of the palpebral fissure due to contraction of the upper and lower eyelids are typically seen in functional HFS.
- Most cases resolve within 2 years of diagnosis.
- Resolution of the spasms by distraction is more typical of functional HFS.
- Both get worse with stress and may get better with BT injections and may not be associated with facial weakness.
- Facial numbness and headache suggest an intracranial pathology.

SUGGESTED READING

Tan EK, Jankovic J. Psychogenic hemifacial spasm. *J Neuropsych Clin Neurosci*. 2001;13:380–384.

NUMBNESS

CASE 23.1: INTERCOSTAL BURNING PAIN

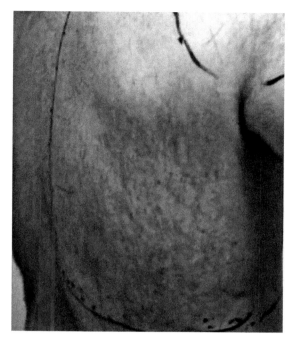

VIDEO 23.1

A 70-year-old man with well-controlled diabetes mellitus (DM) had developed a severe burning sensation and tingling (mostly at rest) along the shown in the video distribution 3 months earlier, which peaked at 5 weeks and plateaued afterward. There was no skin rash, and cervical and thoracic magnetic resonance imaging (MRI) was normal.

These features suggest:

1. Zoster radiculitis
2. Diabetic thoracoabdominal radiculopathy (DTAR)
3. Myelitis
4. Intercostal neuropathy
5. Nonneuropathic pain

DIAGNOSIS

- This syndrome usually occurs in the context of diabetic lumbosacral radiculoplexus neuropathy (DLSRPN), but it may happen in isolation.
- The pathology is similar to that of DLSRPN and involves microvasculitis rather than metabolic etiology. The disorder occurs in patients with well-controlled DM and no significant end organ damage (retinopathy, nephropathy).
- The pain is neuropathic (burning, occurring mostly at rest) and severe.
- Very often, the diagnosis is not made early, and the condition is misdiagnosed as:
  - Zoster radiculitis:
    - Lack of rash 5 days or more after the onset of pain occurs only in rare cases of the zoster.
    - DTAR is bilateral in about 30% of cases, which is vanishingly rare in zoster radiculitis.
  - Acute abdomen: Appendicitis, cholecystitis, diverticulitis, etc. Many patients undergo appendectomy or cholecystectomy before they are diagnosed with DTAR.
  - Coronary heart disease: Cardiac evaluation is usually done before these patients are referred to a neurologist.
- A key diagnostic feature is skin sensitivity to touch, which is not a feature of acute abdomen or coronary artery disease.
- It is important to rule out compressive and intramedullary lesions by appropriate imaging.
- The condition is self-limiting, but it may take 2 years for full recovery.
- Pain management and reassurance are the mainstays of treatment.

CASE 23.2: BURNING PAIN IN A DIABETIC

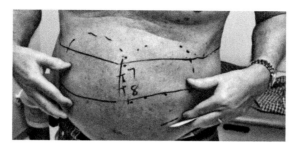

VIDEO 23.2

A 56-year-old man with controlled DM presented with a 6-month history of severe, burning pain that progressively spread in the shown in the video distribution. He used a special elastic T-shirt and bathed with warm water several times a night to reduce pain. His ankle reflexes and foot sensation were normal, and the entire spinal cord MRI was normal.

The pathology of this syndrome is likely due to:

1. Metabolic axonal injury
2. Microvasculitis
3. Compressive neuropathy
4. Drug-induced, intercostal neuropathy
5. Secondary viral infection

DIAGNOSIS

- Pathologically, diabetic neuropathies are classified into those that are caused by:
  - Metabolic and chronic ischemic changes, such as diabetic polyneuropathy.
  - Acute or subacute microvasculitis. This category is characterized by acute or subacute pain and focal or multifocal involvement. The following discussion is about the second category.
- The pain is severe but self-limiting. Electromyography (EMG) usually shows evidence of multifocal axonal neuropathy.
- These patients usually have good diabetes control and no evidence of end organ damage.
- Recovery process may take months to years.
- Examples of this group of diabetic neuropathies include:
  - Diabetic third cranial nerve palsy
  - DTAR
  - DLSRPN
- Detailed pathological studies demonstrated multifocal fiber loss, perineurial thickening, neovascularization, perivascular inflammation, and invasion of small blood vessel walls with mononuclear inflammatory cells, consistent with microvasculitis. The cause of this inflammatory pathology is not clear.

SUGGESTED READING

Dyck PJ, Norell JE, Dyck PJ. Microvasculitis and ischemia in diabetic lumbosacral radiculoplexus neuropathy. *Neurol.* 1999;53:2113–2121.

CASE 23.3: PATCHY SENSORY LOSS

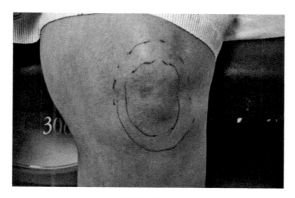

VIDEO 23.3

A 51-year-old woman presented with sequential patchy sensory loss and no evidence of polyneuropathy.

These symptoms are typical of:

1. Psychogenic etiology
2. Diabetic radiculopathy
3. Zoster radiculitis
4. Migrant sensory neuritis of Wartenberg
5. None of the above

DIAGNOSIS

Migrant sensory neuritis of Wartenberg:

- This syndrome is characterized by recurrent episodes of burning pain and subsequent patchy loss of sensation in the distribution of one cutaneous nerve at a time.
- It mostly affects the skin of the extremities, chest, and face.
- These sensory changes are usually induced by movement of a limb or pressure on the skin (e.g., by kneeling), leading to the stretching of a cutaneous nerve.
- It usually affects people in their fourth or fifth decade.
- It is described as a pure sensory mononeuritis multiplex.
- Electrodiagnostic features are that of multifocal axonal sensory loss.
- Biopsy of affected nerves show findings suggestive of an autoimmune vascular process, including:
  - Perineurial scarring
  - Chronic inflammation
  - Axonal loss and regeneration
  - Differential fascicular involvement
  - Endoneurial edema
  - Immunoglobulin deposition
- The effect of immunomodulation on the course of the disease is ill defined, especially as the disorder is purely sensory and does not cause functional impairment other than pain.
- No association is reported between this condition and DM or autoimmune disorders.

CASE 23.4: FOOT NUMBNESS AND NORMAL ANKLE REFLEXES

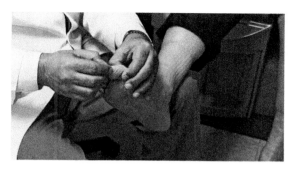

VIDEO 23.4

A 74-year-old healthy man presented with poor balance since age 40 years. Examination is shown in the video. Brain and cervical MRIs are noncontributory.

The most appropriate next diagnostic step is:

1. Thoracic MRI
2. Nerve conduction study/EMG
3. Cerebrospinal fluid (CSF) examination
4. Skin biopsy
5. Nerve biopsy

DIAGNOSIS

Foot numbness and normal ankle reflexes:

- An important clinical scenario commonly seen in neuromuscular clinics is a patient with chronic progressive sensory ataxia with preserved or brisk ankle reflexes.
- Sensory symptoms in the feet are suspected of being neuropathic when ankle reflexes are decreased or absent. In that case, an NCS would be indicated to determine the type and severity of neuropathy.
- However, if the ankle reflexes are brisk or even normal, the following possibilities are to be considered:
  - If foot pain and skin sensitivity to touch are the main features, small fiber neuropathy is an important consideration, and a skin biopsy is indicated.
  - If vibratory and proprioceptive deficits are the main findings, a central lesion is suspected. Cervical myelopathy, whether compressive or not, is the most common cause, but thoracic myelopathy and intracranial lesions are to be considered if cervical MRI is negative.
    - Myeloneuropathy is also possible; therefore, the presence of neuropathy, even if confirmed by NCS, should not preclude investigating the spinal cord in cases where ankle reflexes are brisk or normal in the face of severe foot numbness.
    - Cervical spondylotic myelopathy with diabetic or nondiabetic neuropathy is a common scenario where foot numbness is associated with brisk ankle jerks.
  - Foot numbness with persevered ankle reflexes should always trigger the need to test for Babinski sign, which if positive would support the presence of a central component.
- This patient was found to have moderate cord compression due to a large arachnoid cyst extending from T3 to T6.

CASE 23.5: FOOT PAIN AND ORTHOSTASIS

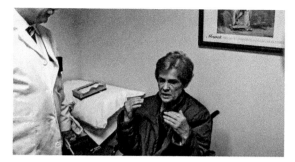

VIDEO 23.5

A 60-year-old woman with no significant past medical history had developed asymmetric progressive pain and numbness of the feet. A month later, she had similar symptoms in the arms and postural hypotension. EMG revealed axonal sensorimotor neuropathy. Autonomic reflex testing revealed moderate dysautonomia. CSF protein was normal. Sed rate was 43 mm/hour. Serum creatinine was 2.3 mg/dl. Immunofixation protein electrophoresis (IFPE) revealed an immunoglobin M (IgM) kappa spike. Left sural nerve biopsy is shown in Figures 23.5.1 and 23.5.2. Family history is remarkable for neuropathy and DM affecting her father.

The likely diagnosis is:

1. Familial amyloidosis
2. Vasculitis
3. Amyloid light-chain (AL) amyloidosis
4. Toxic neuropathy
5. Familial autonomic and sensory neuropathy

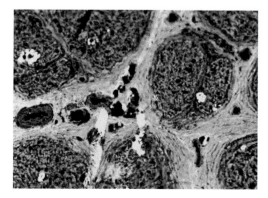

FIGURE 23.5.1 Congo red stain of left sural nerve biopsy viewed under fluorescent light.

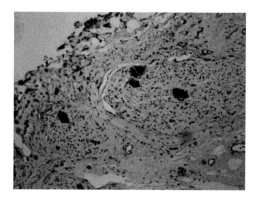

FIGURE 23.5.2 Positive reaction to Kappa chain antibodies.

DIAGNOSIS

- Progressive painful asymmetric or multifocal neuropathy suggests vasculitis or amyloidosis. Dysautonomia is more typical for the latter. Renal impairment is common in both conditions.
- Family history suggests familial amyloid neuropathy (FAP), but monoclonal gammopathy is favorable of AL amyloidosis. Sural nerve biopsy confirmed amyloidosis. The tissue was reacted for different paraproteins, and the reaction was positive for IgM kappa short chain, the same protein found in the serum. Transthyretin (TTR) mutations were negative.
- AL amyloidosis:
  - Amyloid is a misfolded protein in a beta-pleated sheet configuration. It is insoluble and deposited in the extracellular tissue, mostly the nerves (axonal neuropathy), kidneys, heart, tongue, carpal tunnel, and small fiber and autonomic fibers.
- A clinical triad of progressive painful neuropathy, bilateral carpal tunnel syndrome (CTS), and dysautonomia is typical for amyloidosis.
- Monoclonal proteins are precursors of amyloid; therefore, their presence, along with progressive painful neuropathy or dysautonomic symptoms, should raise the possibility of AL amyloidosis, especially if there is renal or cardiac involvement.
- AL amyloidosis consists of kappa or lambda misfolded protein.
- Multiple myeloma may present 1–7 years after diagnosis of AL amyloidosis.
- Clinical syndrome of AL amyloidosis:
  - Painful, distal, symmetric sensory neuropathy.
  - CTS.
  - Dysautonomia: orthostatic hypotension, hyporeactive pupils, anhidrosis, urinary incontinence, and impotence.
  - Myopathy.
  - Cardiac and renal impairment.
  - It may present as mononeuritis multiplex (usually associated with lymphoma); look for lymphadenopathy.
  - It is a progressive disease; survival is 1–10 years.
  - Renal and cardiac involvement is a bad sign.
  - Chemotherapy and peripheral blood stem cell transplantation are the mainstays of therapy.

CASE 23.6: INHALATION FOR FUN

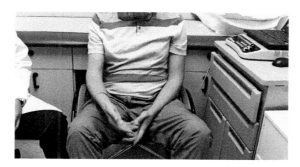

VIDEO 23.6

NCS revealed severe axonal sensorimotor neuropathy. CSF examination was normal. The B_{12} level, copper level, heavy metal screening, IFPE, SR, HbA1c, and antinuclear antibody (ANA) were all negative. The patient was depressed due to the death of his brother. He inhaled the contents of whipped cream chargers (used in cream dispensers) to fight anxiety. He used as many as 100 chargers a day for 2 months. Symptoms started a few weeks later and continued to worsen even though he quit the inhalation 2 weeks earlier.

This progressive neuropathy likely represents:

1. Guillain-Barré syndrome (GBS)
2. Chronic inflammatory demyelinating polyneuropathy (CIDP)
3. Functional B_{12} deficiency
4. Copper deficiency
5. Vasculitic neuropathy

DIAGNOSIS

A 40-year-old man presented with progressive weakness in the arms and legs proceded by severe distal sensory symptoms and ataxia with no pain. Examination revealed severe proximal and distal weakness in the arms and legs, with areflexia and severe sensory impairment to proprioception and vibration in the lower extremities up to the knees. The following are true regarding this case except:

- Most likely, the patient had nitrous oxide toxicity.
- Nitrous oxide inactivates vitamin B_{12} by irreversible oxidation of its cobalt moiety.
- The typical picture of nitrous oxide toxicity is that of subacute combined degeneration of the cord and demyelinating neuropathy.
- It is possible that axonal neuropathy in this case was the end result of severe demyelinating neuropathy.
- This picture is typical for Copper deficiency.

Nitrous oxide toxicity:

- Nitrous oxide is used as an anesthetic (for dentistry, ambulances, childbirth) and appreciated for its antianxiety effect. It is also used to fill whipped cream chargers, which are used as a whipping agent in a dispenser. The gas is usually discharged from a charger into a balloon, from which it is inhaled.
- Recreational use of nitrous oxide is rapidly increasing, especially in the dance and festival scene.
- It is a legal drug that is widely available and cheap.
- Following one inhalation, a euphoric, pleasant, joyful effect is rapidly induced (within 10 seconds) and disappears within minutes.
- Side effects of nitrous oxide include transient dizziness, dissociation, disorientation, loss of balance, impaired memory and cognition, and weakness in the legs.
- Heavy or sustained use of nitrous oxide inactivates vitamin B_{12}, resulting in a functional vitamin B_{12} deficiency and initially causing numbness in the fingers, which may progress further to peripheral neuropathy and megaloblastic anemia. Without the history of inhalation, all the mentioned possibilities should be pursued.
- Nitrous oxide use does not seem to result in dependence.
- Recovery typically occurs after quitting the offensive agent, but it may take months to years depending on the severity and duration of abuse and the resulting neuropathy.

SUGGESTED READING

Van Amsterdam J, Nabben T, van den Brink W. Recreational nitrous oxide use: prevalence and risks. *Regul Toxicol Pharmacol*. 2015 Dec;73(3):790–796. Epub 2015 Oct 22.

CASE 23.7: SEVERE PROPRIOCEPTIVE LOSS

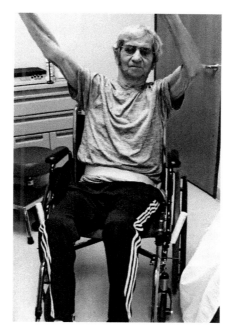

VIDEO 23.7

An 80-year-old man presented with a 6-month history of facial numbness that spread to the left arm and leg a month later, and then the right arm and leg another month later. He lost 30 pounds and became wheelchair bound because of loss of balance. He had no deep tendon reflexes (DTRs), and his strength was normal. CSF protein was 120 mg/dl and IgG synthesis rate was significantly elevated. NCS/EMG revealed sensory polyneuropathy. Examination is shown in the video.

The level of pathology is likely at which of the following?

1. Spinal cord
2. Dorsal root ganglia
3. Peripheral nerves
4. Muscles
5. Nerve roots

DIAGNOSIS

- Video 23.7 showed severe proprioceptive deficit and pseudoathetosis. When his eyes were closed, he could not recognize the position of his face in the space, so he hit his face. He had to open his eyes to direct his finger to his nose.
- Alternating hand movement is disturbed for the same reason. This is different from cerebellar dysfunction, which causes loss of check and intention tremor. He was wheelchair bound due to sensory ataxia.
- Along with asymmetry, areflexia and normal strength suggested dorsal root ganglia (DRG) localization.
- Weight loss and increased CSF protein suggested malignancy. Sjogren syndrome was also an important cause of sensory ganglionopathy, but the age and sex were atypical.
- Anti-Hu antibody titer was significantly elevated.
- Paraneoplastic sensory neuronopathy:
  - Asymmetrical sensory symptoms and loss of proprioception, usually associated with pain.
  - Mostly affects the elderly with a history of smoking and is related to small cell lung cancer (SCLC).
  - Mean survival is 28 months.
  - In 30% of cases, cancer is detected months after the diagnosis of neuronopathy, so periodic surveillance for cancer is important.
  - Chest computed tomography (CT) scan in this case was negative.
  - Other culprit cancers in males may be related to the testicles, esophagus, skin, thymus, and lymph nodes (Hodgkin disease).

SUGGESTED READING

Dropcho, E. Paraneoplastic sensory neuronopathy. *Medlink Neurol*. May 11, 2016.

CHAPTER 24

DEFORMITIES

CASE 24.1: MYALGIA, WEAKNESS, AND HARD BREASTS

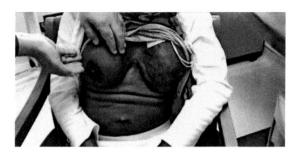

VIDEO 24.1

A 55 year-old woman presented with uremia treated with hemodialysis. She had received a gadolinium-enhanced brain magnetic resonance imaging (MRI) for neurological symptoms and developed a progressive, painful inability to raise her legs and arms, which was confirmed in the examination. She also had severe hardening of the breasts and thigh tissue. The creatine kinase (CK) level and electromyography (EMG) were normal, and nongadolinium MRI of the thighs revealed sclerosis of the subcutaneous tissue with sparing of the muscles.

Which of the following facts are accurate about nephrogenic systemic sclerosis (NSS)?

1. It occurs only in uremic patients who receive gadolinium.
2. It occurs only in dialysis patients.
3. It responds well to cyclophosphamide.
4. It causes fibrosis of the internal organs.
5. It does not cause contractures.

DIAGNOSIS

- NSS is a rare condition characterized by fibrosis of the skin, joints, and internal organs.
- It is associated with exposure to gadolinium, which is used as a paramagnetic contrast in MRIs.
- Different brands of gadolinium may have varying potentials in producing this disorder.
- NSS is more common in patients with renal failure who are on hemodialysis or peritoneal dialysis.
- Gadolinium is contraindicated when the glomerular filtration rate (GFR) is less than 50 ml/min due to the progressively increased risk of NSS.
- No other risk factors are identified, and genetic predisposition is suggested.
- Patients present with severe contractures and joint pain.
- Fibrosis may extend to the liver, lungs, and heart.
- Pathologically, the fibrotic areas show thickened collagen and proliferation of fibroblasts.
- Skin thickening may resemble scleroderma and systemic sclerosis.
- Neuromuscular involvement is difficult to evaluate due to severe joint and skin fibrosis, but fibrosis of the underlying muscles and myopathic changes are demonstrated by EMG and muscle biopsy in a few patients.
- These patients are referred to neuromuscular clinics due to proximal weakness and suspicion of myopathy.
- No treatment is found to be effective in ameliorating the disease.

CASE 24.2: CERVICAL DEFORMITY

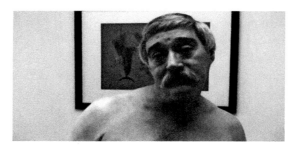

VIDEO 24.2

A 55-year-old man presented with cervical dystonia since childhood, resulting in mechanical cervical deformity confirmed by cervical spine MRI. The patient was referred to the neuromuscular clinic for numbness and spasticity of the legs, which turned out to be due to myelopathy caused by the abovementioned deformity.

Cervical spine mechanical restriction can result from:

1. Long-standing cervical dystonia
2. Periodic familial paralysis
3. Congenital torticollis
4. Head tremor
5. Polymyalgia rheumatica

DIAGNOSIS

- Musculoskeletal deformities (MSDs):
  - Are important markers for hereditary and congenital neuromuscular diseases
  - Can also result from dystonia, contractures, and chronic immobility
  - Can cause neurological dysfunction themselves, regardless of their origin; the patient in this case developed myelopathy due to dystonia-induced cervical spine deformity.
- The most relevant MSDs in neuromuscular disorders are kyphosis, pes cavus, hammertoes, and a high-arched palate.
- Pes cavus is characterized by high foot arches that do not flatten with weight bearing, contrary to the acquired high foot arches that flatten upon weight bearing.
  - A total of 10% of the general population has pes cavus.
  - Pes cavus may represent the earliest manifestations of neuromuscular disorders.
  - Common neuromuscular disorders associated with pes cavus are hereditary motor and sensory neuropathy (HSMN), spinocerebellar ataxia (SCA), hereditary neuropathy with liability to pressure palsy (HNPP), and congenital myopathies.
  - Pes cavus occurs due to imbalance between weak intrinsic foot muscles (lumbricals and interossi) and overactive peroneus and tibialis posterior.
  - Family history of Pes cavus is important to explore because it could be a marker for a hereditary neuromuscular disorder.
- A neuromuscular specialist should make a point to look for MSDs, especially pes cavus, and to ask about family history of these deformities, especially in patients with chronic, idiopathic neuropathies and myopathies.
- Periodic paralysis and tremor are not static disorders and do not cause spinal deformity.
- Polymyalgia rheumatica is a treatable inflammatory disorder characterized by muscle and joint stiffness that usually respond to treatment and does not cause spinal deformity.
- Congenital torticollis is a fixed deformity of the neck position caused by fibrosis of the sternocleidomastoid (SCM), which gradually leads to deformity of the cervical spines.
- Cervical dystonia is a chronic condition that causes positional deformity of the neck, and eventually cervical spines.

CASE 24.3: MULTIPLE MASSES AND PROXIMAL WEAKNESS

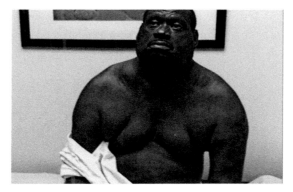

VIDEO 24.3

A 65-year-old man presented with several years' history of chronic progressive proximal weakness, loss of balance, foot numbness, and myalgia. Two benign masses were removed from his upper back a few years earlier. The CK level was 356 U/L, and EMG showed evidence of myopathy and axonal neuropathy. A muscle biopsy and pedigree are shown in Figures 24.3.1 and 24.3.2.

The most likely unifying diagnosis is:

1. Lymphoma
2. Neurofibromatosis
3. Mitochondrial disease
4. Metastatic cancer
5. None of the above

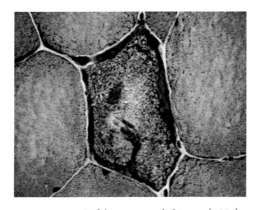

FIGURE 24.3.1 Left biceps muscle biopsy (400x).

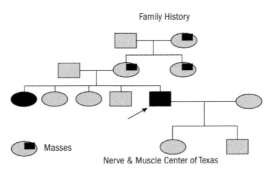

FIGURE 24.3.2 Pedigree of the patient.

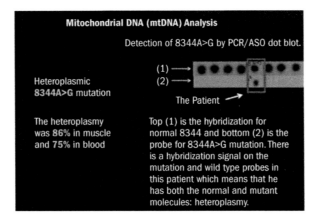

FIGURE 24.3.3 DNA analysis of the patient.

DIAGNOSIS

- These patients are referred to neuromuscular clinics due to proximal weakness and foot numbness.
- Video 24.3 shows several masses in the clavicular area and chest wall.
- Muscle biopsy showed ragged red fibers, suggestive of mitochondrial dysfunction.
- Myopathy, neuropathy, multiple soft masses, and ragged red fibers suggest Madelung disease.
- Genetics is complicated. Most cases are due to mitochondrial mutations, but some are autosomal dominant (AD), while others are sporadic.
- Middle-aged men with a history of alcoholism are typically affected.
- Multiple fatty swelling in the proximal arms and legs, the back of the neck, the side of the neck, around the shoulders, and supraclavicular areas is usually noted.
- Distal symmetric axonal sensorimotor neuropathy is common.
- EMG usually shows nonirritative proximal myopathy and distal axonal neuropathy.
- Autonomic reflexes are abnormal, with evidence of dysautonomia.
- Mild CK elevation is usually seen, and muscle biopsy shows ragged red fibers.
- Surgical removal of lipomas to relieve compression or for cosmetic reasons can be attempted, but recurrence is common.
- The mitochondrial variant is associated with *A8344G* mutation in mitochondrial tRNA^{Lys} (Figure 24.3.3).
- Some families also have myoclonic epilepsy and ragged red fibers (MERRF) syndrome.

SUGGESTED READING

Brunetti-Pierri N, Shaibani A, Zhang S, Wong LJ, Shinawi M. Progressive myopathy with multiple symmetric lipomatosis. *Arch Neurol.* 2009 Dec;66(12):1576–1577.

CASE 24.4: MULTIPLE FAMILIAL MASSES AND FOOT NUMBNESS

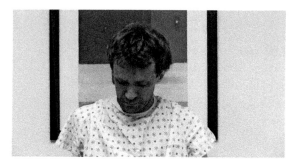

VIDEO 24.4

The patient presented with asymmetric numbness of the feet and a ring enhancing left cerebellar mass, and a brother with similar skin masses.

This clinical picture is typical of:

1. Neurofibromatosis-1 (NF-1)
2. Neurofibromatosis-2 (NF-2)
3. Tuberose sclerosis
4. Schwannoma
5. Hypertrophic neuropathy

The incidence of the following tumors is increased in NF-1 except:

1. Pilocytic astrocytoma
2. Optic glioma
3. Bilateral acoustic neuroma
4. Brainstem glioma
5. Astrocytoma

DIAGNOSIS

NF-1:

- AD disease.
- Prevalence is 1:3,000. New mutations occur in 50% of people.
- Penetrance is complete, with variable manifestations.
- Life expectancy is reduced by 15 years.
- Café-au-lait spots are present in 99% of cases. A careful search may be needed.
- List nodules are present in 50% by age 29 years.
- Scoliosis is common.
- The incidence of the mentioned tumors is increased except for bilateral acoustic neuroma, which is characteristic of NF-2. Astrocytoma is the most common brain tumor in NF-1, which typically causes a ring-enhancing lesion.

SUGGESTED READING

Korf, BR. Malignancy in neurofibromatosis type 1. *The Oncol.* Dec.2000;5(6):477–485.

CASE 24.5: MULTIPLE RUPTURED TENDONS

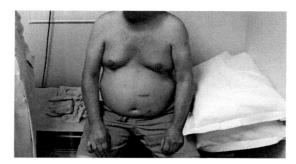

VIDEO 24.5

The following are risk factors for spontaneous multiple tendon ruptures except:

- Chronic medical conditions: chronic renal failure (CRF), diabetes mellitus (DM), hyperparathyroidism
- Systemic steroids
- Neuropathy
- Fluoroquinolones
- Aromatase inhibitors such as anastrazole (estrogen-positive breast cancer).

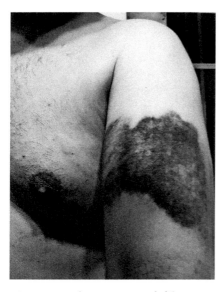

FIGURE 24.5.1 hematoma over left biceps

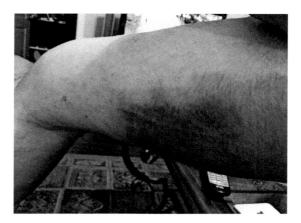

FIGURE 24.5.2 hematoma over the left hamstrings

DIAGNOSIS

- A 50-year-old hairstylist presented who developed sequential, severe pain and hematoma in the shoulders and hips bilaterally over the last several weeks triggered by minimal movement (Figures 24.5.1 and 24.5.2).
- MRI of the biceps muscles showed a complete rupture of the proximal tendon of both biceps and severe attenuation of the supraspinatus and infraspinatus tendons.
- He had no proximal weakness, sensory abnormalities, or reflex asymmetry.
- He had a history of spondylosing arthritis and chronic steroid therapy for Addison disease for 8 years.
- He used several courses of ciprofloxacin over the preceding months for urinary tract infection (UTI).
- This is a rare condition that is predisposed to by:
  - Repeated trauma
  - Chronic medical conditions: CRF, DM, hyperparathyroidism
  - Inflammatory and degenerative arthritides
  - Systemic steroids
  - Fluoroquinolones
  - Aromatase inhibitors: anastrazole (estrogen-positive breast cancer).
  - Genetic factors and collagen disorders, including collagen 6 deficiency and Ehlers-Danlos syndrome (EDS), are associated with ruptured tendons. These rare neuromuscular causes are associated with myopathy, hyperextensible skin and joints, and sometimes cardiomyopathy.

SUGGESTED READING

Seewoodhar J. Multiple, spontaneous tendon ruptures with associated spondylolisthesis and osteoarthritis: A case series. *W Lond Med J*. 2010;2(2):10041–10045.

CASE 24.6: TENDER MASSES

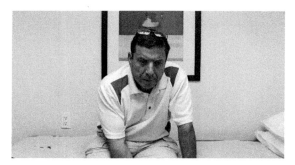

VIDEO 24.6

A 53-year-old pilot presented who had developed acute, severe focal right triceps pain 6 weeks earlier. The pain was constant and spread to his arms and legs in multiple areas of focal pain and tenderness. There was no fever, arthralgia, dysphagia, dyspnea, sensory symptoms, or weakness in the arms or legs. Tramadol did not help, and neither did prednisone at 20 mg/day for 2 weeks. Skin rash was reported 2 weeks before the focal tenderness. Examination revealed exquisite focal tenderness and induration of the right triceps and calves. The CPK level, SR, and eosinophil count were normal. C-reactive protein was 7.8 (upper limit of normal was 4.9), and MRI of the left calf muscles showed enhancing focal lesions (Figs. 24.6.1 and 24.6.2). EMG of the focally tender muscles revealed positive, sharp waves and fibrillation. There were no myopathic units. Needle EMG of other muscles in the legs was normal. Biopsy of the tender nodule in the left gastrocnemius is shown in Figures 24.6.3 and 24.6.4.

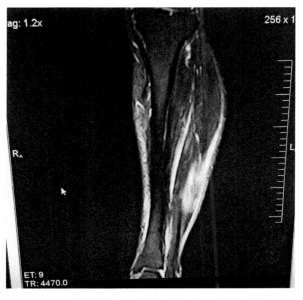

FIGURE 24.6.1 MRI of the right foreleg: longitudinal view.

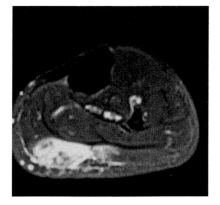

FIGURE 24.6.2 MRI of the right foreleg: coronal view

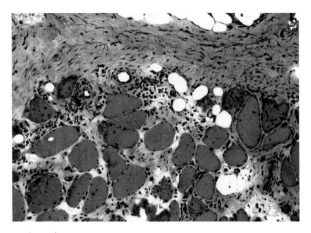

FIGURE 24.6.3 H&E stain (100x).

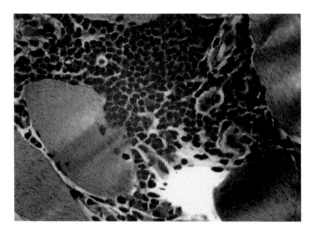

FIGURE 24.6.4 H&E stain (400x)

The most likely diagnosis is:

1. Muscle cysticercosis
2. Nodular myositis
3. Focal myositis
4. Muscle tumor
5. Focal bacterial infection

DIAGNOSIS

Focal myositis:

- Muscle biopsy showed endomysial mononuclear cell infiltration (large clusters of nesting muscle fibers surrounded by thick perimysial fibrosis)

- A rare self-limiting condition usually triggered by a viral infection, as suggested by the abovementioned skin rash in this case.
- Mostly affects females at age 30–50 years.
- Presents with focal enlargement and tenderness of multiple muscles.
- The quads and gastrocnemius are commonly affected.
- Does not evolve into polymyositis.
- CPK is normal or slightly high. EMG of the affected areas shows irritative myopathy.
- MRI shows multiple enlargements and fatty infiltration.
- Nonsteroidal anti-inflammatory drugs (NSAIDs) may be used for pain. Steroids and other immunosuppressive or modulating agents are not needed.
- Resolves spontaneously in months to years.
- Pathologically, focal myositis is characterized by:
  - Inflammatory myopathy
  - Large clusters of nesting muscle fibers surrounded by thick fibrosis

SUGGESTED READING

Smith, AG, Urbanits S, Blaivas M, et al. Clinical and pathological features of focal myositis. *Muscl Nerv.* 2000 Oct;23(101):1569–1575.

FATIGABILITY

CASE 25.1: FATIGABILITY OF SPEECH

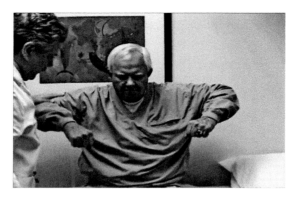

VIDEO 25.1

A 62-year-old man presented with a 6-month history of slurring of speech and undue fatigability of the arm and leg muscles.

Fatigability in myasthenia gravis (MG) affects:

1. Biceps more than triceps
2. Neck extensors more than neck flexors
3. Superior oblique more than superior recti
4. Wrist extensors more than wrist flexors
5. Answers 2 and 4

DIAGNOSIS

- Clinical examination for fatigability is often omitted from the neurological examination. The right deltoid muscle is fatigable in this patient.
- Patients with weakness, fatigue, or both, especially if they have ocular or bulbar symptoms, should always be asked about undue fatigability and worsening of symptoms in the evenings and improvement with rest.
- Occurrence of diplopia with reading and watching television and toward the end of the day is an important diagnostic finding in MG.
- It is important to know that fatigue is a natural phenomenon and increases with age.
- Most neurological motor disorders cause undue fatigability, such as myopathies and amyotrophic lateral sclerosis (ALS).
- The most common medical causes of fatigue are nonneuromuscular and include disorders such as:
  - Anemia
  - Hypothyroidism
  - Obstructive sleep apnea
  - Depression
- MG is an important but rare cause of undue fatigability.
- Problematic cases occur when generalized fatigability is associated with negative myasthenia serology, with no ocular or bulbar symptoms. Chronic fatigue syndrome (CFS) becomes a consideration after medical and psychological causes are ruled out.
  - In CFS, fatigue is almost constant and it does not fluctuate clearly.
- In MG, fatigue affects extensors more than flexors and elevators more than depressors of the eyes.
  - Neck extensors are differentially affected and are much more fatigable than neck flexors, unlike myopathies.
  - Triceps are more affected than biceps, especially in African Americans.
  - Wrist extensors and ankle dorsiflexors can be so severely affected that wrist drop and foot drop may result.
- Fatigue and weakness are used interchangeably by patients. It is important to ask about them separately. Weakness is a motor inability that is present since the start of the movement, and it may or may not fatigue. Fatigability, on the other hand, is weakness that happens only with use and recovers to baseline or close to baseline with rest.
- In severe cases, fatigue may become a fixed weakness; on the other hand, mild weakness may fatigue with use, creating overlap between weakness and fatigue.

CASE 25.2: FATIGABLE NECK MUSCLES

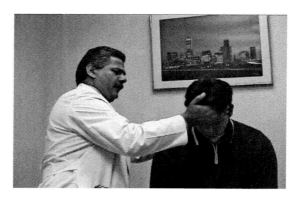

VIDEO 25.2

A 30-year-old man presented with fatigable ptosis and diplopia. Examination is shown in the video. Fatigability of muscles in MG occurs due to:

1. Progressive loss of contractile elements.
2. Reduction of the safety factor.
3. Decreased quantal acetylcholine (ACh) release with successive stimuli at intervals greater than 500 seconds.
4. Blocking of increasing numbers of muscle fibers.
5. MG does not affect the external anal sphincter.

DIAGNOSIS

- Video 25.2 shows right ptosis and fatigability of the neck flexion with restoration after rest.
- Fatigue is a complex phenomenon that is regulated by central and peripheral factors. As far as the neuromuscular junction (NMJ) is concerned, the clinically and neurophysiologically detected fatigue pattern can be understood on the basis of normal physiology.
    - A nerve action potential leads to the fusion of ACh vesicles to presynaptic membrane (docking), followed by release of a neurotransmitter (i.e., ACh) from vesicles into the synaptic cleft and attachment of ACh to postsynaptic ACh receptors (AChRs). This leads to stimulation of the postsynaptic membrane, resulting in a generation of end plate potential (EPP) that usually exceeds 50 mV. This EPP is 3–4 times more than what is needed by a muscle fiber (10–15 mV) to depolarize from its resting membrane potential (safety margin).
    - Repetitive stimulation at frequency of 5 Hz normally depletes ACh-containing vesicles.
    - After four stimulations, the ACh release is resuscitated by newly arriving ACh from the presynaptic terminal.
    - After a minute, the ACh release is reduced due to decreased availability.
- Reduction of postsynaptic AChRs due to antibody reaction leads to reduced amplitude of the EPP safety margin to a level that is barely enough to produce an action potential in the beginning of the exercise, but this cannot be maintained when the normal decline in the release occurs, leading to blocking of muscle fibers and consequently fatigue.
- Quantal release is not affected in MG, but it is in presynaptic neuromuscular disorders.
- The external anal sphincter consists of skeletal muscles, so it is affected by fatigue in MG. Patients, especially female, with pelvic floor weakness may rely on external anal sphincter to prevent leak of urine.
- The right answers are 2 and 4.

CASE 25.3: MYASTHENIA AND ELEVATED CREATINE KINASE (CK) LEVEL

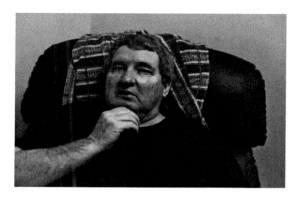

VIDEO 25.3

A 60-year-old man presented with severe chewing difficulty. There was no ptosis or diplopia. He developed subacute proximal weakness. Examination is shown in the video. The acetylcholine receptor antibody (AChR Ab) titer was 25 nml/l, and CK was 5,000 U/L. Electromyography (EMG) revealed 40% short-duration units in the proximal leg and arm muscles and many fibrillations and positive, sharp waves. Computed tomography (CT) of the chest showed a mediastinal mass.

A muscle biopsy will likely show:

1. Lymphorrhagia
2. Granulomatous myositis
3. Caseating granulomata
4. Perimysial inflammation
5. Perifascicular atrophy

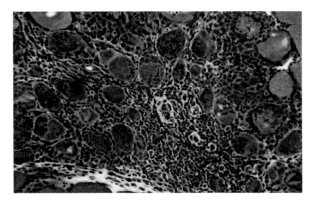

FIGURE 25.3.1 H&E stain (400x): Endomysial non-caseating granuloma with many multinucleated giant cells.

DIAGNOSIS

- Examination showed fatigability of the muscles of mastication and dysarthria.
- Increased CK level, irritative myopathy, and mediastinal mass suggest giant cell myositis.
- Giant cell myositis is a rare form of polymyositis that is usually associated with thymoma and carditis.
- Myositis can occur before or after the diagnosis of MG and thymoma.
- Giant cell myositis has a less favorable prognosis than polymyositis, due to frequent cardiac involvement.
- The formation of granuloma suggests cell-mediated immunity.
- The frequent occurrence of MG suggests humeral immunity.
- The initial presentation of subacute fatigable dysarthria and dysphagia was consistent with MG, but the following factors raised the possibility of polymyositis and promoted a muscle biopsy and CT scan of the chest:
  - HyperCKemia: Mild CK elevation is not inconsistent with MG. More than 5 times the normal CK level is atypical.
  - More severe proximal weakness than expected for MG.
  - More irritaitve myopathic units proximally than expected for MG.
- This patient had a thymectomy 15 years ago, and he continues to enjoy a normal life, but he relapsed every time azathioprine or prednisone was discontinued. Thymoma did not recur.

CASE 25.4: INABILITY TO CHEW A STEAK

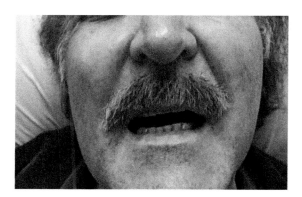

VIDEO 25.4

A 54-year-old man presented with an inability to chew without supporting his chin with his hand. There was no pain.

The most likely diagnosis is:

1. Temporal arteritis
2. Temporomandibular joint (TMJ) dysfunction
3. MG
4. Psychogenic
5. Mandibular dystonia

DIAGNOSIS

- Painless fatigability of the muscles of mastication is characteristic of MG. The patient could not close his mouth completely, and he had left ptosis.
- Sometimes involvement of the jaw muscles is severe enough to cause jaw ptosis.
- Patients may use their hands to support their jaws during mastication, and even talking.
- They cannot keep their mouths shut and their eyes open.
- Jaw claudication, on the other hand, is the inability to chew due to pain, and it is typically caused by temporal arteritis, which can cause ophthalmoplegia as well, adding another layer of diagnostic confusion. Vasculitic changes of the arterial supply of the mastication muscles and extraocular muscles are the pathological explanation of pain and opthalmoplegia.
- Pyridostigmine taken an hour before meals may improve the chewing function.
- Fatigability of the chewing muscles usually improves smoothly, along with the other features of MG, with treatment.

CASE 25.5: CASE 25.4 AFTER TREATMENT WITH PLASMA EXCHANGE (PLEX)

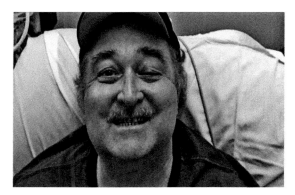

VIDEO 25.5

After five sessions of plasmapheresis (PLEX), the patient in Case 25.4 could close his mouth completely and chew solid food without using his hands.

Plasmapheresis in MG:

1. Is equally effective as intravenous immunoglobulin (IVIG)
2. Is superior to IVIG in the long run
3. Is preferred over IVIG in patients with congestive cardiac failure (CCF)
4. Is less effective than IVIG
5. Is preferred over IVIG in HIV patients

DIAGNOSIS

- Plasmapheresis is shown to be as effective as IVIG in the treatment of MG. A close look at the temporal profile of improvement indicates that plasmapheresis worked faster.
- Due to perceived complications and technical difficulty in obtaining venous access, most experts use plasma exchange (PLEX) for the following indications:
  - Myasthenic crisis
  - To prepare for major surgery
  - Long-term treatment in refractory cases
  - When IVIG is associated with high risk, such as in patients with CCF
- Clinical improvement may appear as soon as the third day of treatment.
- Complications of PLEX occur in 10% of sessions, and they are usually mild and treatable.
- Most complications are related to the vascular access and include obstruction, infection, and thrombosis.
- Procedure-related complications include hypotension, anemia, hypokalemia, and arrhythmia.
- Patients who need a long-term treatment may benefit from arteriovenous fistula (AVF).

SUGGESTED READING

Ebadi H, Barth D, Bril V. Safety of plasma exchange therapy in patients with myasthenia gravis. *Musc Nerv.* 2013;47:510–514.

CASE 25.6: FATIGABILITY OF TRICEPS MUSCLE

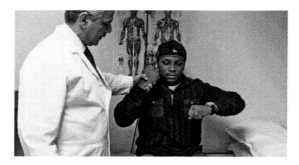

VIDEO 25.6

A 35-year-old man with seropositive generalized MG had responded well to steroids and azathioprine. However, he did not regain the ability to do bench presses, even 3 years later, and he had to give up his favorite sport.

Weakness of the triceps muscles in this case is:

1. Due to MG.
2. Argues against MG.
3. Due to myopathy.
4. Due to C7 radiculopathy.
5. Persistence is against the diagnosis of MG.

DIAGNOSIS

- Weakness of the triceps is common in MG, but is reported only when it is severe or interferes with activity.
- African American myasthenics may have more incidence of triceps weakness than other races.
- It is a good habit for neuromuscular specialists to include the triceps in their examination for weakness and fatigability in patients with MG.
- After treatment, residual weakness of the triceps is not uncommon.

CLINICAL SIGNS

CASE 26.1: EYE MOVEMENT

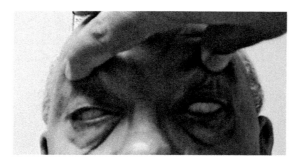

VIDEO 26.1

A 65-year-old man presented with bilateral facial weakness.

The demonstrated in the video upward eye movement is called:

1. Doll's eye movement
2. Bell phenomenon
3. Roving eye movement
4. Oculogyric crisis
5. Leuco-ophthalmia

DIAGNOSIS

- Bell phenomenon is an upward movement of the eye globes with attempted forceful eye closure, or when the cornea is touched. It is a normal defensive function and occurs in about 75% of the population. The rolling of the eyeballs is more readily visible when there is facial weakness, such as in Guillain-Barré syndrome (GBS) or Bell's palsy.

CASE 26.2: SWEATING DURING PREACHING

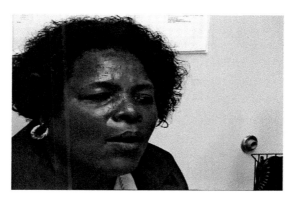

VIDEO 26.2

A 54-year-old preacher had to quit her job due to embarrassing drenching facial sweating that she experienced during preaching. She had no other features of dysautonomia, and her examination was normal.

The following treatments are used for primary facial hyperhidrosis:

1. Anticholinergic medications
2. Sympathectomy
3. Botulinum toxin (BT) injection
4. Steroids
5. Answers 1, 2, and 3

DIAGNOSIS

- Drenching facial sweating provoked by stress is not uncommon, leading to social embarrassment and impairment of ability to work.
- Obesity and female sex are risk factors.
- Focal increase of sweating in the axilla and palms can be disturbing as well.
- To determine the actual dimension of the condition and the area of hyperhidrosis, the patient was asked to re-create the precipitating condition. This also helped define the area that must be injected with BT.
- This case provides a lesson on the importance of reproducing physical signs in the office whenever the physical signs are scarce compared to the symptoms.

CASE 26.3: FACILITATED REFLEXES

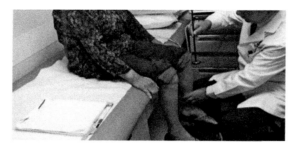

VIDEO 26.3

A 65-year-old woman presented with a 7-month history of fatigue and difficulty arising out of a chair. She lost 20 pounds and developed brownish pigmentation of the skin. Her examination revealed proximal weakness and the abovementioned finding.

The most likely diagnosis is:

1. Myopathy
2. Lambert-Eaton myasthenic syndrome (LEMS)
3. Myasthenia gravis (MG)
4. Proximal motor neuropathy
5. Anxiety

DIAGNOSIS

- Facilitation of reflexes after exercising the related muscles (the quadriceps in this case) is a feature of presynaptic neuromuscular transmission (NMT) disorder. It is similar to facilitation of strength with repeated testing and facilitation of the compound action potential (CMAP) with exercise.
- Areflexia is an important diagnostic criterion of LEMS, besides proximal weakness and fatigue, and only 6% of patients do not display it.
- Transient improvement of strength after exercise is due to accumulation of calcium ions in the presynaptic terminals, resulting in increased acetylcholine (ACh) release.
- This sign is seen in only a third of patients with LEMS; therefore, its absence should not be held against the diagnosis.
- Since LEMS patients usually present with proximal weakness similar to myopathy, the lack of deep tendon reflexes (DTRs) and facilitation of reflexes with exercise should raise the possibility of LEMS in these patients.

CASE 26.4: RESTLESS LEGS

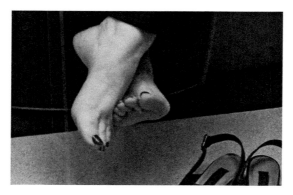

VIDEO 26.4

A 60-year-old woman presented with restlessness and insomnia due to an irresistible desire to move her feet that occurred for decades and responded intermittently to pramipexole. She had no evidence of neuropathy or lumbosacral (LS) radiculopathy. Her hemoglobin was 12 gm/dl. She had two sisters with the same problem.

This is a case of:

1. Parkinson disease
2. Neuropathy
3. Muscle cramps
4. Restless leg syndrome (RLS)
5. Akathisia

DIAGNOSIS

- RLS is a common disorder affecting 5%–10% of the population.
- It is characterized by the urgent and irresistible desire to move the legs, and sometimes arms.
- Patients describe such a desire as tingling or cramping.
- It should be differentiated from other "urge-to-move" disorders like akathisia.
- Differential diagnosis includes polyneuropathy and leg cramps, which can lead to secondary RLS.
- Iron deficiency anemia is commonly associated with RLS. Low brain iron is shown to interfere with the dopaminergic pathway.
- Family members of patients are 7 times more likely to have the disorder than the rest of the population.
- A total of 60% of cases are familial. It is inherited as an autosomal-dominant (AD) disorder with variable penetrance. At least three genetic loci are identified. A genetic control of the dopaminergic system is well established.
- Worsening of leg movement at rest and nighttime and improvement with movement are important diagnostic features.
- A total of 80% of cases are associated with periodic limb movement.
- Dopamine agonists are indicated only in severe cases, and they may cause paradoxical worsening.

CASE 26.5: HYPERREFLEXIA

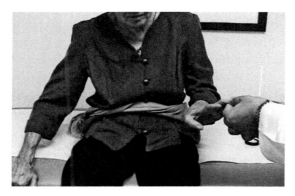

VIDEO 26.5

A 77-year-old woman presented with chronic cervical pain, numbness of the hands, stiffness of the legs, and urinary frequency. She had atrophy and weakness of the hand muscles.

The demonstrated in the video sign is named after:

1. Babinski
2. Hoffmann
3. Lhermitte
4. Uhthoff
5. Chaddock

DIAGNOSIS

- Tapping the nail or flicking the terminal phalanx of the ipsilateral ring finger produces sudden and transient flexion of the thumb and index finger.
- The Hoffmann sign can be normal, especially in hyperreflexic individuals.
- It is more significant if it is unilateral and consistent with upper motor neuron (UMN) injury such as cervical myelopathy and amyotrophic lateral sclerosis (ALS).
- It is called *Babinski sign of the arm,* but it is a deep tendon reflex (DTR; monosynaptic), unlike the Babinski sign, which is a polysynaptic reflex.
- The Babinski sign is always abnormal except in infants.

CASE 26.6: POOR ARM ABDUCTION

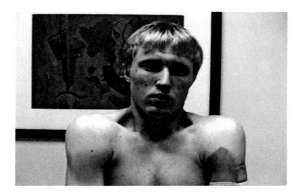

VIDEO 26.6

A 24-year-old man presented with an inability to raise his arms despite good deltoid strength, which he has had since age 15 years.

There are enough clinical findings to strongly suggest:

1. Myotonic dystrophy
2. Facioscapulohumeral muscular dystrophy (FSHD)
3. Duchenne muscular dystrophy (DMD)
4. Bilateral phrenic palsy supraspinatous weakness
5. Severe shoulder arthritis

DIAGNOSIS

- There are several physical findings that suggest FSHD.
- Atrophy of pectoralis is an early sign.
- Normally, the clavicles are pulled down by the pectoralis muscles (shown by the red arrow in Figure 26.6.1), and hence a weak pectoralis leads to "horizontal clavicles."
- The axillary folds are formed by the pectoralis, and they are diagonal lines moving toward the humerus (shown by the black arrow in Figure 26.6.1). When pectoralis is wasted, these folds are "reversed."
- Inability to raise the arms despite preservation of supraspinatus and deltoids is due to scapular instability.
- The presence of pumps and depressions resulting from protruded bones and preserved muscles (deltoid, brachioradialis) alternating with small muscles (biceps and pectoralis) is called the *poly-hill sign.*
- The patient also has mild facial weakness and scapular winging.
- Symptoms of FSHD can be subtle and can escape diagnosis for years.

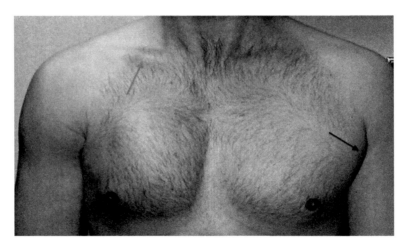

FIGURE 26.6.1 A photo showing the anterior chest wall of a normal person.

CASE 26.7: TENSILON TEST

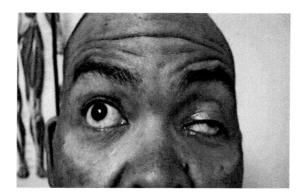

VIDEO 26.7

A 60-year-old man presented with a 6-month history of diplopia. The second half of the recording was taken right after intravenous (IV) injection of 10 mg of edrophonium and shows improvement of the ptosis and left medial rectus (MR) strength.

Improvement of ptosis with edrophonium:

1. Is specific for MG
2. Is 90% sensitive for MG
3. Occurs after 10 minutes of administration
4. Lasts 2 hours
5. None of the above

DIAGNOSIS

- Edrophonium chloride (Tensilon) inhibits ACh esterase. It is short-acting.
- A Tensilon test is used to confirm the diagnosis of MG. It is 90% sensitive but is only 60% specific.
- A false positive test can be seen in LEMS, ALS, and neuropathies, and that is due to increased neuromuscular junction (NMJ) irritability in these conditions.
- The procedure is performed as follows:
  - A vein is cannulated and 2 mg of edrophonium chloride (EC) is injected to test for allergy. Within 2 minutes, 8 mg of the same is pushed.
  - A response is expected in 2–5 minutes. Increased salivation and lacrimation are signs of action.
  - The test is not as valuable if there are no clear outcome measures, such as a significant ptosis or tropia.
  - Some experts advocate for a control arm of the test to rule out a placebo effect.
  - The pulse rate and the blood pressure should be monitored since bradycardia and hypotension can occur. Atropine should be available on standby for emergencies.
  - The duration of action is only a few minutes.
- The use of this test has become limited after the introduction of serological and neurophysiological tests for MG, but it still has a place in ocular myasthenia gravis (OMG), where these tests are not very sensitive.
- In this case, the movement of the left MR and left ptosis improved with edrophonium.

CASE 26.8: SENSORY TRICKS

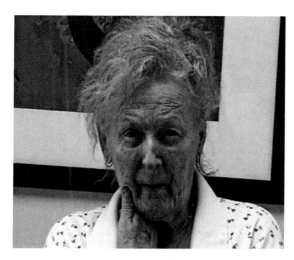

VIDEO 26.8

A 65-year-old woman presented with oromandibular dystonia.

The reason that the patient is touching her face and lips with her finger is:

1. As a random habit
2. To provide tactile stimulation to alleviate dystonia
3. To minimize pain
4. To taste and smell her finger
5. To express shyness

DIAGNOSIS

- Many movement disorders are characterized by amelioration by sensory tricks.
- Cervical dystonia and blepharospasm are more affected by these tricks than hemifacial spasm and writer's cramp.
- Of the sensory tricks, tactile stimulation is the most common. The mechanism is not clear. Somehow, sensory input from the affected area modulates motor output to the involved muscles.

SUGGESTED READING

Loyola DP, Camargos S, Maia D, Cardoso F. Sensory tricks in focal dystonia and hemifacial spasm. *Eur J Neurol.* 2013 Apr;20(4):704–707. doi:10.1111/ene.12054. Epub 2012 Dec 7.

CASE 26.9: OPTIC NEURITIS AND MYELOPATHY

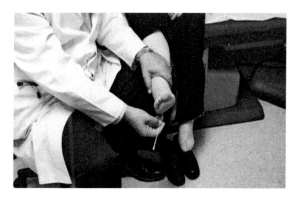

VIDEO 26.9

A 40-year-old woman presented with recurrent transverse myelitis and optic neuritis. The demonstrated in the video signs include all the following except:

1. Babinski sign
2. Chaddock sign
3. Oppenheim sign
4. Hoffman sign
5. Uhthoff

DIAGNOSIS

- There are different ways to trigger an upgoing toe response, which (along with fanning of the other toes) indicates a pyramidal lesion.
- The classical way is to scratch the plantar aspect of the sole of the foot by a rough object starting from the lateral side and making an *L* sign as you get closer to the tarsals (Babinski sign).
- If the sole is ulcerated or wrapped, one can scratch the skin close to the lateral malleolus dorsally and get the same effect (i.e., the Chaddock sign).
- If the foot provides no access to perform either test, then a painful sliding pressure over the shin (tibia) will have the same effect (i.e., Oppenheim sign).
- It is a good practice to strike the sole when sensory impairment of the feet is accompanied by brisk or even preserved ankle reflexes. In that case, a positive Babinski sign would indicate myelopathy, or even encephalopathy, as an explanation for the sensory deficit.

CASE 26.10: TRIPLE HUMP SIGN
AND BULGING ABDOMEN

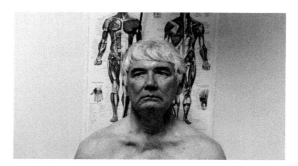

VIDEO 26.10

The demonstrated in the video findings are characteristic of:

1. FSHD
2. Limb-girdle muscular dystrophy (LGMD)
3. Myotonic dystrophy
4. Distal hereditary myopathy
5. Scapuloperoneal muscular dystrophy

The demonstrated in the video bulging of the abdominal wall is:

1. Against the diagnosis of FSHD
2. Common in FSHD
3. More typical for LGMD
4. Represents an incidental finding
5. Is due to eventration of the diaphragm.

DIAGNOSIS

- A 61-year-old man presented with painless, left myopathic foot drop, asymmetrical scapular winging, inverted axillary folds, pectoralis atrophy, and triple hump sign, with similar symptoms in his mother and her brother. These features are very characteristic of FSHD.
- Asymmetry is typical. Focal weakness of the abdominal wall is a common feature.
- Retinal angioma and deafness are also well recognized.
- Inability to raise the arms is not due to deltoid weakness, but rather instability of the scapulae.
- Foot drop with preserved bulk of the extensor digitorum brevis (EDB) is always myopathic.
- FSDH1 is caused by contraction of the *D4Z4* macrosatellite array in chromosome 4q35. It is AD, and 20% of cases result from de novo deletion.
- Life expectancy is not shortened, but 20% of patients eventually require a wheelchair.
- Peripheral blood DNA analysis is used for the diagnosis, and muscle biopsy is not indicated.

CASE 26.11: MOVING UMBILICUS

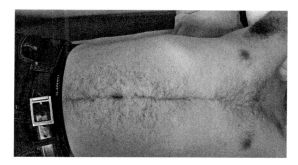

VIDEO 26.11

The demonstrated in the video sign is typically seen in:

1. DMD
2. FSHD
3. LGMD
4. Diabetes mellitus (DM)
5. Paramyotonia congenital (PMC)

DIAGNOSIS

- "When a patient sits up or raises the head from a recumbent position, the umbilicus is displaced toward the head. This is the result of paralysis of the inferior portion of the rectus abdominis, so that the upper fibers predominate, pulling upwards the umbilicus." Charles Edward Beevor (1854–1908).
- This is called *Beevor's sign*. It is caused by a disease that leads to preferential weakness of the lower abdominal muscles, causing upward movement of the umbilicus upon flexion of the torso in a recumbent position.
- Typically, it is noted in FSHD. It is also reported with T9–T10 spinal cord injury and ALS.

SUGGESTED READING

Awebuch GI, Nigro MA, Wishnow R. Beevor's sign and facscioscapulohumeral dystrophy. *Arch Neurol.* 1990;47:1208–1209.

CHAPTER 27

SKIN SIGNS

CASE 27.1: CHRONIC INFLAMMATORY DEMYELINATING POLYNEUROPATHY (CIDP) WITH HYPOGONADISM

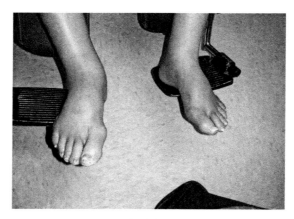

VIDEO 27.1

A 52-year-old man with refractory chronic inflammatory demyelinating polyneuropathy (CIDP) had developed recurrent, severe ascites. Computed tomography (CT) scan of the abdomen revealed splenomegaly. He also developed hypogonadism, which required testosterone replacement. Gradually, he developed the shown in the video skin lesions. Immunofixation protein electrophoresis (IFPE) showed immunoglobin A (IgA) monoclonal gammopathy.

The elevation of the following factor in the serum would confirm the diagnosis:

1. Nerve growth factor (NGF)
2. Vascular endothelial growth factor (VEGF)
3. Hepatocyte growth factor (HGF)
4. Brain-derived growth factor (BGF)
5. Human chorionic gonadotropin (hCG)

DIAGNOSIS

- Polyneuropathy is the most common manifestation of polyneuropathy, organomegaly, endocrinopathy, monoclonal gammopathy, and skin changes (POEMS) syndrome.
- Cutaneous manifestations of POEMS are diverse, and none is pathognomonic. They include:
  - Hemangiomas
  - Hyperpigmentation (the most common skin feature)
  - Skin thickening
  - Acrocyanosis
  - Hypertrichosis (associated with endocrine disorders)
  - Facial lipodystrophy
  - Leukonychia
  - Livedo reticularis
- VEGF plays an important role in the pathogenesis of POEMS, but its role in the genesis of the skin lesions is less clear and its level is not significantly different in patients with skin lesions than in those without.
- Patients with refractory CIDP should be watched for skin lesions and organomegaly, and VEGF should be checked. VEGF is very sensitive, but not specific. In POEMS, levels are often very high.
- Peripheral edema, ascites, and pleural effusion are common and carry a bad prognosis.
- Serum M-protein is present in 85% of cases; therefore, its absence does not exclude POEMS.
- The paraproteins of POEMS syndrome are typically immunoglobin G (IgG) or IgA with lambda light chains, but immunoglobin M (IgM) may occur as well.
- Mild elevation of VEGF occurs in inflammatory neuropathies.
- VEGF is increased early in scleroderma.

SUGGESTED READINGS

Barete S, Mouawad R, Choquet S, et al. Skin manifestations and vascular endothelial growth factor levels in POEMS syndrome: impact of autologous hematopoietic stem cell transplantation. *Arch Dermatol.* 2010;146(6):615–623.

Dispenzieri A. POEMS syndrome: update on diagnosis, risk stratification, and management. *Am J Hematol.* 2012 Aug;87(8):804–814.

CASE 27.2: SKIN RASH AND WEIGHT LOSS

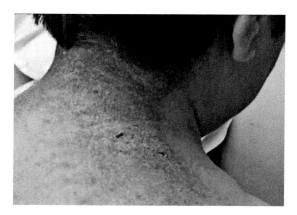

VIDEO 27.2

A 54-year-old woman presented who had developed weight loss and dysphagia over 6 weeks. The abovementioned symptoms and signs are consistent with:

1. Scleroderma
2. Systemic lupus erythematosus (SLE)
3. Dermatomyositis
4. Psoriasis
5. Polymyositis

DIAGNOSIS

- Cutaneous manifestations of dermatomyositis are diverse.
- Skin lesions are not required for the diagnosis of dermatomyositis, which has a characteristic muscle pathology.
- Skin lesions precede myopathy in most cases, and they may never be accompanied by myopathic changes (amyopathic dermatomyositis).
- Skin eruption of dermatomyositis is usually itchy and scaly.
- Common skin signs are:
  - Heliotropes and lilac discoloration of the eyelids with periorbital swelling.
  - Gottron papules.
  - Malar erythema.
  - Poikiloderma.
  - Photosensitivity.
  - Violaceous erythema.
  - Periungual telangiectasia.
  - Macular rash on the face, upper trunk, anterior neck (V sign), back and shoulders (shawl sign), knees, elbows, and neck.
  - Thickening and hyperpigmentation are common in chronic cases.
  - In dark skin, diagnosis of skin rash may be delayed.
- It is important that patients with proximal weakness, elevated creatinine kinase (CK), or both are examined for skin lesions and their nail beds examined with a magnifying lens such as an ophthalmoscopic lens.
- In severe cases, skin lesions coalesce and cover a wide surface area and become very erythematous and itchy. Bullous eruption is also reported.
- Skin lesions usually resolve along the myopathic features with treatment.
- In this case, the knuckle skin, which is typically affected in dermatomyositis, was spared and the rash mostly appeared on the upper back.
- Skin biopsy usually shows chronic inflammatory changes.

CASE 27.3: PUFFY EYES AND SKIN RASH

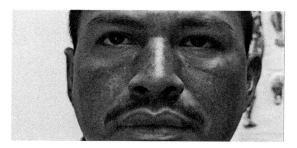

VIDEO 27.3

A 33-year-old man presented with an 8-month history of puffiness around the eyes and rash around the elbows and knees, followed by difficulty climbing stairs. Electromyography (EMG) was myopathic and the creatine phosphokinase (CPK) level was 670 U/L.

The muscle biopsy in this case will likely show:

1. Endomysial inflammation
2. Noninflammatory myopathy
3. Perifascicular atrophy (PFA)
4. Cytoplasmic inclusion bodies
5. Red-rimmed vacuoles

Dermatomyositis is shown in Figure 27.3.1).

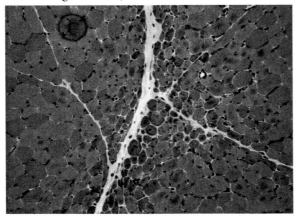

FIGURE 27.3.1 H & E stain (100x): perifascicular atrophy.

DIAGNOSIS

- The pathology shows perifascicular atrophy (PFA). This feature is very highly characteristic of dermatomyositis, but it is not pathognomonic. PFA also occurs in other vasculopathies, like SLE and scleroderma.
- There is erythematous violaceous rash affecting the knuckles, forehead, and malar areas of the face. This is typically seen in dermatomyositis.
- Pathological changes in dermatomyositis are very characteristic and can be used to make the diagnosis of dermatomyositis even in the absence of skin rash.
- These changes reflect the vascular nature of the disease, as opposed to the actual myopathic nature of polymyositis and inclusion body myositis (IBM). The number of the intramuscular blood vessels is reduced.
- The target antigen is located on the intramuscular endothelium, and the primary inflammation is perivascular, with less prominent invasion of nonnecrotic muscle fibers than in polymyositis.
- The inflammatory infiltrate mainly consists of CD4, confirming the humoral nature of the disease as opposed to the cell-mediated immunity of polymyositis and IBM (increased CD8 count).
- The periphery is the watershed area of these fascicles, and it reflects ischemic changes more than the central areas, leading to atrophy and degeneration of several layers of muscle fibers located on the margin of the fascicles. This feature is called perifascicular atrophy (PFA) and is very highly characteristic of dermatomyositis (DM) but not pathognomonic. PFA also occurs in other vasculopathies like SLE and scleroderma.
- PFA occurs in 60% of cases; therefore, its absence is not against the diagnosis of dermatomyositis.
- Myopathic features such as variation of muscle size and shape and muscle fiber necrosis and phagocytoses are less pronounced than in polymyositis.
- Increased vacuolation and glycogen contents of some affected fibers are also commonly reported.
- Major histocompatibility complex (MHC) class I expression occurs in 95% of cases.
- Deposition of the membrane attack complex of the intramuscular microvasculature differentiates dermatomyositis from polymyositis and IBM.

CASE 27.4: FOOT ULCER

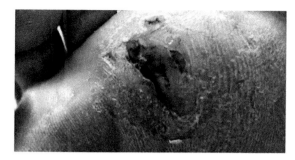

VIDEO 27.4

A patient presented with poorly controlled diabetes mellitus type 2 (DM2) for 20 years. She has neuropathy and peripheral vascular disease (PVD).

The following factors contributed to this ulcer:

1. Neuropathy
2. PVD
3. Callus formation
4. Trauma
5. Hyperglycemia

DIAGNOSIS

- During their lifetime, 50% of diabetics develop foot ulcers.
- Having diabetic feet is the major cause of hospitalization among diabetics.
- Every year, 85,000 limb amputations occur due to diabetes in the United States.
- Untreated foot ulcers lead to amputation in 85% of cases.
- The skin over the metatarsal heads is vulnerable to pressure due to lack of subcutaneous fat.
- Repeated pressure leads to callus formation, an area with poor circulation that often ulcerates.
- Lack of pain due to neuropathy, poor circulation due to PVD, and hyperglycemia, which create a favorable environment in which bacteria can flourish, all contribute to the appearance and progression of a diabetic foot ulcer.
- Minor trauma may cause significant tissue destruction with little pain.
- Osteomyelitis is a common complication.
- Tissue infection spreads quickly and may be life-threatening.
- A nonresponsive ulcer to therapy should be debrided, the foot should be rested, and intravenous (IV) antibiotics should be administered.
- Wearing special wide shoes is helpful.
- Educated patients who inspect their feet every night are less likely to develop diabetic foot ulcers.

CASE 27.5: SKIN RASH AND NEUROPATHY

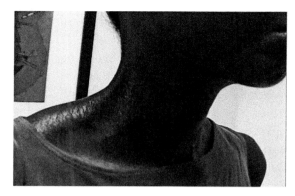

VIDEO 27.5

A 31-year-old woman presented with a 3-year history of dysphagia and skin rash. She then developed severe proximal arm, leg, and neck extensor weakness. The creatinine kinase (CK) level was 250 U/L. EMG revealed findings of nonirritative myopathy. Nerve conduction study (NCS) revealed evidence of axonal neuropathy. She had been on cyclophosphamide and prednisone for a year when this examination was done. Muscle biopsy revealed endomysial inflammatory changes.

The following occurs in scleroderma, but not dermatomyositis:

1. Proximal weakness
2. Skin rash
3. Dysphagia
4. Neuropathy
5. Progressive course

DIAGNOSIS

- Patients with scleroderma present to the neuromuscular clinic due to skin rash and muscle weakness, thus mimicking dermatomyositis.
- This serious autoimmune illness has a spectrum of presentations; the most serious is progressive widespread sclerosis of the skin and internal organs.
- Raynaud phenomenon is common.
- It targets females at age 30–50 years.
- Skin lesions: The skin is thick, shiny, and adherent. It is different from the violaceous erythematous rash and periorbital discoloration and edema that are typical of dermatomyositis.
- The arms, trunk, and face are mostly affected. Difficulty in mouth opening and contracture of extremities are typical features.
- Gastrointestinal (dysphagia, diarrhea), cardiac (pericarditis), and pulmonary (fibrosis) involvement is common.
- Neuropathies are common in scleroderma but are not a feature of dermatomyositis. They include:
  - Trigeminal neuropathy
  - Asymmetric painful sensorimotor axonal neuropathy (vasculitic)
  - Entrapment neuropathies
- Polymyositis (overlap syndrome) is not uncommon. Polymyositis-scleroderma (PM-Scl) antibodies are usually positive.
- VEGF level is increased.

SUGGESTED READINGS

http://neuromuscular.wustl.edu

Ringel RA, Brick JE, Brick JF, Gutmann L, Riggs JE. Muscle involvement in the scleroderma syndrome. *Arch Intern Med*. 1990 Dec;150(12): 2550–2552.

CASE 27.6: HARD SKIN IN A UREMIC PATIENT

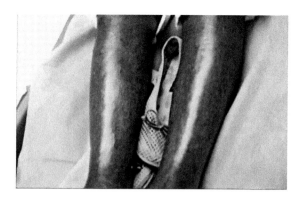

VIDEO 27.6

A 70-year-old woman on hemodialysis for 5 years had magnetic resonance imaging (MRI) of the neck for radicular symptoms. She developed pain and stiffness of the legs 2 weeks after the MRI, and she could not walk anymore. Her skin was very tight and firm and was attached to the under-lying structures.

The most likely diagnosis is:

1. Scleroderma
2. Systemic sclerosis
3. Dermatomyositis
4. Nephrogenic systemic fibrosis (NSF)
5. SLE

DIAGNOSIS

- These patients are referred to neuromuscular clinics due to muscle weakness and hardening of the skin, leading to suspicion of scleroderma or dermatomyositis.
- NSF is due to fibrosis of the skin and other structures like heart, lung, and muscle in hemodialysis patients who receive gadolinium.
  - A total of 5% of patients with renal impairment who received gadolinium developed NSF.
- Excessive exposure of renal patients to gadolinium is damaging to the tissue.
- Avoidance of gadolinium in high-risk patients leads to a dramatic drop in reported cases.
- Pathological features are due to proliferation of fibrocyte and histiocytes and collagen bundles. CD34 + dermal dendrites are abundant.
- The latent period between exposure and disease is 2–4 weeks.
- Typical lesions are focal, edematous, and tender and turn into hard, confluent lesions in the legs and arms, and then the chest and abdomen, while sparing the head.
- Muscle fibrosis, confirmed by MRI and biopsy, is reported with minimal weakness and significant joint contracture.
- Sed rate and eosinophil count are usually high, but CK is usually normal. EMG is myopathic or shows decreased insertional activity due to fibrosis.
- The disease is progressive, but 40% of cases go into remission after the dialysis is stopped.
- Gadolinium should be avoided when the glomerular filtration rate (GFR) is less than 50 ml/min.
- Renal transplantation is the best hope. Plasma exchange (PLEX) is reported to be beneficial.

SUGGESTED READING

Levine JM, Taylor RA, Elman LB, et al. Involvement of skeletal muscle in dialysis-associated systemic fibrosis (nephrogenic fibrosing dermopathy). *Muscl Nerve.* 2004;30(5):569.

CASE 27.7: POLYMYOSITIS AND EAR EROSION

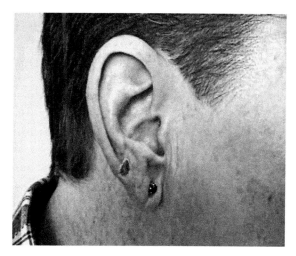

VIDEO 27.7

A 65-year-old woman presented with a history of polymyositis with bilateral ear pain and trachitis. These lesions are typically seen in:

1. Relapsing polychondritis (RPC)
2. Scleroderma
3. Vasculitis
4. POEMS syndrome
5. NSF

DIAGNOSIS

- RPC is an autoimmune inflammation of the cartilaginous structures (ears, nose, joints, eyes, respiratory tract).
- At least one-third of the cases are associated with systemic inflammatory conditions such as vasculitis and polymyositis.
- Auricular involvement is the most common feature, and it is the presenting finding in 40% of cases.
- Recurrent attacks lead to deformity of the ears and nose (saddle nose).
- Hoarseness, aphonia, stridor, dyspnea, and cough indicate respiratory tract involvement.
- Polyarthritis, heart valvular disease, renal involvement, gastrointestinal (GI), and skin involvement are usual.
- Encephalopathy (seizures, hemiplegia, dementia), myelopathy, and inflammatory neuropathy are well reported.
- Different types of systemic vasculitis occur in 25% of cases and are associated with poor prognosis.
- Other autoimmune diseases, such as Graves' disease, rheumatoid arthritis (RA), SLE, ulcerative colitis, and polymyositis, are reported.
- There are no specific serological markers or pathological findings for this condition. The diagnosis is made mostly based on the inflammation of multiple cartilaginous structures.
- The disease is generally responsive to steroids and steroid-sparing agents, but it is occasionally fatal, and most of the time, recurrent attacks lead to cumulative disability.
- Neuromuscular patients with cough, wheezes, progressive neuropathy, and/or myopathy and hematuria should be investigated for RPC as well as other possibilities such as Wagner granulomatosis and Churg strauss disease.

CASE 27.8: DILATED CAPILLARIES AND PROXIMAL WEAKNESS

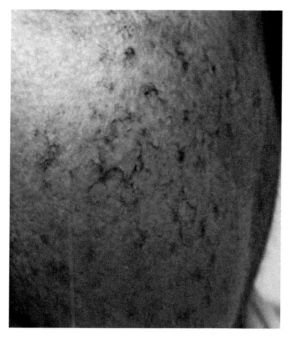

VIDEO 27.8

A 62-year-old woman presented with scleroderma, proximal weakness, and skin lesions.
These skin lesions are:

1. Telangiectasias
2. Varicose veins
3. Spider nevi
4. Hemangiomas
5. None of the above

DIAGNOSIS

- *Telangiectasia* means small, dilated loops of blood vessels, usually capillaries.
- It usually develops on the face and legs, and less commonly on other parts of the body.
- It may occur in normal people due to sun damage to the skin and aging.
- Neurological and neuromuscular associations:
  - Congenital:
    - Ataxia telangiectasia
    - Sturge-Weber syndrome
  - Acquired:
    - Cushing syndrome, including chronic steroid therapy
      - Carcinoid syndrome
    - Scleroderma
- Laser therapy and sclerotherapy are usually effective.
- The most common causes of proximal weakness and telangiectasia are chronic steroid therapy and scleroderma.

CASE 27.9: PROXIMAL WEAKNESS, ASTHMA, AND SKIN RASH

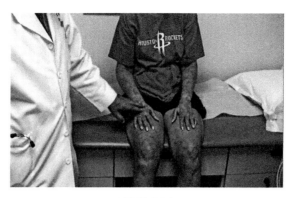

VIDEO 27.9

A 50-year-old woman presented with weight loss, bronchial asthma, muscle weakness, and skin rash that had evolved over a few months. CPK level was 450 U/L. Peripheral eosinophil count was 34%. EMG revealed findings of irritative myopathy and axonal polyneuropathy. Erythrocyte sedimentation rate (ESR) was 87 mm/hour. The nerve biopsy is shown in Figure 27.9.1.

The most likely diagnosis is:

1. Dermatomyositis
2. SLE
3. Vasculitis
4. Scleroderma
5. POEMS syndrome

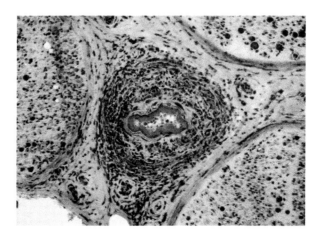

FIGURE 27.9.1 Nerve biopsy; H & E stain: 400x.

DIAGNOSIS

- The nerve biopsy image shows invasion of vascular walls with inflammatory cells.
- Progressive, asymmetrical, axonal, painful neuropathy and erythematous and purpuric skin rash are very suggestive of vasculitis. Proximal weakness suggests myositis; high ESR and CK levels support the diagnosis of vasculitis, which is confirmed by nerve biopsy.
- Skin rash is one of the important manifestations of systemic vasculitis, and it is due to inflammation of the cutaneous blood vessels.
- Cutaneous vasculitis may be the only feature of vasculitis, although more frequently, it is part of a systemic picture, with involvement of the peripheral nervous system (PNS).
- Pathology of skin lesions does not always reflect the picture of the systemic vasculitis; for example, it may not show granuloma in Wegner or Churg-Struass vasculitis. Therefore, skin biopsy is usually inadequate for the diagnosis, and muscle biopsy, nerve biopsy, or both are more likely to provide more specific information.
- Skin lesions usually show fibrinoid necrosis and perivascular neurotrophilic infiltration.
- Palpable purpura:
  - Is very characteristic of cutaneous vasculitis.
  - Maculopapular rash usually precedes palpable purpura.
  - These purpuras do not blanch by pressure, unlike simple purpura.
  - They are caused by extravasation of erythrocytes through damaged blood vessels.
  - They are more common in the legs and buttocks because the increased hydrostatic pressure predisposes the body to their formation.
  - Purpura has many other causes, such as thromboembolism due to hyperviscosity, malignancy, etc.
  - Antiphospholipid syndrome may produce purpura that can be confused with vasculitis, but the former usually is associated with livedo reticularis in the legs.
- Cutaneous vasculitis may affect the scalp, causing alopecia.
- Exacerbation of the skin lesions usually correlates with the exacerbation of systemic vasculitis, and they heal together.

CASE 27.10: INSENSITIVE FEET TO ANT BITES

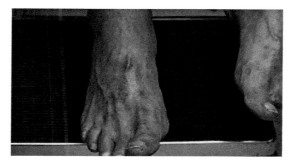

VIDEO 27.10

A 50-year-old diabetic patient noticed red spots on his feet every time he worked in the back-yard. Some of these lesions became infected. He had no foot pain. Examination is shown in the video. During examination, he was found to have a lesion on the left side of his forehead, and he recounted a history in the video of seizures.

The following statements are true regarding the foot lesions:

1. They are likely a manifestation of diabetic neuropathy.
2. They are related to the port wine stain on the forehead.
3. They may lead to gangrene and amputation.
4. They are vascular in nature.
5. This is a normal response to a specific kind of ants.

DIAGNOSIS

- Diabetes mellitus (DM) is the most common cause of neuropathy in the United States (leprosy is the leading cause internationally).
- Diabetic vascular and neuropathic complications are the most common cause of nontraumatic amputations.
- Diabetes is associated with 10 types of neuropathies, the most common of which is distal symmetrical predominantly sensory polyneuropathy, which evolves gradually and may precede the diagnosis of DM by up to 2 years.
- Sensory neuropathy may present with pain, but more often, it presents with numbness of the feet that usually does not get attention until unnoticed injuries, such as shoe-induced trauma or insect bites, occur repeatedly.
- These skin lesions are vulnerable to spreading infection due to the associated hyperglycemia and vascular insufficiency, and they may lead to gangrene.
- Diabetics should always be instructed to inspect their feet every night for skin lesions.
- The left forehead lesion is a port wine stain. This birthmark may occur anywhere on the skin and is usually an isolated and benign condition.
- Port wine stain may be associated with cerebral vascular abnormalities (Sturge- Weber syndrome), leading to seizures.
- Neuropathy is not a feature of Sturge-Weber syndrome, but it may be a feature of other phacomatoses (neurocutaneous syndromes), such as neurofibromatosis.
- Phacomatoses are disorders of the central nervous system (CNS), skin, and sometimes eye due to shared ectodermal origin of these structures. They include:
  - Neurofibromatosis
  - Tuberous sclerosis
  - Ataxia telangiectasia
  - Sturge-Weber syndrome
  - von Hippel–Lindau disease
  - Incontinentia pigmenti
  - Nevoid basal cell carcinoma syndrome
  - Wyburn-Mason syndrome

CHAPTER 28

ELECTROMYOGRAM (EMG) FINDINGS

CASE 28.1: DYSARTHRIA AND PARASPINAL SPONTANEOUS ACTIVITY

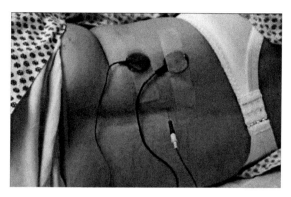

VIDEO 28.1

A 65-year-old woman presented with a 7-month history of slurring of speech and swallowing difficulty. She noticed heaviness and twitching of the arms. The creatine kinase (CK) level was 530 IU/ml. Among other findings, the thoracic paraspinal (TPS) muscles and tongue showed the demonstrated in the video activity.

These discharges are:

1. Specific for amyotrophic lateral sclerosis (ALS).
2. Specific for inflammatory myopathies.
3. Irregular.
4. Not visible by physical examination.
5. Single-fiber electromyography (SFEMG) of an affected muscle may show an increased jitter.

DIAGNOSIS

- Fibrillations are spontaneous, regular discharges of single muscle fibers, and they are typically seen in denervation, but also in inflammatory myopathies.
- Fibrillation is not visible via physical examination, unlike fasciculation.
- The initial positivity (negative deflection) differentiates fibrillation from end-plate potentials.
- TPS muscles are very sensitive for fibrillation, and they should be tested routinely, especially if motor neuron disease (MND) or inflammatory myopathies are suspected. They are preferred over lumbar and cervical paraspinal muscles, which are common targets for radiculopathies.
- It may take up to 2 weeks for fibrillation to appear after an insult, depending on how far the affected muscle is from the injured nerve. TPS muscles are affected early in ALS due to their proximity to the motor neurons, and therefore El Escorial criteria (EEC) count the thoracic regions as one of four important regions (cervical, lumbar, and bulbar) where denervation should be looked for in suspected ALS cases.
- Fibrillation does not resolve immediately after the cause is treated, and it may stay for years or even permanently. Often, fibrillation potentials from a long-standing injury become very low amplitude. Therefore, paraspinal muscles in a surgically treated lumbar or cervical spine lose their value as indicators of new denervation, although some studies suggest that if you see large-amplitude fibrillation potentials in the lumbar paraspinal muscles in a patient with prior lumbar surgery, it may reflect more recent denervation.
- SFEMG is a very sensitive test for myasthenia gravis (MG). A negative test in a weak muscle excludes MG.
- SFEMG is not specific and is positive in early reinnervation due to remodeling of the motor unit. Such changes can be seen in MND, polyneuropathies, radiculopathies, and polymyositis.

CASE 28.2: LEG PAIN AND SPONTANEOUS FAST ACTIVITY

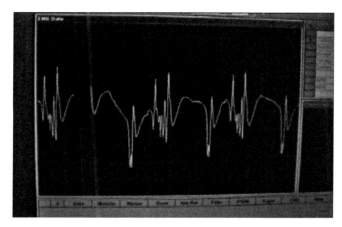

VIDEO 28.2

A 72-year-old woman presented with chronic lower back pain radiating to the right calf and numbness of the lateral aspect of the right foot. She had absent right ankle reflex and history of L5 laminectomy 7 years earlier, with pain relief for a year. EMG showed the demonstrated in the video finding in the right gastrocnemius.

These discharges are:

1. Specific for myopathy
2. Specific for radiculopathy
3. Specific for chronic denervation
4. Specific for ALS
5. Nonspecific

DIAGNOSIS

- Complex, repetitive discharges (CRDs) are regular, spontaneous discharges of groups of muscle fibers that occur in nonrhythmic bursts.
- The fibers are activated ephaptically.
- The usual firing rate is 30–40 Hz.
- Abrupt onset and abrupt end differentiate them from the waxing and waning myotonic discharges.
- CRDs are not specific and occur in chronic neurogenic and myopathic conditions.

CASE 28.3: SKIN RASH
AND SHORT-DURATION UNITS

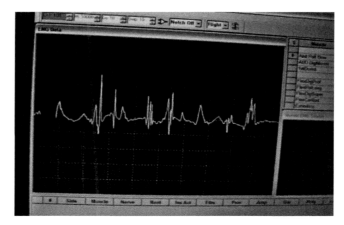

VIDEO 28.3

A 36-year-old woman presented with a 6-month history of difficulty climbing stairs and fatigue. She had symmetrical proximal weakness of the legs and arms and a CK level of 800 IU/L. Skin lesions are shown in the video.

The abovementioned findings suggest:

1. Dermatomyositis
2. Polymyositis
3. ALS
4. Inclusion body myositis (IBM)
5. Systemic lupus erythematosus (SLE)

DIAGNOSIS

EMG is a useful tool to diagnose myopathies, but with the following limitations:

- Some myopathies, such as mitochondrial and metabolic myopathies, do not usually cause EMG abnormalities except late in the course of the disease.
- A well-trained operator is needed to detect the subtle changes in some myopathies since low-amplitude, very brief, short-duration motor unit potentials (MUPs) interspersed with normal MUPs are hard to detect.
- In chronic myopathies, mixed short- and long-duration potentials may lead to diagnostic confusion. Observing the recruitment rate of MUPs can help sort this out.

The following findings are seen in myopathies:

- Short-duration, low-amplitude, polyphasic units with early recruitment. Proximal muscles are the first to demonstrate such units in most myopathies.
- Spontaneous discharges (fibrillation and sharp waves), especially in TPS muscles, are commonly seen in inflammatory, metabolic, and toxic myopathies. Irritative myopathy is commonly used to describe myopathies with spontaneous discharges.

The proximal weakness, skin rash, elevated CK level, and irritative myopathic findings in the demonstrated case were very consistent with dermatomyositis.

CASE 28.4: FAMILIAL NEUROGENIC FIRING

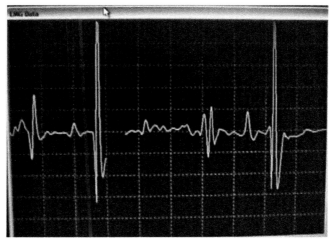

VIDEO 28.4

A 40-year-old Hispanic man presented with a 20-year history of dysarthria and muscle twitching. He had a brother with the same problems. He had tongue fasciculation and diffuse areflexia, with mild sensory impairment in the feet. The CK level was 1,300 IU/L. The shown in the video finding was seen in all the tested muscles in the arms and legs.

He most likely has:

1. Androgen receptor (AR) mutation
2. Superoxide dismutase (SOD) mutation
3. Polymyositis
4. Sporadic ALS
5. TAR DNA-binding protein 43 mutation (TDP43 mutation)

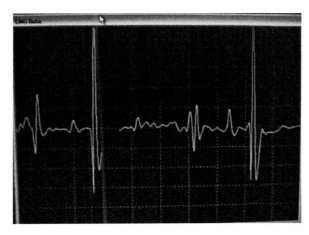

FIGURE 28.4.1 A still screen of an EMG showing motor unit potentials.

DIAGNOSIS

- Chronic denervation is usually associated with reinnervation. The reinnervated motor units produce high-amplitude (20 mv in this case; Normal level: 4) and long-duration potentials (normal level is 5–15 milliseconds). Due to loss of synchrony, polyphasicity occurs (normal value is up to three phases).
- The frequency of firing of motor units increases to compensate for the neuronal loss; therefore, this finding is one of the hallmarks of denervation.
- There are different ways to calculate firing frequency:
  - ◆ Set the sweep at 1,000 and count the number of times that a specific single MUP appears in the screen at the time that a second unit starts firing.
  - ◆ Count the number of seconds between two identical MUPs and divide 1,000 by that number to convert to milliseconds. In this case, there are 5 squares between the two units (50 milliseconds), and therefore, the firing frequency is 20 Hz (normal level is 10) (Figure 28.4.1).
- *Recruitment pattern* is a term used to measure the amount of units recruited with maximum contraction. If there are not enough units to fill the screen, recruitment is said to be decreased. Due to potential for muscle injury and pain during contraction, this method is obsolete.
- There are occasions when recruitment is decreased but firing frequency is normal. This is typically seen in central causes such as stroke, myelopathy, and hysterical weakness or poor effort. When the problem is of a lower motor neuron (LMN) nature, fast firing of normal-appearing MUPs also can be an important clue that muscle weakness is caused by a demyelinating process due to a partial conduction block proximally.
- Kennedy disease is a chronic hereditary LMN disease that affects both bulbar and spinal muscles. EMG is very important in order to reveal the chronic, widespread denervation and to rule out myopathy that is suspected due to elevated CK level, which is common in this disease. The very stable, chronic-appearing MUPs with fairly symmetric findings helps differentiate Kennedy disease from ALS, where MUPs are usually very polyphasic and unstable and (initially at least) asymmetric. The presence of abnormal sensory nerve action potentials (SNAPs) helps distinguish Kennedy disease from ALS and spinal muscular atrophies (SMAs).
- In this case, the chronic, diffusely denervating process with a family history, elevated CK level, and abnormal sensory responses strongly suggested Kennedy disease, which is caused by mutation of the *AR* gene.

CASE 28.5: SPONTANEOUS ACTIVITY AFTER RADIOTHERAPY

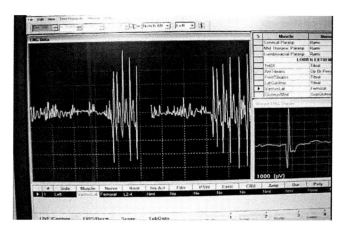

VIDEO 28.5

A 65-year-old woman with a history of rectal cancer 8 years earlier presented with progressive, asymmetrical, painless leg weakness. She had normal sensation and absent knee reflexes and normal sural responses. The demonstrated in the video activity is obtained from the right thigh adductors.

These findings represent:

1. Myokymia
2. Myotonia
3. Neuromyotonia
4. CRDs
5. Artifacts

DIAGNOSIS

- Radiation is toxic to the motor neurons, and the neurotoxic effect may not appear until several years after the exposure.
- Slowly progressive, painless weakness and atrophy in the regions distal to the irradiated area are the first symptoms.
- Symptoms may progress for a few months and then plateau. The exact cause is not clear. Vascular injury and DNA repair malfunction have been proposed.
- Recurrence of the tumor is typically associated with more pain and a progressive course.
- Myokymia is highly characteristic of this syndrome, but it also can be seen in focal nerve injury such as multifocal motor neuropathy with conduction block (MMNCB), carpal tunnel syndrome (CTS), brainstem glioma, and multiple sclerosis (MS). The presence of myokymia in a weak limb that had prior radiation treatment for cancer very strongly suggests that the weakness is from postradiation changes rather than from recurrent tumor, especially if the weakness is painless.
- Myokymia is a rhythmic, spontaneous discharge of the same motor unit and is repeated every 0.1–3 seconds (of bursts)
- Frequency of the potentials is 5–70 Hz. Each burst may have 2–7 potentials.

CASE 28.6: CHRONIC FAMILIAL WEAKNESS

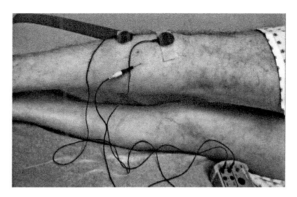

VIDEO 28.6

A 51-year-old man presented with chronic weakness and atrophy of the bilateral distal leg muscles and areflexia. His mother had similar symptoms.

The shown in the video discharges:

1. Have high amplitude
2. Have a firing rate below 10 HZ
3. Indicate chronic denervation
4. Are myopathic
5. Indicate acute denervation

DIAGNOSIS

- The recorded MUPs have an amplitude of 10 mV (gain is 1,000 mV) and a firing frequency of 25 Hz. These are reinnervated large units and indicate chronic denervation.
- Chronic denervation with normal sensory responses suggest:
  1. Radiculopathy
  2. MND
  3. Rarely, motor neuropathy
- Chronic and diffuse denervation with a positive family history suggests chronic familial MND, such as SMA.
- Reinnervation units are responsible for fiber-type grouping in muscle biopsy.

CASE 28.7: DECELERATING MOTORCYCLE ENGINE

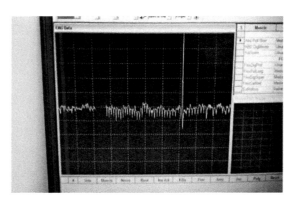

VIDEO 28.7

A 55-year-old woman presented with muscle stiffness for several years. Her father had a premature Christmas tree cataract. The patient has a pacemaker.

The following mutation is responsible for this condition:

1. Cytosine-thymine-guanine (CTG) repeat expansion
2. CTG repeat contraction
3. A mutation in the coding region of the dystrophia myotonica-protein kinase (*DMPK*) gene
4. Stable mutation
5. Autosomal recessive (*AR*) gene

DIAGNOSIS

- Myotonic discharges are spontaneous muscle fiber discharges noticed by needle EMG.
- They appear, as do many fibrillations, as positive, sharp waves with waxing and waning frequency and amplitude.
- Firing frequency 20–40 Hz.
- Accelerating and decelerating motorcycle engine (in military terms, a *dive bomber*).
- Neuromyotonia: Frequency is more than 150 Hz and CRDs have abrupt onset and abrupt outset.
- Myotonic discharges correlate with slow muscle relaxation clinically.
- They occur in myotonic disorders, dystrophic and nondystrophic, and in metabolic, toxic, and inflammatory myopathies.
- They are more prominent in distal muscles.
- CTG repeat expansion correlates with severity and age of onset, but it is not clear if it is correlated with the severity of electrical myotonia, which varies from one muscle to another.
- CTG repeat expansion varies among different tissues, but not among different muscles, despite variability in strength.

SUPPLEMENT FOR CASE 15.8

Classification and diagnostic criteria for IBM:

  I. Characteristic features: inclusion criteria
   A. Clinical features
       • Duration of illness: greater than 6 months
       • Age of onset: greater than 30 years
       • Muscle weakness
           ◆ Must affect proximal and distal muscles of arms and legs
           ◆ Patient must exhibit at least one of the following features:
               ▪ Finger flexor weakness
               ▪ Wrist flexor more than wrist extensor weakness
               ▪ Quadriceps muscle weakness [equal to or less than grade 4 medical research council (MRC)]
   B. Laboratory features
       • Serum CK less than 12 times normal.
       • Muscle biopsy.
           ◆ Inflammatory myopathy characterized by mononuclear cell invasion of nonnecrotic muscle fibers
           ◆ Vacuolated muscle fibers
           ◆ Either:
               ▪ Intracellular amyloid deposits (must use the fluorescent method of identification before excluding the presence of amyloid) or 15–18-nm tubulofilaments by electron microscopy (EM)
       • EMG must be consistent with features of inflammatory myopathy; however, long-duration potentials are commonly observed and do not exclude diagnosis of sporadic IBM (sIBM).
 II. Diagnostic criteria for IBM
   A. Definite IBM
       • The patient must exhibit all muscle biopsy features, including invasion of nonnecrotic fibers by mononuclear cells, vacuolated muscle fibers, and intracellular (within muscle fibers) amyloid deposits or 15–18-nm tubulofilaments.
       • None of the other clinical or laboratory features is mandatory if muscle biopsy features are diagnostic.
   B. Possible IBM
       • If the muscle biopsy shows only inflammation (invasion of nonnecrotic muscle fibers by mononuclear cells) without other pathological features of IBM, then a diagnosis of possible IBM can be given if the patient exhibits the characteristic clinical and laboratory features.

INDEX